POPULATION DYNAMICS OF SUB-SAHARAN AFRICA

Demographic Change
in Sub-Saharan Africa

Demographic Effects of Economic Reversals
in Sub-Saharan Africa

Effects of Health Programs on Child Mortality
in Sub-Saharan Africa

Factors Affecting Contraceptive Use
in Sub-Saharan Africa

Population Dynamics of Kenya

Population Dynamics of Senegal

Social Dynamics of Adolescent Fertility
in Sub-Saharan Africa

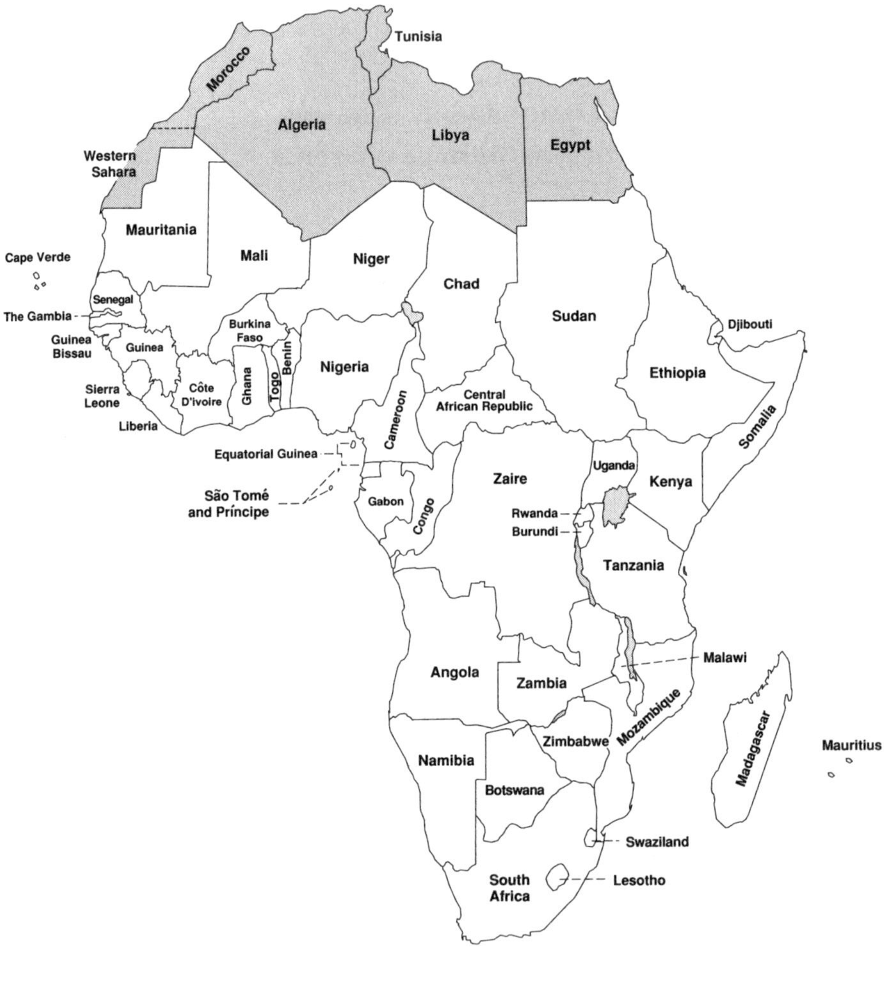

NOTE: This map, which has been prepared solely for the convenience of readers, does not purport to express political boundaries or relationships. The scale is a composite of several forms of projection.

POPULATION DYNAMICS OF SUB-SAHARAN AFRICA

POPULATION DYNAMICS OF SENEGAL

Gilles Pison, Kenneth H. Hill, Barney Cohen, and Karen A. Foote, Editors

Working Group on Senegal

Panel on the Population Dynamics of Sub-Saharan Africa

Committee on Population

Commission on Behavioral and Social Sciences and Education

National Research Council

NATIONAL ACADEMY PRESS
Washington, D.C. 1995

NATIONAL ACADEMY PRESS • 2101 Constitution Avenue, N.W. • Washington, D.C. 20418

NOTICE: The project that is the subject of this report was approved by the Governing Board of the National Research Council, whose members are drawn from the councils of the National Academy of Sciences, the National Academy of Engineering, and the Institute of Medicine. The members of the committee responsible for the report were chosen for their special competences and with regard for appropriate balance.

This report has been reviewed by a group other than the authors according to procedures approved by a Report Review Committee consisting of members of the National Academy of Sciences, the National Academy of Engineering, and the Institute of Medicine.

Library of Congress Catalog Card No. 95-68873
International Standard Book Number 0-309-05280-7

Additional copies of this report are available from: National Academy Press, 2101 Constitution Avenue, N.W., Box 285, Washington, D.C. 20418. Call 800-624-6242 or 202-334-3313 (in the Washington Metropolitan Area).

B546

Printed in the United States of America

WORKING GROUP ON SENEGAL

GILLES PISON (*Chair*), Muséum National d'Histoire Naturelle, Paris, France
ANOUCH CHAHNAZARIAN,† Johns Hopkins University and Institut Français de Recherche Scientifique pour le Développement en Coopération (ORSTOM), Dakar, Senegal
PHILIPPE HUGON, Université de Paris X, Paris, France
CHEIKH MBACKE, Rockefeller Foundation, Nairobi, Kenya
AWA THIONGANE, Direction de la Prévision et de la Statistique, Dakar, Senegal

BARNEY COHEN, *Staff Officer*
PATRICIA A. DeFRISCO, *Senior Project Assistant*
KAREN A. FOOTE, *Staff Officer*
JOAN MONTGOMERY HALFORD, *Senior Project Assistant**
PAULA J. MELVILLE, *Senior Project Assistant***
SUSAN L. SHUTTLEWORTH, *Senior Project Assistant****

† deceased December 1993
* through July 1992
** through April 1994
***through April 1995

PANEL ON THE POPULATION DYNAMICS OF SUB-SAHARAN AFRICA

KENNETH H. HILL (*Chair*), Department of Population Dynamics, Johns Hopkins University
ADERANTI ADEPOJU, Institut de Développement Economique et de la Planification (IDEP), Dakar, Senegal
JANE T. BERTRAND, School of Public Health and Tropical Medicine, Tulane University
CAROLINE H. BLEDSOE, Department of Anthropology, Northwestern University
WILLIAM BRASS, Centre for Population Studies, London School of Hygiene and Tropical Medicine, England
DOUGLAS C. EWBANK, Population Studies Center, University of Pennsylvania
PHILIPPE FARGUES, Centre d'Etudes et de Documentation Economique, Sociale et Juridique (CEDEJ), Cairo, Egypt
RON J. LESTHAEGHE, Faculteit van de Economische, Sociale en Politieke Wetenschappen, Vrije Universiteit Brussel, Belgium
PATRICK O. OHADIKE, Regional Institute for Population Studies (RIPS), Accra, Ghana
ANNE R. PEBLEY, RAND, Santa Monica, California
DANIEL M. SALA-DIAKANDA, Economic Commission for Africa, Addis Ababa, Ethiopia

COMMITTEE ON POPULATION

RONALD D. LEE (*Chair*), Department of Demography, University of California, Berkeley
CAROLINE H. BLEDSOE, Department of Anthropology, Northwestern University
JOSE-LUIS BOBADILLA, World Bank, Washington, D.C.
JOHN BONGAARTS, The Population Council, New York
JOHN B. CASTERLINE, The Population Council, New York
LINDA G. MARTIN, RAND, Santa Monica, California
MARK R. MONTGOMERY, The Population Council, New York
ROBERT A. MOFFITT, Department of Economics, Brown University
ANNE R. PEBLEY, RAND, Santa Monica, California
RONALD R. RINDFUSS, Carolina Population Center, University of North Carolina, Chapel Hill
JAMES P. SMITH, RAND, Santa Monica, California
BETH J. SOLDO, Department of Demography, Georgetown University
MARTA TIENDA, Population Research Center, University of Chicago
AMY O. TSUI, Carolina Population Center, University of North Carolina, Chapel Hill

JOHN G. HAAGA, *Director*
BARNEY COHEN, *Research Associate*
PATRICIA A. DeFRISCO, *Senior Project Assistant*
KAREN A. FOOTE, *Program Officer*
JOEL A. ROSENQUIST, *Project Assistant*
JOYCE E. WALZ, *Administrative Associate*

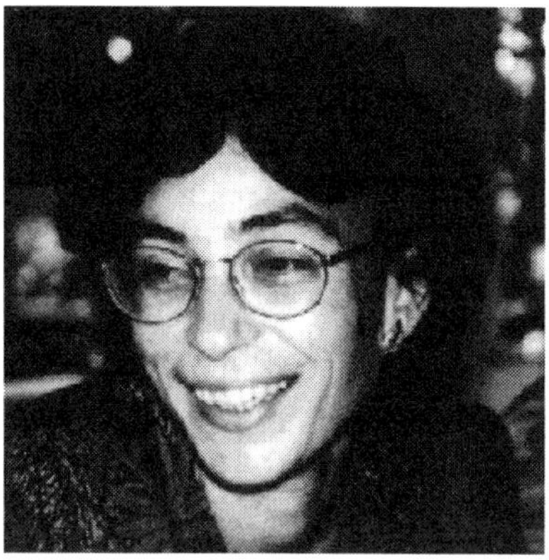

This report is dedicated to the memory of Anouch Chahnazarian, Ph.D., who died on December 26, 1993, at the tragically early age of 40, cutting short a distinguished career. Dr. Chahnazarian was an active member of the Working Group on Senegal until her final illness. Her enthusiasm, energy, and intellectual rigor combined to make an enormous contribution to the preparation of this report.

Dr. Chahnazarian grew up in Belgium, obtaining a B.A. in social sciences from the Free University of Brussels and a master's degree in demography from the Catholic University of Louvain. She then came to the United States to pursue her graduate training, obtaining a Ph.D. in sociology/demography from Princeton University in 1986.

From Princeton, Dr. Chahnazarian joined the Department of Population Dynamics at The Johns Hopkins University, first as a research associate, and then in 1988, as an assistant professor. Her initial work at Johns Hopkins consisted largely of responsibility for all aspects of a child health survey in Haiti, but on joining the faculty, she took on teaching responsibilities and acquired a devoted group of doctoral advisees. While at Princeton, she had been involved in a child mortality study in Zaire, and she returned there in 1989 to design and conduct a follow-up survey of the same area. Her lifelong interest in Africa, where she had lived as a child, led her to take a leave of absence from Johns Hopkins in 1991 to join the Institut Français de Recherche Scientifique pour le Développement en Coopération (ORSTOM), working as the demographer for the population observatory in Niakhar, Senegal. She concentrated her work on systematizing the data collection, processing, and analysis procedures for the observatory, to provide a sound basis for future use of the data for research purposes. Tragically, she was unable herself to take advantage of the important improvements she introduced. She was taken ill in March 1993.

Dr. Chahnazarian's contribution to this report, both intellectual and inspirational, was enormous. She is sorely missed by her colleagues and friends on this working group, the Panel on Population Dynamics of Sub-Saharan Africa, the Committee on Population, and throughout the demographic community.

Preface

This report is last in a series of studies carried out under the auspices of the Panel on the Population Dynamics of Sub-Saharan Africa of the National Research Council's Committee on Population that were initiated during my term as chair. The National Research Council has a long history of examining population issues in developing countries. In 1971 it issued the report *Rapid Population Growth: Consequences and Policy Implications*. In 1977, the predecessor Committee on Population and Demography began a major study of levels and trends of fertility and mortality in the developing world that resulted in 13 country reports and 6 reports on demographic methods. Then, in the early 1980s, that committee undertook a study of the determinants of fertility in the developing world, which resulted in 10 reports. In the mid- and late 1980s, the Committee on Population assessed the economic consequences of population growth and the health consequences of contraceptive use and controlled fertility, among many other activities.

No publication on the demography of sub-Saharan Africa emerged from the early work of the committee, largely because of the paucity of data and the poor quality of what was available. However, censuses, ethnographic studies, and surveys of recent years, such as those under the auspices of the World Fertility Survey and the Demographic and Health Survey programs, have made available data on the demography of sub-Saharan Africa. The data collection has no doubt been stimulated by the increasing interest of both scholars and policymakers in the demographic development of Africa and the relations between demographic change and socioeconomic developments. In response to this interest, the Committee on Population held a meeting in 1989 to ascertain the feasibility and desirability of a major study of the demography of Africa, and decided to form the Panel on the Population Dynamics of Sub-Saharan Africa.

The panel, which is chaired by Kenneth Hill and includes members from Africa, Europe, and the United States, met for the first time in February 1990 in Washington, D.C. At that meeting, the panel decided to set up six working groups, composed of its own members and other experts on the demography of Africa, to carry out specific studies. Four working groups focused on cross-national studies of substantive issues: the social dynamics of adolescent fertility, factors affecting contraceptive use, the effects on mortality of child survival and general health programs, and the demographic effects of economic reversals. The two other working groups were charged with in-depth studies of Kenya and Senegal, with the objective of studying linkages among demographic variables and between those variables and socioeconomic changes. The panel also decided to publish a volume of papers reviewing broad topics across sub-Saharan Africa: levels and trends of fertility; the proximate determinants of fertility, nuptiality, child mortality, adult mortality, internal migration, and international migration; and the demographic consequences of the AIDS epidemic.

This report, one of the two in-depth country studies, analyzes the population dynamics of Senegal. Senegal was chosen for two key reasons. First, it provided an interesting comparison with the case study on Kenya: in contrast with Kenya, demographic changes have not been apparent in Senegal. Second, Senegal has an abundance of national- and local-level data, not all of which had previously been analyzed.

This report is the result of the joint efforts of the working group members and staff and represents a consensus of the members' views on the issues addressed. The Committee on Population and the Panel on the Population Dynamics of Sub-Saharan Africa appreciate the time and energy devoted by all the working group members to the study. Gilles Pison wrote the first drafts of Chapter 1 and the child mortality portion of Chapter 5; Ken Hill wrote the first draft of the adult mortality section in Chapter 5; Philippe Hugon wrote the first draft of Chapter 2; Karen Foote, Philippe Hugon, and Awa Thiongane wrote the first draft of Chapter 3; and Anouch Chahnazarian and Barney Cohen wrote the first draft of Chapter 4. As noted above, however, this report represents the views of the working group as a whole, and considerable effort by all the members and staff went into the refinement of the early drafts.

The working group would like to acknowledge the help of the Statistical Division of the government of Senegal in releasing tables and data from the 1988 census. In addition, Papa Thiécouta Ndiaye, Ibrahim Sarr, and

Boubacar Sow worked with members of the working group in analyzing the 1988 census data on fertility. We would also like to thank Emmanuel Lagarde, Nathalie Paquet, and Ely Sene for their valuable research assistance, and Barbara McKinney for writing a valuable background paper on fertility in Senegal. Most specially, we wish to express our sincere appreciation to Anouch's colleagues who were very supportive of Anouch's efforts on this working group both before and during her illness.

As is the case for all of the panel's work, this report would not have been possible without the cooperation and assistance of the Demographic and Health Surveys (DHS) Program of Macro International, Inc. We are grateful to the DHS staff for responding to our inquiries and facilitating our early access to the survey data.

We are also most grateful to the organizations that provided financial support for the work of the Panel on the Population Dynamics of Sub-Saharan Africa: the Office of Population and the Africa Bureau of the Agency for International Development, the Andrew W. Mellon Foundation, the William and Flora Hewlett Foundation, and the Rockefeller Foundation. Besides the funding provided, the representatives of these organizations were a source of information and advice in the development of the panel's overall work plan.

Special thanks are also due to Paul Hurwit for translating portions of the manuscript that were originally written in French; to Joan Montgomery Halford and Paula Melville for providing superb administrative and logistical support to the working group; to Paula Melville, Trish DeFrisco, and Susan Shuttleworth for meticulous assistance in the preparation of the report manuscripts; to Rona Brière and Elaine McGarraugh for skillful editing of the report; and, last but not least, to Eugenia Grohman for guidance and extraordinary patience through the review and production process.

SAMUEL H. PRESTON
Chair (through November 1993)
Committee on Population

Contents

EXECUTIVE SUMMARY 1

1 INTRODUCTION 7

2 GEOGRAPHIC AND SOCIOECONOMIC SETTING 9

Geographic Overview, 9
Historical Overview, 10
Education, 13
Economic Background, 13
Notes, 29

3 POPULATION GROWTH AND DISTRIBUTION 30

Overview of National Population Trends, 30
Overview of Regional Trends, 34
Migration, 35
Notes, 43

4 FERTILITY 45

Introduction, 45
Levels and Trends of Fertility, 46

Proximate Determinants of Fertility, 77
Summary and Conclusions, 106
Notes, 108

5 MORTALITY 113

Introduction, 113
Child Mortality, 114
Adult Mortality, 157
Appendix: Health Infrastructure and Programs, 185
Notes, 194

6 CONCLUSIONS 196

Fertility, 196
Mortality, 197
The Demographic Transition in Senegal in an African Context, 198
Notes, 201

APPENDIX A: Data Sources 203
APPENDIX B: Correcting the Fertility Estimates in the 1988 Census 208
APPENDIX C: Methodology for Analysis of Child Mortality 220
APPENDIX D: Growth Balance Methods for Estimating Coverage of Adult Deaths 222

REFERENCES 225

INDEX 237

Executive Summary

This report examines recent changes in the demographic situation of Senegal, particularly those related to fertility and mortality rates. Although the data reviewed for this study vary quite substantially in quality and level of coverage, on careful analysis they produce a rather consistent story of demographic change over the last 30 years.

The population of Senegal, estimated at 6.9 million in 1988, increased by 2.7 percent per year between 1976 and 1988. This rapid growth can be attributed to both sustained high fertility—on average each woman bears approximately six children—and declining mortality. The United Nations estimates that the population will more than double between 1988 and 2015, to 14.3 million and that it will reach close to 17 million by 2025 (United Nations, 1991).

FERTILITY

According to the latest large-scale national demographic survey in Senegal—the Demographic and Health Survey of 1992-1993 (DHS-II)—if fertility rates were to remain constant, women entering their reproductive lives today could expect to bear, on average, 6.1 children over the course of their lives. However, it is doubtful that young women starting their reproductive lives today will actually achieve this level of fertility, which would require no change in fertility behavior over 35 years. National demographic surveys indicate that fertility declined by over one child per woman between 1975-1978 and 1989-1992.

The decline in fertility in Senegal has occurred almost entirely among women under age 30. A comparison of age-specific fertility rates between 1975-1978 and 1989-1992 reveals that the decline in fertility among women aged 15-19 is approximately twice as large as that among women aged 20-29 (32 versus 17 percent). Furthermore, the decline among women aged 20-29 is twice as large as that among women over age 30 (17 versus 8 percent).

Fertility decline in Senegal is also strongly associated with differing levels of urbanization and education. Even in the late 1970s, the World Fertility Survey (WFS) reported that fertility was lower among urban and literate women. However, both of these groups were relatively small and overlapped considerably, so that the net effect on the national total fertility rate estimates was small. These subgroups have now become larger and their effect on the general level of fertility more noticeable. A decline in fertility first appeared in Dakar in the early 1980s, and, to date, still appears to be limited to urban areas. The total fertility rate in Dakar, the most densely populated region, has fallen from 6.8 children per woman in 1975-1978 to 4.9 children per woman in 1989-1992. All surveys indicate that women with some education report lower fertility than women with no education, and an ever-increasing fraction of the school-aged female population is going to school (World Bank, 1988).

The driving force behind the changes in the level and pattern of fertility has been a trend towards later marriage. Of course, in some areas of Senegal, such as Casamance, women have always married relatively late. However, the more general trend towards later marriage probably began in Dakar in the 1980s and has been spreading to the interior of the country ever since. The pattern of later marriage is also strongly linked to formal education, although signs of change are emerging even among women who have never attended school.

Little of the fertility decline in Senegal appears to be attributable to either a decrease in ideal family size or an increase in the use of modern contraception. There has been a trend towards wanting fewer children, which stretches across all parities and all age groups of women. However, current preferences still lie very close to the physiological maximum level, assuming a continued regime of delayed marriage and long birth intervals. The proportion of women using modern contraception has increased over the recent past. Nationally, use of modern contraception among currently married women has increased from less than 1 percent in 1978 to a little under 5 percent in 1992-1993. However, use is almost entirely restricted to certain subgroups of the population, particularly women in urban areas and women with at least a primary-level education, so that the absolute number of users is still very low.

In summary, the above features suggest that Senegal's small fertility decline is unlike those that have occurred recently in other sub-Saharan African countries. In Botswana, Kenya, and Zimbabwe—usually considered to be the three countries in the vanguard of African fertility transition—fertility declines are associated with increases in the use of modern contraception. Botswana, Kenya, and, to a lesser extent, Zimbabwe, have also experienced a decline in teenage marriages, but they have also experienced a greater separation of teenage marriage and teenage fertility, consequently leading to an increase in nonmarital fertility. This separation of marriage and fertility has had the effect of reducing the influence of marriage on fertility rates (Working Group on the Social Dynamics of Adolescent Fertility, 1993). In Senegal, fertility has fallen because marriage has been delayed, and marriage and fertility have remained linked.

On the other hand, the Senegalese pattern matches more closely, but not exactly, the pattern found in certain northern African countries during the first phase of their fertility declines. For example, most of the initial decline in fertility observed in countries such as Algeria, Egypt, and Tunisia can be attributed to later age at first marriage (Fargues, 1989; National Research Council, 1982). In these countries, the initial phase of fertility decline was immediately followed by a second phase linked to a substantial decline in the demand for children and a corresponding increase in modern contraceptive use among married women. Whether Senegal follows this pattern and experiences a second phase of fertility decline immediately following the first will depend on what happens to the demand for children. As noted, this report documents a small decline in women's "ideal" family size, but that decline is achievable with later age at first marriage and is too small to increase the demand for modern contraception.

Assuming Senegal achieves further increases in primary and secondary school enrollment for women, as well as greater urbanization, further fertility declines can be expected to occur in the near future. In rural areas, further declines in actual fertility can be achieved through the mechanism of later marriage. However, in urban areas, particularly Dakar, most of the decline in actual fertility that is achievable solely by an increase in age at marriage has already occurred, so that future fertility reductions must await greater coverage of modern contraception.

If the government of Senegal wishes to foster fertility decline, strong policies targeting both girls and women of reproductive age are needed. For girls, policy should aim at increasing formal education. For women, action should be taken to promote the availability of contraception while increasing women's functional literacy and reducing their domestic burden. These policies, combined with interventions aimed at improving maternal and child health, should have a good chance of making women more receptive to the use of modern contraceptives.

MORTALITY

Both child and adult mortality have undergone substantial declines over the past several decades in Senegal.

Child Mortality

Senegal has undergone a continuous decrease in child mortality since World War II. In 45 years, from 1945-1990, child mortality—measured by the probability of dying before age 5—fell substantially, declining from approximately 400 to 130 per 1,000. This decrease accelerated toward the end of the 1970s and the beginning of the 1980s.

The difference between child mortality rates in urban and rural settings is sharp. Between the mid-1960s and 1986, child mortality declined at a relatively slow pace in Dakar, from about 150-200 to about 100 per 1,000. By contrast, until the early 1970s, child mortality ranged between 350 and 400 per 1,000 in the rural areas; as noted above, the mortality decline in the rural areas, which was by no means homogenous, began only in the late 1970s in most areas. The probability of dying decreased from 370 per 1,000 in the early to mid-1970s to 230 per 1,000 a decade later. Because of the relatively rapid decline in child mortality in the rural as compared with the urban areas, the differential between the two narrowed from three to one during 1960-1975 to two to one at the beginning of the 1980s.

Regional differences in child mortality are marked and have been consistent over time. Since the late 1960s, the probability of dying before age 5 has been far lower in the western grand region[1]—where it fell from 183 per 1,000 in 1968 to 111 per 1,000 in 1988-1992—than in any of the other three grand regions. In general, the second-lowest child mortality has been in the northeastern region, where it fell from 253 to 183 between 1968-1972 and 1988-1992, followed by the central region, where it fell from 304 to 170 in the same time period. Child mortality has remained the highest in the southern region, where it has consistently been almost twice that found in the west.

Ironically, the study area of Mlomp, a rural area in the south, experienced the earliest and one of the most rapid declines of all the small-scale study areas reviewed in this report. The pattern of mortality decline in Mlomp—where the decline in infant mortality occurred before that in child mortality—was also slightly different from that recorded elsewhere. Mlomp's early and rapid mortality decline and the unusual pattern of that decline are likely the result of the establishment of a private dispensary and a maternity clinic in 1961, which soon after their establishment were providing high-quality health services to a large majority of the residents in the area.

The acceleration of the mortality decline in rural areas beginning in the late 1970s can be linked to the improved infrastructure of health programs in Senegal, which until that time had been located almost exclusively in the urban area of Dakar. Two initiatives had a large impact on the rural areas: (1) the new primary health care policy, which, starting in 1978, led to the construction of a large number of maternity clinics in rural areas, and (2) the World Health Organization's Expanded Programmme on Immunization (EPI), which, when implemented in 1981, had as one of its goals better services for children in rural areas. By the beginning of the 1990s, vaccination had increased substantially throughout Senegal. Fifty-five percent of children aged 12-23 months were completely vaccinated in 1990, up from 18 percent in 1984. The improvement in rural areas greatly exceeded that in urban areas, narrowing the gap that had earlier existed between the two. Since the early 1990s, however, greater emphasis has been placed on the EPI services in urban areas than in rural areas. Therefore, the rural-urban gap is likely widening again, and greater emphasis on EPI services in rural areas is needed.

Surprisingly, the period of economic stagnation and the implementation of the structural adjustment policies did not produce the large adverse effects on child mortality that might have been expected.

Differences in mother's level of education and urban/rural residence are the two socioeconomic variables most strongly related to differentials in child mortality in Senegal. A child whose mother has attended school is almost one-third less likely to die, regardless of other factors, underscoring the importance of female education not only for fertility, as suggested above, but also for child mortality. Likewise, living in an urban area is associated with a risk of death one-third to one-half lower than that in rural areas.

Adult Mortality

Adult mortality has also been falling in Senegal. The expectation of life at age 15 for males increased from 48.3 to 49.9 years of age between 1976 and 1988, and that of females from 47.1 to 51.5 years between 1972 and 1988. These national-level declines are supported by results from local surveys.

As with child mortality, adult mortality levels are not uniform throughout the country. Survivorship data from the 1988 census indicate that in the early to mid-1970s, adult mortality ranged from very high levels in the southeastern part of the country to relatively low levels in the west. In the southeastern regions of Tambacounda and Kolda, the likelihood of someone aged 15 dying before reaching age 60 was 50 percent. In the five more centralized regions of Diourbel, Fatick, Kaolack, Louga, and Ziguinchor, however, the likelihood of dying between the ages of 15 and 60 was around 35 percent. In the western regions of Thiès and Dakar and in Saint-Louis, the probability of dying between the ages of 15 and 60 was around 20 percent.

As with child mortality, adult mortality is negatively related to socioeconomic status—as indicators of wealth increase, adult mortality decreases. In all cases, the negative relationship is stronger for female adult mortality than for male adult mortality.

NOTE

1. The term "grand region" is used throughout this report in reference to the four WFS and DHS regions, as opposed to the ten administrative regions used in discussions of the 1988 census. (Figure A-1 shows the geographic area included in each of the "grand" regions. Figure 2-2 shows the 10 administrative regions and the 30 administrative departments.)

1

Introduction

Sub-Saharan Africa has experienced rapid demographic changes over the course of the past several decades, the most notable being a decline in mortality. Fertility has also begun to decline in some areas. Where these changes have taken place, they have not occurred simultaneously throughout the continent. In contrast with southern and eastern Africa, the decline in mortality in western Africa has been relatively late and the decline in fertility, until recently, nonexistent.

Against this background, the Panel on the Population Dynamics of Sub-Saharan Africa selected two countries, Kenya and Senegal, as case studies to try to shed light on the determinants of the demographic transition under way in Africa. Kenya was selected primarily because it was clear that demographic changes were taking place there, and because the country's social and economic development exceeded that of other countries in the region (see Working Group on Kenya, 1993).

This study on the population dynamics of Senegal was chosen for two key reasons. First, it seemed to provide an interesting contrast to the case study of Kenya. Demographic changes were not as apparent in Senegal as in Kenya, and there did not seem to be much economic and social development in Senegal. In addition, Senegal and Kenya are geographically and linguistically distinct; Senegal is a francophone country in western Africa, while Kenya is an anglophone country in eastern Africa. Second, Senegal has an abundance of available national- and local-level data, not all of which had been analyzed. These available data have made it possible and rewarding to undertake an indepth demographic study of the country.

This report describes the demographic situation in Senegal, focusing in particular on fertility and mortality and the socioeconomic factors associated with the levels and trends of these demographic phenomena. It is both a review of earlier research of demographic topics in Senegal and a presentation of original analysis from recent data. It attempts to trace long-term demographic trends in Senegal and to look in detail at the present and very recent past. It presents demographic levels and trends for the whole country, as well as at the departmental and regional levels, and examines whether the geographic variations in demographic phenomena are linked with differences in socioeconomic characteristics.

The report is based primarily on existing data sets, including several major national demographic surveys conducted in Senegal (the Demographic Survey in 1960-1961, the National Demographic Survey in 1970-1971, the World Fertility Survey in 1978, the Demographic and Health Surveys in 1986 [DHS-I] and in 1992-1993 [DHS-II]), and the two Senegal censuses in 1976 and 1988. The report also relies heavily on various smaller-scale studies, including longitudinal studies in the rural areas of Bandafassi, Niakhar/Ngayokhème, and Mlomp, which provide high-quality data over long periods of time for these areas. Throughout the report, the various surveys are referenced with bracketed numbers ([1], [2], [3], etc.) that correspond to the listing in Appendix A, which describes and provides the reference information for each survey.

The report is organized as follows: Chapter 2 presents a brief summary of Senegal's geography and socioeconomic history and of the geographic variations in socioeconomic characteristics at the departmental and regional levels. Chapter 3 presents the country's general demographic trends. Chapter 4 examines the levels, trends, and proximate determinants of fertility in Senegal and describes the nuptiality patterns and their changes that are likely to be responsible for a portion of the observed changes in fertility. This chapter also explores the geographic variations in fertility and its determinants and their relationships to differing socioeconomic characteristics. Chapter 5 presents levels and trends in child and adult mortality, examines the health policies and programs that are likely to have affected mortality, explores geographic variations in child mortality, and attempts to relate these variations to differences in socioeconomic characteristics and public-sector service provision. Chapter 6 offers some conclusions and attempts to place the demographic transition in Senegal in the wider African context.

2

Geographic and Socioeconomic Setting

GEOGRAPHIC OVERVIEW

Senegal is a mid-size African country located on the western coast of the continent. It is bordered by Mauritania to the north, Mali to the east, Guinea to the southeast, and Guinea-Bissau to the south; The Gambia forms an enclave along the Gambia River. Senegal has a surface area of 196,722 square kilometers (km^2), which supports a population estimated at 6.9 million in 1988, making the average density 35 inhabitants/km^2.

Senegal is a relatively flat country and exhibits few pronounced topographical features, although the southeastern part of the country, on the Guinean border, contains small massifs.

The climate varies greatly between the northern and southern portions of the country. Rainfall ranges from less than 400 mm per year in the northern half of the country, which forms part of the Sahel, to more than 1,000 mm per year in parts of the southern half (Moore et al., 1992, data from 1980-1987). Senegal has been experiencing progressively less and less rainfall since early in the century (see Figure 2-1). The rainy season, which takes place roughly between the months of July and November, lasts up to 6 months in the southern part of the country and 3 months in the north. The daily temperature can reach 110 degrees Fahrenheit during the day and fall to 60 degrees at night.

Senegal is currently divided into ten administrative regions, each of which is further subdivided into three departments (see Figure 2-2). The

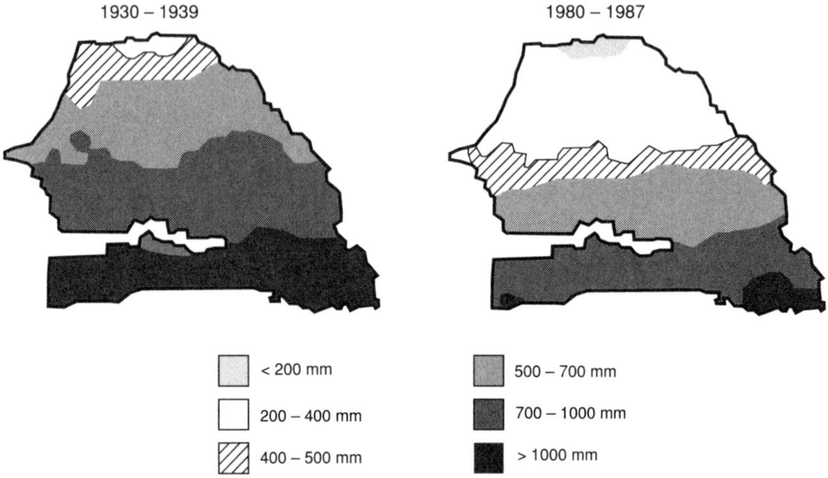

FIGURE 2-1 Annual average rainfall in Senegal, 1930-1939 and 1980-1987. SOURCE: Moore et al. (1992).

subdivisions within Senegal have changed twice since 1960 when there were seven regions: Dakar, Thiès, Saint-Louis, Tambacounda, Diourbel, Sine-Saloum, and Casamance;[1] the last three of these regions have each split into two since 1960. In 1976, Diourbel was divided into Louga and Diourbel, so that there were eight regions during the 1976 census. In 1984, Casamance was divided into Kolda and Ziguinchor, and Sine-Saloum was divided into Fatick and Kaolack.

HISTORICAL OVERVIEW

Based on the findings from many archaeological sites, archaeologists have discovered that the geographic area of Senegal was already quite populated 500-1,000 years ago. The distribution of the population was quite different, however, with the interior of the country being relatively more populated than today. The current distribution of the population, which is more heavily concentrated along the Atlantic coast, emerged only after a series of migrations over the last 300 years (see Becker and Mbodji, 1994).

Senegal's history is rich with international contacts. As early as the tenth century, the people of Senegal had links with Arab traders from North Africa. In the following century, Islam entered Senegal, and to this day it remains the predominant religion. The Portuguese, the first Europeans to explore Senegal, arrived in 1445, followed shortly thereafter by the French, the Dutch, and the British. During the seventeenth and eighteenth centu-

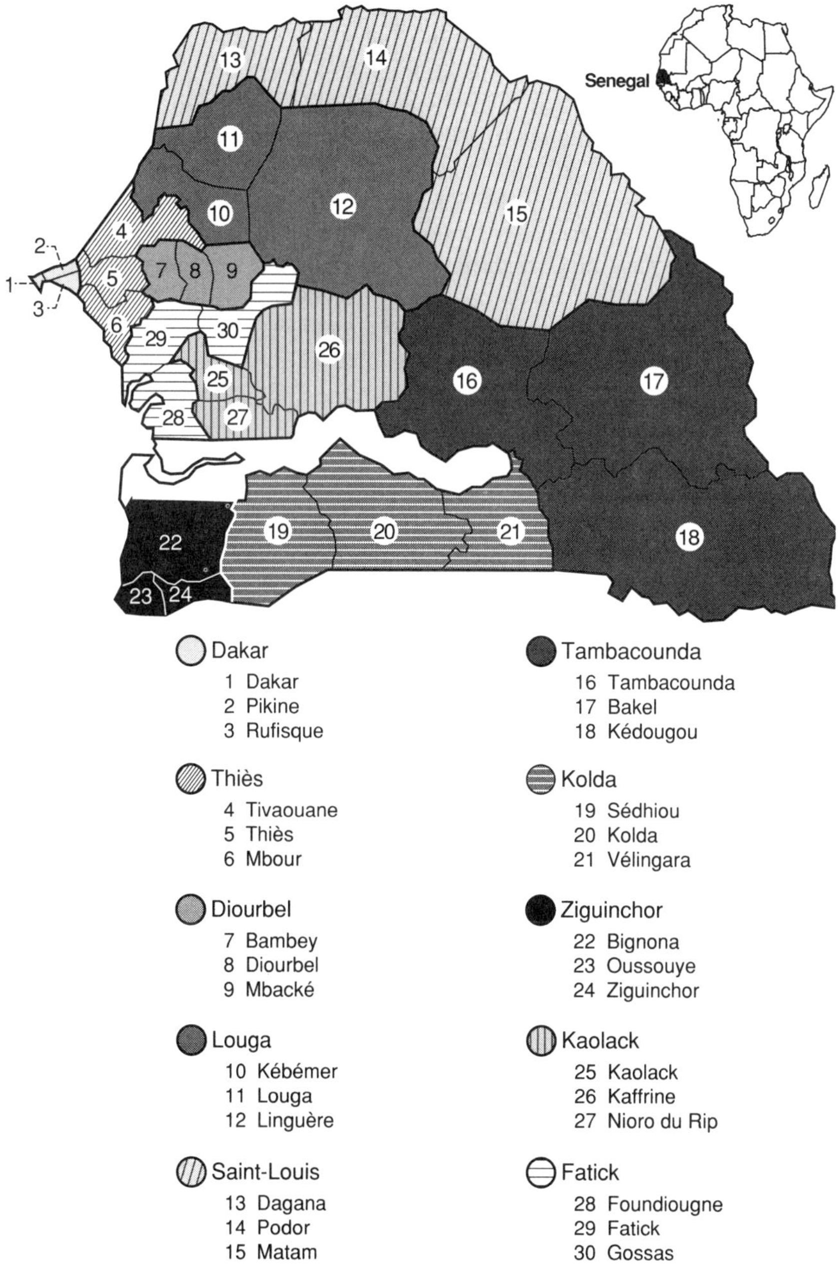

FIGURE 2-2 Administrative divisions in Senegal. NOTE: The white area of the map is The Gambia.

ries, the Europeans were responsible for the export of slaves, ivory, and gold; the export of slaves was outlawed in 1848.

By 1840, the French had gained enough control of the area to establish Senegal as a French possession. As the French penetrated the Senegalese hinterland, they came into conflict with the Tukulor Empire of Seku Ahmadu, who ruled in the mid- to late nineteenth century, and the Wolof (Gordon, 1988). The final struggle of the Senegalese against French domination was by the peoples of Casamance in the southern part of the country. This struggle lasted into the twentieth century (Gordon, 1988). In addition, France fought the British for control of the mouth of the Gambia River. Inability to oust the British led to a settlement of boundaries in 1889 between French-controlled Senegal and British-controlled Gambia.

Near the end of the nineteenth century, France became increasingly desirous of taking over additional parts of western Africa, which they did using Senegal as a base. By the beginning of the twentieth century, France had control of much of western Africa; this area became known as French West Africa in 1895.

There are virtually no demographic data available for Senegal from this period. However, long-term vital registration systems for the cities of Dakar and Saint-Louis were established and have been maintained to the present (Garenne, 1994). The vital registration data indicate that mortality began to decline in these areas in the second decade of the twentieth century (see Diop, 1990, and Garenne et al., 1993, as cited in Garenne, 1994). Administrative counts of the whole population are also available from the beginning of the century, although they tend to be of doubtful quality (see Becker and Mbodji, 1994). The French also conducted a census in these areas and in Rufisque and the island of Gorée in 1907 (Verrière, 1965:17).

After World War II, the Senegalese were given additional rights and representation, partly in appreciation of their support for the de Gaulle government during the war (Gordon, 1988). Moreover, during the early part of the twentieth century, political groups began organizing in Senegal. The combination of increased rights and the growing strength of these political groups led to Senegal's eventual independence from France, which was achieved on April 4, 1960.

One of the political groups that was active prior to Senegalese independence was formed in 1948 by Léopold Sédar Senghor, who became the country's first president in 1960 and served in that position until December 31, 1980, when he voluntarily resigned. In accordance with the Senegalese constitution, the Prime Minister, Abdou Diouf, became the president upon Senghor's resignation. Two years later, in February 1983, Diouf was elected president in his own right. He was reelected in 1988 and again in 1993 and remains Senegal's president today.

Senegal has had a relatively stable government since independence, unlike many of its neighbors. This has made the country relatively attractive to foreign investors; it continues to benefit from substantial foreign investment, particularly from France, with which Senegal has maintained close ties.

EDUCATION

Educational statistics point to a successful history of educational expansion in Senegal. Between 1960 and 1983, primary school enrollment quadrupled from 129,00 to approximately 533,000 (World Bank, 1988). Gross primary school enrollment rose from 27 percent in 1960 to 53 percent in 1983. Although girls still lag far behind boys, their gross primary enrollment ratios rose impressively from 18 percent in 1960 to 42 percent in 1983; the comparable figures for boys were 37 and 63 percent, respectively (World Bank, 1988).

Secondary school expansion has been equally impressive. The total number of children in secondary school rose from a meager 13,000 in 1960 to over 113,000 in 1983. Here, females made less significant gains: females as a percentage of total enrollment increased from 27 to 33 percent over this 23-year period (World Bank, 1988).[2]

The above rapid gains may have been achieved partly at the expense of the quality of education offered. Recent data indicate that Senegal spends only $3.60 per pupil on educational materials, although the World Bank recommends that a minimum of $5 is necessary (World Bank, 1988).

Unfortunately, the gains in enrollment rates are now being threatened. Recent predictions indicate that gross primary enrollment rates in Senegal will fall from around 50 percent in 1983 to around 40 percent by the year 2000. A combination of demographic, fiscal, and social factors is responsible. Rapid population growth has placed strong demographic pressures on a system that is feeling the fiscal constraints of structural adjustment policies. In addition, some African parents may be becoming increasingly disillusioned about the quality of education being offered and its usefulness for their children, given the reduced prospects of obtaining employment in the formal sector after graduation (International Labour Organization, 1989).

ECONOMIC BACKGROUND

Overview

Like most African countries, Senegal has undergone a series of economic reversals and changes of policy in the last three decades. The overall picture is one of stagnation in personal income. The gross domestic product (GDP), expressed in constant Communauté Financière d'Afrique (CFA) francs,

TABLE 2-1 Senegal Population Size and Growth Rates at Various Points over Time

Year	Population	Interval	Average Annual Growth Rate
1960	3,110,000	—	—
1970	3,906,000	1960-1970	2.3
1976	4,998,000	1970-1976	4.2
1988	6,897,000	1976-1988	2.7
—	—	1960-1988	2.9
—	—	1970-1988	3.2

NOTE: See Appendix A for description of surveys.

SOURCES: 1960: République du Sénégal (1964)
1970: République du Sénégal (1974)
1976: 1976 census (unpublished tables)
1988: 1988 census (unpublished tables)

increased at a rate of 3.5 percent per year during the 1960s and 2.2 percent per year between 1970 and 1990 (Duruflé, 1994). Population growth kept pace at an average annual rate of 2.9 percent between 1960 and 1988 (see Table 2-1). The per capita gross national product (GNP) was not much higher in 1991, when it was estimated to be US $720 (World Bank, 1993b), than it had been in 1965, just after independence (Duruflé, 1994). Despite this weak performance in 1991, Senegal's per capita GNP was still more than twice the average for sub-Saharan African countries (see Table 2-2).

This long-term stagnation masks considerable short-term fluctuation. There was some growth in the early 1960s, followed by a decline in GDP per capita in 1968-1973. Favorable prices for groundnuts and phosphates (the country's chief exports) helped produce a short-lived boom in the mid-1970s, followed by a deterioration in 1978-1981 due in large part to drought and the rapid increase in oil prices (Montalieu and Plane, 1993).

While overall GDP growth has been weak since the 1960s, there has been an increase through most of the period in public-sector expenditures, private consumption, and imports. The result has been persistent deficits in the public-sector budget and the balance of payments (Rouis, 1994; World Bank, 1993b).

During the 1980s and 1990s, Senegal implemented structural adjustment and stabilization policies aimed at liberalizing markets, reducing public-sector employment and the role of government in the economy, and reducing subsidies on inputs such as fertilizers. These policies have resulted in a reduction in the public-sector deficit and in urban-rural income differentials, but virtually no growth in per capita GNP (Berg, 1990; Montalieu and Plane, 1993; World Bank, 1993b). During 1980-1991, real GNP per capita grew by only 0.1 percent per year. This was a higher rate of increase than for sub-Saharan Africa as a whole, but lower than for other countries classified by the World Bank as "middle-income" (see Table 2-2). One consequence of the economic downturn has been that the government has had to cut back in the health sector. Despite an increase in real health spending between 1975 and 1987, government expenditures on health as a percentage of total government expenditures dropped from 5.9 percent in 1975-1979 to 3.3 percent in 1986-1987 (Ogbu and Gallagher, 1992). These changes were partly offset by an increase in health care from the private sector.

The Structure of Production

The share of services in Senegal's domestic production has grown over time, from 56 percent of GDP in 1970 to 62 percent in 1991 (Duruflé, 1994). Industry's share has been roughly constant during the same period, at 19-20 percent. The share of agriculture has fallen from 24 to 20 percent (Duruflé, 1994). However, the amount of land cultivated has increased somewhat since independence, and the agricultural sector still employs the majority of the labor force (60 percent of working adults according to a recent World Bank [1993a] estimate).

Groundnuts are Senegal's main cash and export crop, providing inputs for processing industries and accounting for a significant portion of export earnings. Yields have been very erratic, varying from 1.4 million tons in 1975-1976 to 0.2 million in 1980-1981, and 0.7 million in 1990-1991 (Figure 2-3) (Caicedo, 1990; Duruflé, 1994).

Millet and sorghum are Senegal's main food crops; their production (now around 700,000 tons per year) has been expanding on average by 1 percent per year (Berg, 1990). About one-third to one-half of the rice consumed in Senegal is produced locally, although imports have been increasing. Vegetable production has been increasing rapidly, as has small animal husbandry around the urban centers. Cattle production is erratic because of the country's climatic fluctuations.

Senegalese agriculture has suffered from deteriorating soil quality, erratic rainfall, and low prices to producers (Duruflé, 1994). These problems have been exacerbated by a decline in the use of fertilizer, which has fallen to one-third of its level in 1980, as well as decreased use of other inputs (World Bank, 1993a). Since 1986, as part of the adjustment program discussed above, the country has announced new agricultural policies intended to free prices, liberalize markets, and eliminate subsidies for inputs such as fertilizers.

The fishery sector makes up only 2.3 percent of GDP but contributes

TABLE 2-2 Social, Economic, and Demographic Indicators for Senegal and Other Countries and Regions

Indicator	Senegal	Côte d'Ivoire	Low Income[a] Economies Excluding China and India	Middle Income[b] Economies	Sub-Saharan Africa
Population (in millions), 1991	7.6	12.4	1,111.2	1,401.0	488.9
Total fertility rate, 1991	6.1	6.6	5.2	3.2	6.4
Infant mortality rate, 1991	81	95	91	38	104
GNP per capita					
(1980 dollars)[c]	450	1,150	230	1,400	—
(1991 dollars)[d]	720	690	350	2,480	350
World Bank ranking[d]	43	42	—	—	—
Average annual growth rate of GNP per capita, 1980-1991[d]	0.1	–4.6	1.0	0.3	-1.2
Annual change in real wages (%) (1980-1985)[e,f]	–6.9	–4.4	—	—	—
Total external debt as percentage of GNP[d]					
1980	50.5	58.8	33.5	31.9	28.6
1991	63.1	222.6	85.7	41.2	107.9
Percentage living in urban areas[d]	39	40	28	62	29

Females per 100 males in primary school, 1990[d]	72	71	76	91	76
Primary school net enrollment, 1990[d,g]	48	—	72	89	46
Primary pupil/teacher ratio, 1990[d]	58	36	39	25	41
Secondary school enrollment, 1990[d,h]	16	—	28	126	17
Tertiary school enrollment, 1990[d,h]	3	—	4	16	2

[a]The World Bank defines low-income economies as those with a GNP per capita of US $635 or less in 1991 (World Bank, 1993b).

[b]The World Bank defines middle-income economies as those with a GNP per capita of more than US $635, but less than US $7,911 in 1991 (World Bank, 1993b).

[c]Data from World Bank (1982).

[d]Data from World Bank (1993b).

[e]Data from Vandemoortele (1991).

[f]Data for Côte d'Ivoire refer to 1980-1988.

[g]Percentage of school-age children enrolled in school, 1990.

[h]Percentage of age group enrolled in education.

SOURCES: World Bank (1982, 1993b); Vandemoortele (1991)

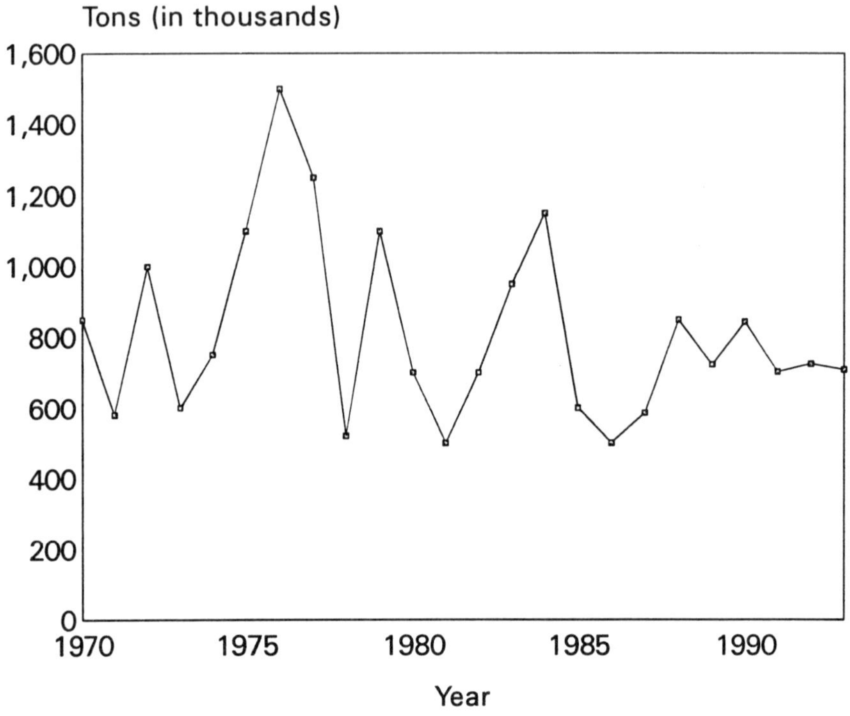

FIGURE 2-3 Groundnut production (in thousand tons) in Senegal, 1970-1993. SOURCE: Duruflé (1994).

substantially (22 percent) to Senegal's merchandise export earnings (World Bank, 1993a). The rate of growth in the quantity of fish caught has declined over the past decade from 3.9 percent per year in the 1980s to 2.5 percent in the early 1990s. This decline is due in part to overfishing off the coast of Senegal and has resulted in the closing of five fish-canning factories since 1988 (World Bank, 1993a).

Senegal has a relatively diversified industrial sector that is geographically concentrated in the Dakar region (Boone, 1993; Valette, 1991). Manufacturing consists mainly of food and agricultural processing (groundnut oil mills, sugar mills, seafood processing), textiles, and petroleum products. The industrial sector grew an average of 5.3 percent per year during 1970-1980 and 3.8 percent per year during 1980-1991 (World Bank, 1993b). Phosphates, the most important product of the mining sector, accounted for 7 percent of Senegal's exports of goods in 1991 (International Monetary Fund, 1993a).

Import-substituting industries still benefit from considerable government protection, despite measures undertaken since 1986 to liberalize trade and exchange rates. The overvaluation of the CFA franc, until the 50 percent devaluation in January 1994, increased costs for import-using industries and hurt the competitiveness of Senegalese manufacturers. A new industrial policy includes subsidies to exports, relaxation of some provisions of the labor code, and managerial reform (Barro, 1991; Logeay, 1990).

Officially, Senegal's service sector produced 62 percent of the GDP in 1991 (World Bank, 1993b). Figures for informal-sector output in particular are very unreliable, but there is evidence that an increasing proportion of new entrants to the labor force in Senegal work in small-scale informal service enterprises in the cities (Barro, 1991). In 1986, there were 173,000 workers in the "modern private sector," compared with 537,000 in the "informal sector," mainly in services and retail trade (Barro, 1991).

Dependency, External Shocks, and Adjustment

In the years following World War II and for a time after independence, Senegal's exports expanded rapidly, and their structure changed as the proportion of manufacturing increased from 3 percent in 1965 to 22 percent in 1990 (Hugon, 1993). Dependence on groundnuts fell from 44 percent of exports in 1966-1973 to 16 percent in 1989-1991 (International Monetary Fund, 1993a).

However, deterioration in the terms of trade and a failure to maintain the competitiveness of exports have resulted in a chronic trade deficit, which has been financed by grants and loans, membership in the CFA franc zone, and remittances from abroad (Duruflé, 1994). Official development assistance made up 12 percent of the GDP in 1991 (Rouis, 1994). Total official development assistance increased by 7.4 percent per year during the decade 1980-1989, and on a per capita basis was two-thirds higher than for other sub-Saharan African countries between 1984 and 1988 (World Bank, 1993a). In 1991, "official unrequited transfers," as measured in balance-of-payments statistics, equaled US$374 million (of which $105 million was represented by cancellation of debt), or about $50 per inhabitant (International Monetary Fund, 1993a). Before the mid-1980s, remittances from Senegalese abroad appeared to roughly balance remittances from foreigners working in Senegal. (Remittances are typically one of the most difficult elements to measure in balance-of-payments statistics.) However, remittances from Senegalese abroad have since increased—to $83 million in 1991, compared with $51 million remitted out of Senegal (International Monetary Fund, 1993a).

In 1980, Senegal's external debt was 50.5 percent of GNP. This proportion rose to 63.1 percent in 1991 (see Table 2-2). Debt service amounted to 20 percent of the value of goods and services exported in 1991, which was down somewhat from 29 percent a decade earlier (World Bank, 1993b).

At the end of the 1970s, the economic situation in Senegal had deteriorated to the point that significant economic reforms were considered necessary. Between 1978 and 1981, the rate of GDP growth slowed to 0.8 percent per year. Two reasons posited for this decline are that (1) during 1978-1981 there were two major droughts in Senegal, and (2) the world price for groundnuts, Senegal's most important export, declined (Rouis, 1994). At the same time, the public-sector deficit was 12.5 percent of GDP, savings were negative, inflation was at 12 percent, and debt service represented 18.5 percent of total exports.

In December 1979, economic reforms were announced. The goals of these reforms were to raise public savings, increase investment in the productive sector, liberalize trade, and reduce the government's role in the economy. Funds to implement the reforms were provided by the International Monetary Fund (IMF) and the World Bank; however, they were withdrawn when implementation of the reforms was judged unsatisfactory (Rouis, 1994).

Since 1986, there have been renewed efforts to implement reforms, with mixed results. Either none of the announced reforms were implemented, or those that were implemented were later halted or changed in mid-course. Lack of government commitment to the reforms has also been a problem, particularly since the 1988 election (Rouis, 1994).

Fiscal policy reform was one of the primary goals of the economic reforms. There were attempts to reform the tax system and widen the tax base and to control public expenditures, primarily by reducing public-sector employment and transfers to public enterprises. As a result, 21 public enterprises were closed and 26 others partially or fully privatized; however, these firms represented only 19 and 11 percent, respectively, of government assets and equity (Rouis, 1994). The number of civil servants was reduced from 69,000 in 1986 to approximately 62,000 in 1992 (the figure in 1973 had been 40,000). These measures met with some success, as the public-sector deficit fell from 8 percent in 1982 to 1 percent a decade later, though there was criticism that the revenue increases were due not to taxes, but to windfalls from petroleum, and that the expenditure decreases came from cuts in investment and maintenance (Rouis, 1994:302-303, 328).

Monetary policy has also been a target of reform. Senegal is a member, with six other West African nations, of the West African Monetary Union, established in 1962. Each member country uses the same currency (the CFA franc), which is tied to the French franc at a fixed rate of exchange. Interest rates in member countries are uniform. In 1989, the Monetary Union countries adopted a plan to decrease the administrative controls of the economy and increase the role of the markets. In Senegal, banking reforms since 1989 have led to the closing of some insolvent banks, privatization of other banks, and steps to curb abuses of government-guaranteed loans.

Interest rate controls have been removed. Financial-sector reform has been considered a success, with a stronger banking system, and inflation rates averaging less than 3 percent in recent years (Guillaumont, 1992).

In January 1994, the CFA franc was devalued by 50 percent. The devaluation decreased purchasing power for consumers of imported goods, primarily among the urban salaried population.

Trade policies have also been revised to reduce protection for import-competing industries and increase the competitiveness of Senegal's exports. These policies were implemented in two phases between 1986 and 1988, the main objectives being to eliminate most of the quantity restrictions on imported goods and to decrease tariffs. Under pressure from industry, the government reintroduced some protective measures in 1989, but the effective rate of protection averaged across commodities is still down from 165 percent in 1985 to 98 percent in the early 1990s (Rouis, 1994:308).

Policies have also been implemented to reduce government intervention in the domestic economy. By the end of 1988, progress had been made toward reducing or phasing out government subsidies for agricultural inputs. Producer prices for cash crops were reduced somewhat, but the price for groundnuts is still controlled (Rouis, 1994). At the same time, prices for consumer goods were decontrolled for all but 16 goods (those goods remaining under control included such staples as sugar, salt, tea, flour, tomatoes, and cooking oil) (Rouis, 1994).

The most effective reforms dealing with the civil service were implemented in 1990. The number of ministries was cut from 23 to 15, and almost 3,800 civil service jobs were eliminated (Rouis, 1994).

The macroeconomic outcomes of the adjustment policies indicate only mixed success (see Table 2-3). The greatest macroeconomic success of the decade was the reduction of the inflation rate to 2.7 percent, down from 9.1 percent and 10.0 percent during the crisis and stabilization periods, respectively. Growth of GDP increased from 2.3 percent per year during the precrisis period to 3.2 percent per year during 1986-1991. However, with the population growing at an annual rate of 2.9 during the same period, GNP per capita increased by only around 0.3 percent per year. Gross domestic investment and savings still accounted for a smaller proportion of the GDP during 1986-1991 than during the precrisis period 1970-1978 (Rouis, 1994).

Data on the distribution of income among social classes, between rural and urban residents, and across regions are very deficient. Earnings in the informal sector and subsistence farming, especially, are difficult to measure; most published studies refer only to earnings of formal-sector workers and cannot readily be generalized or compared over time. The gap between urban and rural incomes probably narrowed during the adjustment period. The minimum wage in the formal sector (SMIG)[3] was about at the same

TABLE 2-3 Selected Macroeconomic Indicators, 1970-1991

Indicator	Precrisis 1970-1978	Crisis 1979-1981	Stabilization 1982-1985	Partial Adjustment 1986-1991
GDP growth (%)	2.3	1.8	4.3	3.2
Gross domestic investment/GDP (%)	17.7	13.9	11.9	12.8
Gross domestic savings/GDP	10.5	–1.2	0.6	7.6
Growth in exports (%)	6.0	–0.7	5.5	3.3
Inflation rate (%)	7.4	9.1	10.0	2.7
Real effective exchange rate (1985 = 100)[a]	101.8	100.1	93.7	122.6
Current account deficit/GDP[b]	–10.4	–19.3	–18.2	–10.0

[a]An increase indicates appreciation.
[b]Excluding official transfers.

SOURCE: Rouis (1994)

level in real terms in 1990 as it was in 1972. Average wages of civil servants fell relative to the SMIG from a ratio of 5.2 in 1969-1970 to 4.7 in 1988-1989. There is some evidence that the economic crisis has led to decreases in monetary transfers from young people to older family members (Antoine and Mbodji, 1991).

Regional Disparities in Socioeconomic Indicators

Socioeconomic levels vary greatly from one region to another in Senegal. This section examines regional and departmental differences in six indicators of socioeconomic status, based on data from the 1988 census:

- percentage of the population aged 6 and older with some schooling;
- school enrollment rates for children aged 7-12;
- percentage of households obtaining their water supply from a faucet or standpipe, whether placed inside or outside the home;
- percentage of households with electricity;
- percentage of households with toilets or latrines; and
- percentage of households whose houses have been built using good construction techniques.[4]

A final indicator, the arithmetic mean of the last four indicators, termed the "composite facilities indicator," provides a crude measure of overall living conditions by administrative department. These indicators are presented in Table 2-4. Their associations with fertility and mortality rates are discussed in Chapters 4 and 5, respectively.

Some geographic differences are clear. The socioeconomic contrasts between the relatively populated west and the less populous east—or between the regions surrounding Dakar and those farther from the capital—exist to a greater or lesser degree for all of these socioeconomic indicators.

The percentage of the population aged 6 and older with some schooling ranges from 17 to 56 percent, depending on the region (see Figure 2-4). Two regions—Dakar and Ziguinchor—have rates that are clearly higher than the national average. School enrollment rates for children aged 7-12 show similar geographic variations (see Figure 2-5). Three regions do not fall within the general pattern that delineates between the western areas close to Dakar and the eastern regions farther from the capital: Ziguinchor, despite its distance from Dakar, has high rates of school attendance; and Louga and Diourbel, though relatively close to Dakar, have low attendance rates.

Whereas census data on educational differences are available only at the regional level, indicators measuring access to running water, electricity,

TABLE 2-4 Selected Socioeconomic Indicators, Senegal, 1988 (in percent)

Region and Department	Households with Good Construction[a]	Households with Electricity	Households with Latrines	Households with Access to Running Water[b]
Dakar	88	63	75	92
Dakar	89	80	79	95
Pikine	88	49	77	88
Rufisque	84	49	50	90
Diourbel	38	11	26	51
Bambey	31	4	11	24
Diourbel	35	17	23	43
Mbacké	45	11	39	75
Fatick	30	4	12	23
Fatick	32	5	11	19
Foundiougne	34	3	16	15
Gossas	23	5	10	34
Kaolack	29	11	22	32
Kaffrine	14	1	9	18
Kaolack	49	25	38	55
Nioro du Rip	20	3	17	13
Kolda	16	4	23	4
Kolda	13	6	25	3
Sédhiou	19	2	18	5
Vélingara	12	4	29	3
Louga	24	9	16	36
Kébémer	20	5	14	32
Linguère	17	4	9	31
Louga	34	15	23	43
Saint-Louis	37	14	25	29
Dagana	60	30	40	50
Matam	25	3	15	21
Podor	15	4	13	6
Tambacounda	14	7	22	9
Bakel	20	5	24	14
Kédougou	6	4	5	6
Tambacounda	15	10	27	8
Thiès	58	20	25	47
Mbour	57	17	22	43
Thiès	69	30	33	60
Tivaouane	44	11	18	36
Ziguinchor	34	9	14	12
Bignona	26	3	6	3
Oussouye	19	4	6	14
Ziguinchor	47	17	25	21

[a]A composite indicator combining proportion of houses with permanent floor, wall, and roof materials.

[b]Running water wither within the house or outside.

[c]Average of water, electricity, latrine, and good construction indicators.

Composite Indicator[c]	Population in Urban Areas	Population Aged 6 and Older That has had Some Schooling	School Enrollment Rate for Males Aged 7-12	School Enrollment Rate for Females Aged 7-12
79	97	56	79	64
86	96			
75	100			
68	90			
31	22	17	35	16
18	8			
29	42			
42	17			
17	10	24	45	35
17	9			
17	8			
18	14			
24	23	25	43	28
11	5			
42	53			
13	6			
11	11	18	39	19
12	19			
11	5			
12	11			
21	15	17	34	18
18	6			
15	7			
29	27			
26	27	24	39	25
45	56			
16	8			
9	5			
13	16	18	26	17
16	7			
5	15			
15	21			
37	34	32	55	38
35	34			
48	50			
27	13			
17	38	45	81	65
10	12			
11	11			
27	70			

SOURCE: 1988 census (unpublished tables)

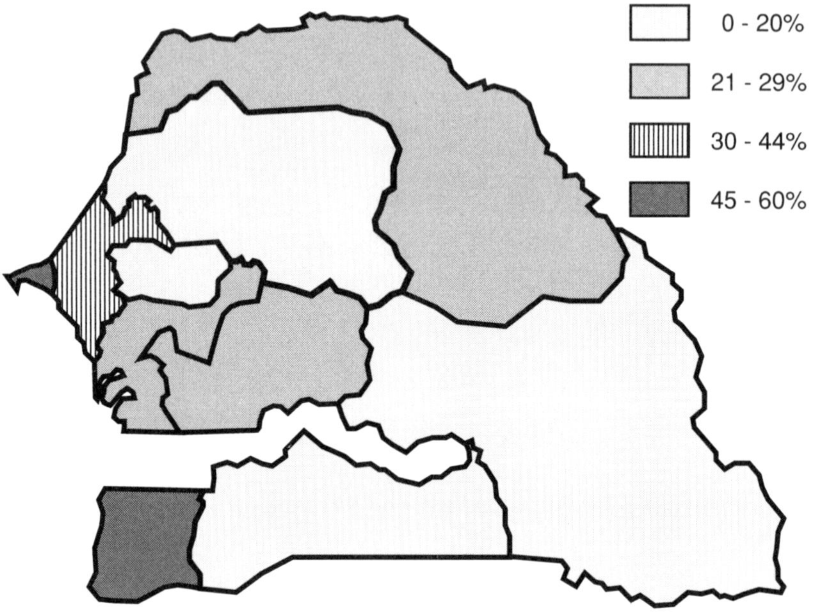

FIGURE 2-4 Percentage of population aged 6 and older with some schooling, Senegal, 1988. SOURCE: 1988 census (unpublished tables).

toilets or latrines, and well-constructed housing are available for each of the 30 administrative departments within Senegal.

There is great variation throughout Senegal in access to running water and electricity (see Table 2-4). Urban dwellers have the greatest access to running water and electricity. More than 90 percent of households in the region of Dakar have access to clean water, compared with only 4 percent in the Kolda region. Likewise, over 60 percent of households in Dakar have access to electricity, but no other region exceeds 20 percent.

The disparity between east and west in the percentage of households with toilets or latrines is not as great as that for the other socioeconomic indicators; however, the gradient reappears when we analyze the good construction indicator. Over 85 percent of the houses in the region of Dakar are considered to be of good construction, but less than 15 percent in Tambacounda. The quality of housing construction is better in urban than in rural areas (see Table 2-4).

The composite facilities indicator makes it possible to see the overall socioeconomic status of the regions (see Figure 2-6). As expected, in general the departments with higher socioeconomic status are those closest to Dakar. The most underprivileged regions are Kolda and Tambacounda,

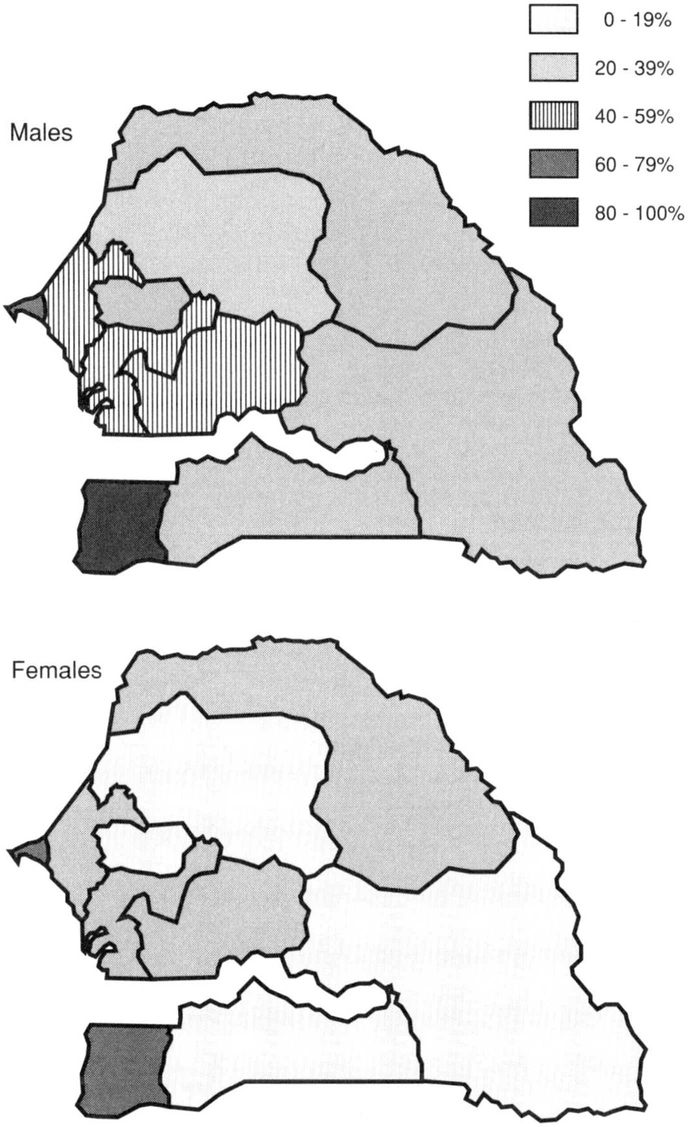

FIGURE 2-5 Percentage of males and females aged 7-12 enrolled in school, Senegal, 1988. SOURCE: 1988 census (unpublished tables).

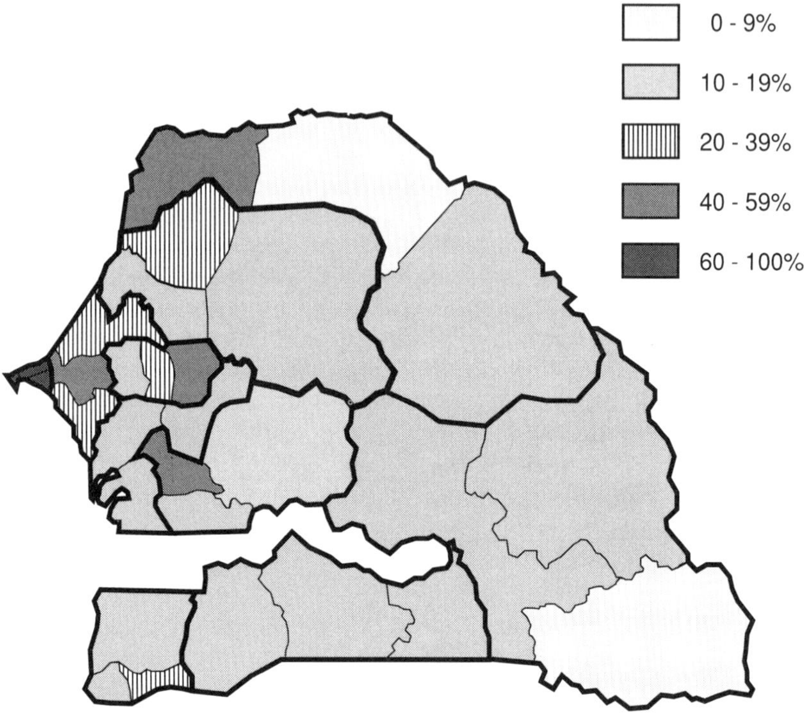

FIGURE 2-6 Composite facility indicator (average of percentage of houses with good construction, electricity, toilet, and access to water), Senegal, 1988. SOURCE: 1988 census (unpublished tables).

which have indicators of less than 15 (see also Table 2-4). The three regions with the highest indicators are Dakar (79), Thiès (37), and Diourbel (31), all located in the western part of the country.

In summary, geographic variations in socioeconomic status seem to be linked primarily to distance from the capital. Overall, the regions most distant from Dakar are those least densely populated, least urbanized, least developed, and with the lowest school-attendance rates. People living in these regions are less likely to have access to running water, electricity, and good housing. This finding must, however, be qualified. First, among those regions equidistant from the capital, the northern regions are better served with water and electricity than those in the south. Second, despite its distance from Dakar, the Ziguinchor region to the south has one of the highest school-enrollment rates in the country. Furthermore, it has the most effective health-care system, particularly in the areas of child health and vaccinations (see Chapter 5). Finally, although relatively close to Dakar, the regions of Louga and Diourbel have relatively low levels of school enrollment.

NOTES

1. The names of some of the regions have changed. In this report we use the current names to eliminate confusion.

2. Though not strictly comparable because they cover different age groups, the 1976 and 1988 census figures show that school enrollment probably stagnated during the period between the two censuses. In 1976, 44.7 percent of males aged 5-14 were enrolled in school; this proportion increased to 45.7 percent of males aged 6-14 in 1988. In 1976, 28.4 percent of females aged 5-14 were enrolled in school; this increased to 30.7 percent of females aged 6-14 in 1988.

3. SMIG stands for "salaire minimum garanti," the lowest salary authorized by the law.

4. "Good construction" is the arithmetic mean of the percentage of households having cement brick walls; tiled or cement floors; and a concrete, zinc, tile, or slate roof.

3

Population Growth and Distribution

As in other parts of Africa, the population of Senegal has been increasing rapidly over the past several decades. This chapter traces the growth and distribution of the population of Senegal over the last 30 years and discusses briefly both interregional and international migration. From administrative counts, which probably underestimate the true size of the population, it is estimated that Senegal's population increased from about 1.1 million in 1904 to 2.3 million in 1958, or at an annual rate of 1.3 percent over the period 1904-1958 (Becker and Mbodji, 1994). Estimates of the total population based on data from the 1960-1961 Demographic Survey [1], the 1970-1971 National Demographic Survey [2], as well as from the 1976 [17] and 1988 [18] censuses, allow us to analyze this growth at both the national and regional levels.

OVERVIEW OF NATIONAL POPULATION TRENDS

Between 1960 and 1988, the population of Senegal more than doubled from 3.1 to 6.9 million. The annual growth rate between these dates was 2.9 percent. Growth rates for the periods 1960-1970, 1970-1976, and 1976-1988 are shown in Table 3-1. The erratic nature of the series, increasing from 2.3 to 4.2 percent, then decreasing to 2.7 percent, may be due to the unreliability of survey data (see the section Overall Levels and Trends under Levels and Trends of Fertility in Chapter 4 and Sources and Quality of Data in Chapter 5 for general discussions concerning the sources and qual-

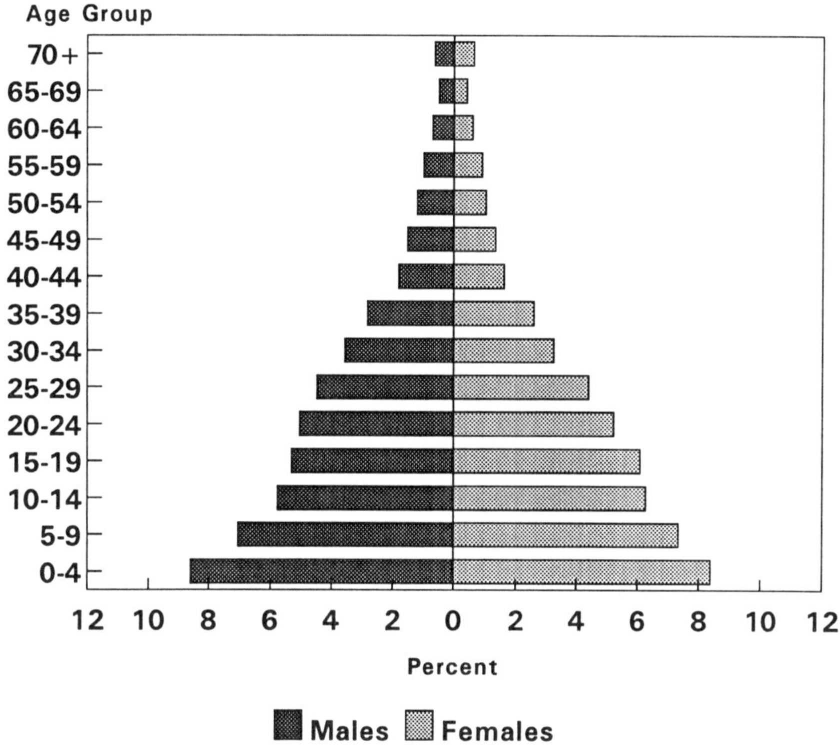

FIGURE 3-1 Population pyramid, Senegal, 1988. SOURCE: 1988 census (unpublished tables).

ity of data used in this report), and therefore should be interpreted with caution. When longer intervals, such as 1960-1988 or 1970-1988, are taken into consideration, the annual average growth rate remains close to 3 percent.

The importance of Dakar in terms of population growth and population distribution within Senegal cannot be overestimated. Dakar, which has the smallest geographic area of any of the ten administrative regions, had the largest population in 1988, the highest growth rate since the 1976 census, and it was the only region that recorded more than 1 million inhabitants in the 1988 census.

The relatively young age structure of the national population is apparent in Figure 3-1. Over the past several decades, the proportion of the population in the younger ages has been increasing slowly. In 1960, 42.7

TABLE 3-1 Regional Populations and Growth Rates, Senegal, 1960, 1970, 1976, 1988

	Population Size			
Region	1960	1970	1976	1988
Dakar	444,000	681,000	941,000	1,489,000
Kolda and Ziguinchor	530,000	618,000	731,000	990,000
Diourbel and Louga	503,000	630,000	843,000	1,109,000
Saint-Louis	345,000	389,000	515,000	660,000
Tambacounda	151,000	244,000	287,000	386,000
Kaolack and Fatick	727,000	798,000	1,006,000	1,321,000
Thiès	410,000	547,000	675,000	941,000
Total	3,110,000	3,906,000	4,998,000	6,897,000

NOTE: Selected regions are grouped so that the geographic areas are comparable over time. 1960 data dated July 1, 1960; 1970 data assumed to be dated July 1, 1970; 1976 census date April, 1976; 1988 census date May, 1988.

percent of the population was under the age of 15; this proportion had increased to 47.2 percent in 1988.

The structure of the population by gender reveals some possible bias in age reporting. In general, one would expect the sex ratio (number of males per 100 females) to be close to 104-106. However, sex ratios for Senegal indicate that there is a deficit of males aged 15-49, followed by a deficit of females above age 50 (see Figure 3-2). These deviations may be explained by the fact that African adult men tend to overstate their age and understate that of their wives. Such over- and understatement of the respective sexes would lead to the pattern described above. These biases are apparent to a greater or lesser extent in each of the regions in Senegal. The smallest difference is in Dakar, where because of higher levels of education and better civil registration, age misreporting is likely to be lower than in other regions.

There are five major ethnic (language) groups in Senegal: Wolof (42.7 percent), Poular[1] (23.7), Serer (14.9), Mandingo (7.6),[2] and Diola (5.3). Another ten groups comprise the remaining 5.7 percent of the population. Wolof is the most prominent group in five of the regions in the western and central part of the country—Louga, Diourbel, Kaolack, Thiès, and Dakar.[3] The Serer are the most prevalent in Fatick. The Poular are the most prevalent in the two southeastern regions, Tambacounda and Kolda, and in the northern region of Saint-Louis. Finally, the Diola form a majority in Ziguinchor (unpublished tables, 1988 census).

Growth Rate			
1960-1970	1970-1976	1976-1988	1960-1988
4.3	5.5	3.8	4.3
1.5	2.9	2.5	2.2
2.2	5.0	2.3	2.8
1.2	4.8	2.1	2.3
4.8	2.8	2.4	3.4
0.9	4.0	2.2	2.1
2.9	3.6	2.7	3.0
2.3	4.2	2.7	2.9

SOURCES: 1960: République du Sénégal (1964); 1970: République du Sénégal (1974); 1976: République du Sénégal (1982a-h); 1988: 1988 census (unpublished tables)

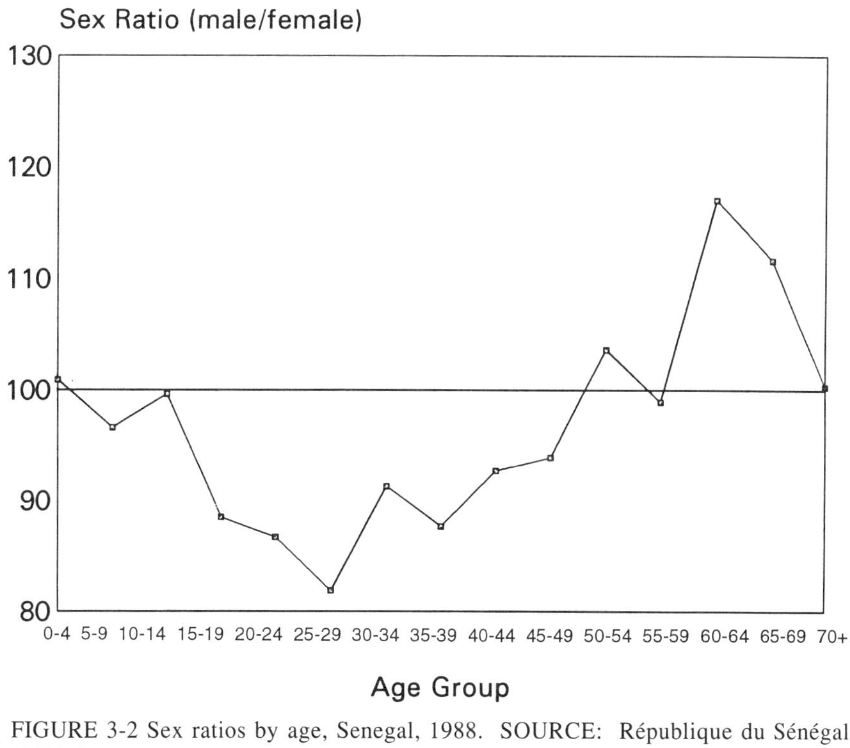

FIGURE 3-2 Sex ratios by age, Senegal, 1988. SOURCE: République du Sénégal (1992a).

OVERVIEW OF REGIONAL TRENDS

As suggested above, population growth has not taken place uniformly throughout the country. Regional differences are due to differences both in natural growth (births minus deaths) and in migration patterns. Over the last century, two major migrations have modified quite substantially the distribution of the population: the rural exodus, which is partly responsible for the accelerated growth of Dakar as well as many other smaller urban areas; and a general movement away from the north of the country towards the south, which has resulted in a relative decline in the northern regions to the advantage of the regions in the center and the south of the country (see Becker and Mbodji, 1994). Aside from Tambacounda during 1960-1970, data indicate that Dakar has had the most rapid population growth of any region over the past several decades (see Table 3-1). Between 1960 and 1988, the population of Dakar grew an average of 4.3 percent per year. The combined regions of Kaolack and Fatick had the slowest population growth, 2.1 percent per year. The combined regions of Kolda and Ziguinchor, and Saint-Louis, also grew relatively slowly over this time period—2.2 and 2.3 percent per year, respectively.

The most notable change in the distribution has taken place in the region of Dakar. In 1960, just over 14 percent of the population resided in Dakar. This proportion increased in both 1970 and 1976. In 1988, over 21 percent of the population lived in Dakar. Four of the six remaining regions (as shown in Table 3-1) lost relative population over the same period.

Historical rates of regional population growth and redistribution have created a situation where regional densities are extremely varied. Dakar is by far the most densely populated: it is estimated that there are 2,707 inhabitants per square kilometer (km^2) in that region. The next most densely populated is Thiès, where there are 143 inhabitants per km^2. Diourbel follows closely. The remaining regions are much less densely populated. The most sparsely populated region is Tambacounda, where there are a mere 6.5 inhabitants per km^2. It is clear from Figure 3-3 that the population is densest in the western region and sparsest as one moves east.

The level of urbanization also varies by region quite substantially within Senegal, as can be seen in Table 2-4. The western part of the country is by far the most urbanized. The most urban region is Dakar (97 percent), followed by Ziguinchor (38 percent). Six of the ten regions have fewer than 25 percent of their population in urban areas. The least urbanized region is Fatick, where only 10 percent of the population lives in an urban setting.

Because of high levels of in-migration of people aged 15-59, the age structure of the population in Dakar (see Figure 3-4) differs from that of the country as a whole (see Figure 3-1).

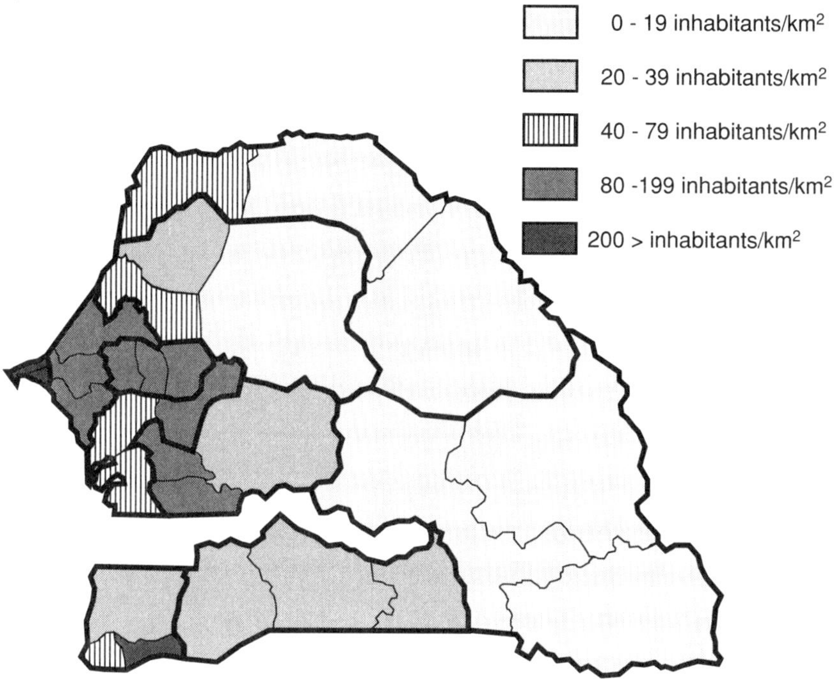

FIGURE 3-3 Population density (inhabitants per km^2) by department, Senegal, 1988.
SOURCES: République du Sénégal (1992c-k); 1988 census (unpublished tables).

MIGRATION

People migrate for various reasons, the most common being economic or family reasons, or education. The study of migration is of interest for several reasons. Because migrations exhibit age- and sex-based selectivity, they affect the demographic structures of the source and destination areas. As a component of population dynamics, migrants contribute directly to population increase or decline in both source and destination areas. Furthermore, migrants often have different rates of childbearing than their nonmigrant counterparts due, among other things, to the postponement of marriage, spousal separation, and exposure to new ideas and norms.

For this study, internal migrants are defined as those people who move within national borders, but across regional boundaries. In general, knowledge about internal migration remains fragmentary, though limited information is available from the national demographic surveys in 1960-1961 [1] and 1970-1971 [2] and the 1976 [17] and 1988 [18] censuses, which asked

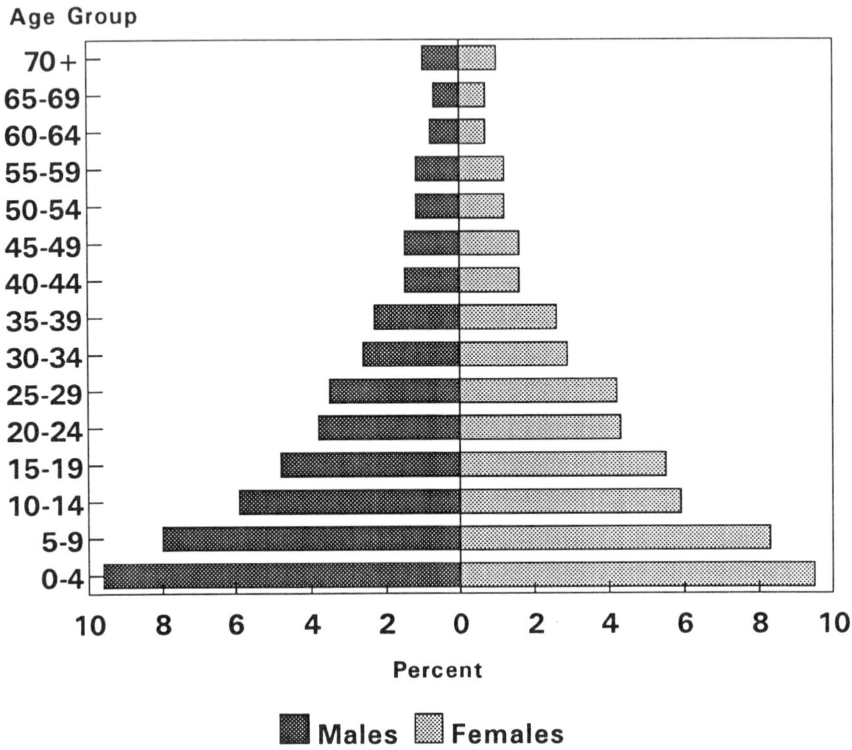

FIGURE 3-4 Population pyramid, Dakar, 1988. SOURCE: 1988 census (unpublished tables).

for place of birth. From these data, we are able to obtain a measure of lifetime migration.

The proportion of persons residing in a region other than that containing their place of birth varies according to source. But all of the sources indicate that the proportion of the population living in a region other than their region of birth is highest for the Dakar region, where at each observation more than one-third of the population was born in another region. The highest proportion of Dakar residents born elsewhere—46 percent—was recorded in 1960.

Three types of internal migration are discussed briefly below: (1) lifetime migration, which includes individuals who have migrated since birth; (2) migration of individuals who have moved within the past 5 years;[4] and (3) temporary migration, which includes individuals who at the time of the 1988 census had resided in a region for a period of less than 6 months.[5]

Temporary migration includes circular migration, particularly seasonal migration. In addition, this section briefly addresses international migration.

Lifetime Migrants

The proportion of lifetime migrants living in other regions varies markedly from one source to another, probably reflecting both data quality and time-based in-migrant/out-migrant variations among the regions. Despite these inconsistencies, several trends can be noted. First, some regions exhibit very low migration over the entire period; among them are eastern Senegal (Tambacounda), Saint-Louis, Louga, and, to a lesser extent, the Casamance areas (Kolda and Ziguinchor). Other regions occupy an intermediate position, showing fluctuations from time to time. This is the case in Sine-Saloum (Fatick and Kaolack) and the regions of Thiès and Diourbel.

Migration Within the Last 5 Years

Information on migration in the last 5 years is available from the 1979 Labor Force Survey and the 1988 census. During the 5 years preceding the census, all regions in Senegal had both in-migrants and out-migrants, though the magnitude of these flows was different. Three regions experienced net in-migration during the 5 years preceding the census (Dakar, Ziguinchor, and Tambacounda); the others (except Diourbel and Kolda) experienced net out-migration (see Table 3-2). The importance of migration for Dakar is apparent; in-migration, out-migration, and net in-migration are far higher for Dakar than for any of the other regions. In most regions, the migration for both males and females was mostly among young adults. Females exceeded males in terms of in-migration within the last 5 years in Dakar, Diourbel, and Ziguinchor, the latter of which also reported more female than male out-migrants. Fatick, Louga, and Thiès also reported more female than male out-migrants.

Analysis of migration flows by type of residence reveals that among migrants moving within the 5 years preceding the census, migration from one urban area to another was most common. Migrants moving from rural to urban areas were the next most prevalent. Movements into rural areas were the least typical (see Figure 3-5). Clearly, since most migrants moved into urban areas, there was a net urban gain, which can be seen in Figure 3-6. It is clear from both of these figures that most of the movement has taken place among the younger ages.

More recent information on migration is available from the 1991-1992 Enquête Sur les Priorités [6], which asked respondents to list their last place of residence. A preliminary analysis of these data indicates that there has been little change in the pattern of migration since the 1988 census.

TABLE 3-2 Net Migration Within the 5 Years Preceding the 1988 Census, by Region

Region	In-Migration	Out-Migration	Net In-Migration
Dakar	69,000	49,000	20,000
Diourbel	18,000	18,000	0
Fatick	12,000	14,000	-2,000
Kaolack	18,000	20,000	-2,000
Kolda	9,000	9,000	0
Louga	7,000	19,000	-12,000
Saint-Louis	11,000	18,000	-7,000
Tambacounda	8,000	7,000	2,000
Thiès	23,000	29,000	-6,000
Ziguinchor	22,000	15,000	7,000

SOURCE: République du Sénégal (1992d)

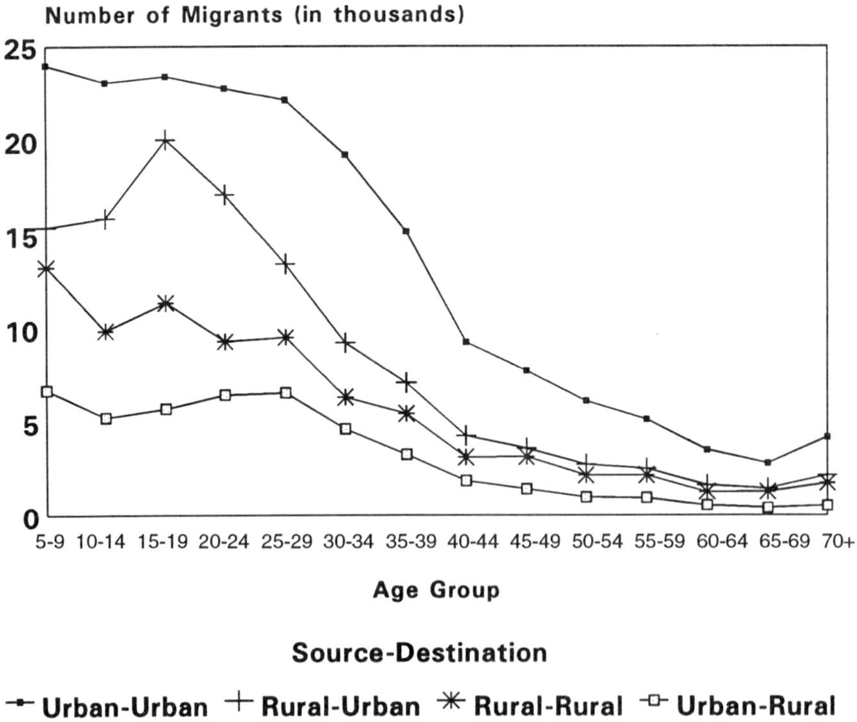

FIGURE 3-5 Internal migration by urban or rural source and destination, Senegal, 1988. SOURCE: 1988 census (unpublished tables).

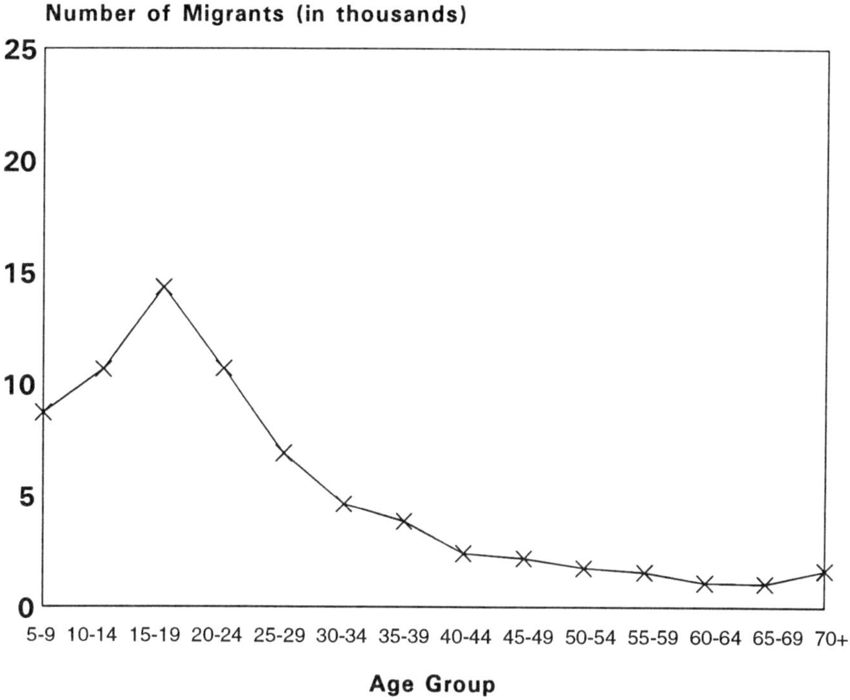

FIGURE 3-6 Net rural-urban gain, Senegal, 1988. SOURCE: 1988 census (unpublished tables).

Temporary Migration

Senegal has a long tradition of seasonal migration of agricultural laborers from the southern and southeastern regions to the groundnut fields, in central Senegal. In the past, seasonal migration has been linked predominantly to the very limited use of agricultural equipment, making human labor an important factor in production. Recently, however, this type of migration has been decreasing gradually as a result of increasing mechanization in rural areas, as well as crop diversification in the areas of outmigration.

Emigration of household labor concerns the movement of domestic workers coming mainly from the Basse Casamance (Ziguinchor) and the Sine (Fatick and Kaolack), and traveling to the regional capitals, in particular Dakar. These population shifts begin in October, at the end of the heavy agricultural season. The workers return at the beginning of the rainy season (May-June).

Because the 1988 census was taken at the end of the dry season, a time when a portion of the temporary migrants are away from home, those not living in the region of their usual residence can serve as a proxy for temporary migrants. Such temporary migrants comprised just over 5 percent of the entire population at the time of the census (see Table 3-3). By region, this proportion varied between 2.7 percent in Dakar and 8.4 percent in Ziguinchor.

Not only was Ziguinchor different from the other regions in terms of magnitude, but this region was the only one to have more female than male temporary migrants. In fact, over 52 percent of the temporary migrants were female.

Comparison of male and female temporary migrants by age reveals that it is not uncommon for temporary migrants to be predominately female in the younger age groups. Between the ages of 10 and 14, females exceed males in terms of temporary migration in six regions. In Fatick and Ziguinchor, females also exceed males between the ages of 15 and 19. After the early adult years, however, male migration surpasses that of females.

Though female migrants in the older ages in Fatick and Ziguinchor do not exceed males, the proportion of female migrants in these two regions is

TABLE 3-3 Percentage of Temporary Out-Migrants by Region and Distribution by Sex, Senegal, 1988

Region	Total Population	Out-Migrants Residents (%)		
		Percent of Total	Male	Female
Dakar	1,489,000	2.7	63.5	36.5
Diourbel	619,000	5.8	67.2	32.7
Fatick	510,000	7.0	53.6	46.3
Kaolack	811,000	3.6	60.8	39.2
Kolda	592,000	4.7	57.7	42.3
Louga	490,000	6.9	65.5	34.5
Saint-Louis	660,000	7.0	65.4	34.6
Tambacounda	386,000	4.6	59.6	40.4
Thiès	941,000	5.4	60.5	39.5
Ziguinchor	398,000	8.4	47.4	52.6
Total	6,896,000	5.1	60.5	39.5

NOTE: Temporary out-migrants, or absent residents, are those individuals who at the time of the 1988 census were absent from their region of residence and had been absent for a period of less than 6 months (see footnote 5 in this chapter for exceptions to this definition).

SOURCE: 1988 census (unpublished tables)

consistently higher than in the other regions for every age group 10-14 through 45-49. The proportion of female migrants is the highest in Ziguinchor and second highest in Fatick. The implications of high female migration for fertility are discussed in Chapter 4.

Ziguinchor comprises mostly Diola (61 percent), and Fatick comprises mostly Serer (55 percent). These two ethnic groups are more likely than others to take part in seasonal labor migration to find domestic work in urban areas before they marry (Sy, 1991). Hence, the relatively high levels of female seasonal migration in Ziguinchor and Fatick can be explained in part by the ethnic composition of those regions.

The repercussions of these migration movements for demographics, labor, and the financial inflows coming from the areas of in- and out-migration appear to be among the most intensely analyzed aspects of migration. Diop and Dieng (1985) examined the effects of population outflows on the agricultural work force. Their overall conclusion is that any migration of youth from an area of agricultural undermechanization draws away labor and affects the effective performance of agricultural activities. However, this effect is attenuated by the seasonal timing of the departures and returns, which often coincide with the end and resumption of heavy agricultural labor, respectively. This situation is true for young Diola and Serer women in Casamance (Ziguinchor and Kolda) and Sine (Fatick and Kaolack). During the period of absence, the supply of domestic labor increases in the cities.

International Migration

The number of international migrants living in Senegal is estimated to be 213,656, or 3.1 percent of the population (unpublished tables, 1988 census). The greatest proportion live in Dakar (37 percent), followed by Kolda (21 percent), while the smallest proportion live in Louga (0.9 percent).

Most of the immigrants (78 percent in 1976 and 86 percent in 1988) come from within Africa. "Push" factors have been the major driving force for international migrants to Senegal: Three out of Senegal's four immediate neighbors have had internal problems in the recent past (e.g., Guinea-Bissau and Guinea in the 1970s and 1980s and Mauritania in the 1990s). Guinea was the primary source country at the time of the last two censuses in 1976 and 1988, respectively (see Table 3-4). Guinea-Bissau was the second most important source country in each of these two years and Mauritania the third.

The record of Senegalese emigrants is more difficult to ascertain because one must rely on censuses and vital records from other countries. New censuses are available for Burkina Faso (1985) and Mauritania (1988), but they did not report foreign-born population by source, so we are unable

TABLE 3-4 Immigrants to Senegal by Source, 1976 and 1988

Source	1976	1988
The Gambia	3,000	25,000
Guinea	39,000	65,000
Guinea-Bissau	24,000	32,000
Mali	9,000	19,000
Mauritania	11,000	27,000
Other Africa	7,000	17,000
Europe	15,000	9,000
France	—	8,000
Middle East and Asia	7,000	2,000
Americas	1,000	1,000
Undetermined and other countries	2,000	17,000
Total	118,000	214,000

NOTE: The definition of an immigrant for the purpose of this table is a person who has crossed an international boundary into Senegal, regardless of the reason or duration of stay (Russell, 1993).

SOURCES: Data for 1976 adapted from Russell (1993:Tables 8-2, 8-7); data for 1988 from 1988 census (unpublished tables).

to know how many came from Senegal. In fact, not having recent data, or having data that are not completely disaggregated are common problems with African censuses, especially in western Africa. Data are often incompletely analyzed and when they are analyzed, the results are not published or are published with great delay. Nevertheless, such data are highly uncertain and provide just an idea of what are the main streams of migration. Data on the number of Senegalese in selected African countries is available from respective censuses, most of which took place in the 1970s (Russell, 1993). Côte d'Ivoire was the destination of 40,000 migrants from Senegal in 1988 (see Table 3-5). The only other countries having a Senegalese immigrant population over 15,000 (for which there are data) are The Gambia and Mauritania.

Not surprisingly, because of its former strong ties with Senegal, France also has a substantial Senegalese emigrant population. In the 1982 census there were 32,336 Senegalese emigrants enumerated in France. In 1990, that number had risen to over 45,000.

TABLE 3-5 Senegalese Emigrants by Selected African Destinations

Destination Country	Year	Senegalese Emigrants
Burkina Faso	1975	2,000
Congo	1984	3,000
Côte d'Ivoire	1988	40,000
The Gambia	1973	27,000
Guinea-Bissau	1979	6,000
Mali	1976	4,000
Mauritania	1977	18,000

SOURCE: Data from Russell (1993:Tables 8-2, 8-6); data for Côte d'Ivoire from United Nations (personal communication, 1995).

Conclusion

Migration has become an important part of population dynamics in Senegal. Despite the substantial migration from Senegal to France documented above, the vast majority of migration takes place internally. Migration is selective as a function of age, sex, and type of residence. Typically, the migration process accelerates as the development process advances, such that the number of migrants tends to increase over time. As discussed in Chapter 2, recent economic downturns have necessitated the implementation of structural adjustment programs in Senegal. A great deal more research will be needed before we know how these economic downturns have affected migration flows.

NOTES

1. Contains the Peul and Toucouleur ethnic groups.

2. Contains the Bambara, Malinké, Mandingo, Soce, and Sarakhole ethnic groups.

3. The influence of the Wolof extends beyond these boundaries, however. An additional 40 percent of the population speaks Wolof, and (together with French) Wolof serves as an informal lingua franca throughout the country (World Bank, 1988:153).

4. An indepth treatment of migration between urban and rural areas is not presented here because rural/urban differentiation has not been consistent over time. In 1988, rural/urban differentiation was not by population size, but by administrative classification. In 1988, there were two administrative classifications—com-

munes and rural communities. Communes were reported as urban areas and rural communities as rural areas. An example of two cities—Touba in Diourbel and Oussouye in Ziguinchor—shows how the use of these administrative classifications instead of population size has made the classification of areas as urban and rural inconsistent. Touba, in Diourbel, is classified as part of a rural community. This rural community had 138,604 inhabitants in 1988, most of whom likely lived in Touba. Since Touba was classified as part of a rural community, however, it was designated as rural. By contrast, Oussouye, in Ziguinchor, is classified as a commune and therefore was considered to be an urban area in the census, despite a population of only 3,849 inhabitants.

5. Exceptions to this definition are government employees who were assigned to a region within the past 6 months, women who married within the past 6 months, and infants less than 6 months of age who have lived in the same region for their whole life. These individuals were considered to be de jure residents.

4

Fertility

INTRODUCTION

The average growth rate of the population in sub-Saharan Africa has been around 3 percent per year since the 1960s, higher than in any other major region in the world. If these rates remain constant, the population will double in the next 23 years. The reason for Africa's rapid rate of population growth is well known: while mortality and fertility rates fell substantially in Latin America and Asia between 1965 and 1985, only mortality fell in sub-Saharan Africa; fertility remained relatively stable, well above the level required to replace the population.

The existing demographic regime in sub-Saharan Africa is unlikely to remain in effect for very long. According to data from the Demographic and Health Surveys (DHS), the level of fertility has already fallen by more than 10 percent in seven sub-Saharan African countries (Kenya, Botswana, Senegal, Zimbabwe, Zambia, Burundi, and Malawi). Not all of these fertility declines are completely plausible, but fertility certainly appears to have fallen in at least three DHS countries at the national level (Kenya, Botswana, and Zimbabwe), as well as in South Africa, for which DHS-type data suggest a substantial decline. Furthermore, fertility declines appear to have occurred in several other countries at the subnational level (e.g., southwestern Nigeria, southern Namibia, northern Tanzania). These changes were documented in a chapter on fertility trends in sub-Saharan Africa in a recent volume by the Committee on Population (see Cohen, 1993).

This chapter examines levels, trends, and determinants of fertility in Senegal. The next section combines recent census and survey results to build a general description of the pattern of fertility in Senegal and how it has changed over the last 20 years. This is followed by a section on explanations for these patterns, focusing on marriage, breastfeeding, and contraception, some of the most important determinants of fertility change.

LEVELS AND TRENDS OF FERTILITY

Overall Levels and Trends

The standard measure of fertility used here is the total fertility rate (TFR).[1] Despite dramatic improvements in the quantity and quality of population data for Senegal since the early 1960s, our knowledge and understanding of fertility levels and trends in the country still relies mainly on findings from ad hoc single-round surveys. Since 1960, five surveys have furnished information that permits the estimation of fertility in Senegal at the national level: the Demographic Survey (DS) of 1960-1961 [1]; the National Demographic Survey (NDS) of 1970-1971 [2]; the World Fertility Survey (WFS) of 1978 [3]; and two rounds of the DHS (DHS-I, DHS-II) in 1986 [4] and 1992-1993 [7].[2] The data from each of these sources are not all of comparable quality. For example, the 1960-1961 DS data are generally thought to have suffered from an underenumeration of births and deaths (Cantrelle et al., 1986) and to be of lower quality than the data from the other sources.

In addition to these surveys, fertility estimates are available from two censuses, conducted in 1976 [17] and 1988 [18]. The 1976 census questionnaire did not collect information on births, so fertility estimates for 1976 have been derived from the age distribution using stable population theory. The 1988 census contained a single question on births in the last 12 months. Unfortunately, because of mistakes in the coding and processing of the data, the TFR estimates produced at the time the official report of the 1988 census was being prepared were implausibly low. Consequently, fertility estimates were not included in official reports on the 1988 census, and to this day, fertility estimates from the 1988 census remain unpublished. In this report we have remedied the situation by adopting a simple correction procedure to estimate total and age-specific fertility rates (ASFRs) for 1988 that takes these data problems into account. (See Appendix B for a detailed explanation of the procedure used.)

Finally, there are a number of subnational studies [8-16] in which accurate birth registers have been maintained over several years. Although these small study areas are not representative of the entire country, they yield fertility estimates that may be more accurate than those derived from large-scale surveys and censuses. Hence, small-scale studies can provide a useful independent check on the accuracy of the other estimates.

In all, seven observations of the national TFR are available for the period 1960-1993. In principle, by putting these observations in sequence we can observe the trends in fertility over the last 30 years. However, since the quality of the data varies among the surveys, some estimates are considerably more reliable than others. Tests of internal and external consistency show that the quality of the data from several sources is often mediocre to poor. Furthermore, the methodology used to collect the information was not the same across all surveys. For example, the WFS and the DHS collected complete birth histories from all women, while the 1988 census only asked women about births in the last 12 months. This latter method is more prone to omission of births, particularly of children who died, so that it almost invariably produces lower estimates of the TFR.[3] One needs to bear in mind such issues of varying data quality and methodology when comparing across survey instruments, and to remain reasonably cautious when interpreting small fluctuations in the overall rate.

Table 4-1 provides a summary of the available estimates of the TFR for the period 1960-1992 at the national level and for various subpopulations. Figure 4-1 shows national-level TFR estimates for the age range 15-34 (this age range has been used so that estimates of fertility from the three birth history surveys, WFS, DHS-I, and DHS-II can be used for periods up to 15 years prior to the survey dates) plotted against calendar time. Figure 4-2 shows the national age patterns of fertility, as the proportion of total fertility contributed by each age group.

The Brass P/F ratio technique—whereby current fertility rates are cumulated and compared with reported lifetime fertility—provides a check of the internal consistency of each survey and a sensitive test for changing fertility. For cross-sectional surveys where fertility rates have not changed in the recent past, average parity equivalents (F) should be roughly equivalent to reported average parities (P). If fertility is rising, lifetime fertility will be lower than cumulated current fertility, particularly at higher age groups which have had more time for differences to emerge, and P/F ratios will fall with age. If fertility is falling, on the other hand, the opposite will be the case, and P/F ratios will rise with age. Figure 4-3 shows P/F ratios for the 1960-1961, 1970-1971, 1978, 1986, and 1992-1993 surveys.

The fertility estimates shown in Figure 4-1 come from different sources and data collection methodologies. The 1960-1961 DS [1] included questions on births and deaths over the preceding 12 months, as well as on live births and child survivorship during a woman's entire life. The TFR based on data for births during the preceding 12 months was estimated to be 5.4 children per woman. This figure may have underestimated the true TFR as a result of the omission of certain vital events.[4] However, fertility rates and age-specific parities for the 1960-1961 DS are fairly consistent, at least above age 25 (see P/F ratios in Figure 4-3). If the P/F ratios are used to

TABLE 4-1 Levels and Trends in the Total Fertility Rate, 1960-1992

Year	Source	Subgroup	TFR
National Level			
1960-1961	DS	n.a.	5.4
1970-1971	NDS	n.a.	6.4
1976	Census	n.a.	7.0
1975-1978	WFS	n.a.	7.2
1983-1986	DHS-I	n.a.	6.6
1987-1988	Census	n.a.	5.9
1989-1992	DHS-II	n.a.	6.1
WFS and DHS Regions			
1975-1978	WFS	West	7.1
		Center	7.3
		Northeast	7.2
		South	7.4
1983-1986	DHS-I	West	5.9
		Center	7.1
		Northeast	6.6
		South	7.0
1987-1988	Census	West	5.5
		Center	6.0
		Northeast	6.0
		South	6.4
1989-1992	DHS-II	West	5.6
		Center	6.4
		Northeast	6.6
		South	6.5
Administrative Regions			
1967-1971	Ferry (1976)	Cap-Vert	6.6
1975-1978	WFS	Dakar	6.8
1983-1986	DHS-I	Dakar	5.5
1987-1988	Census	Dakar	5.0
		Thiès	6.2
		Saint-Louis	6.2
		Tambacounda	5.9
		Louga	5.7
		Diourbel	5.6
		Fatick	6.9
		Kaolack	6.1
		Ziguinchor	6.8
		Kolda	6.3
1989-1992	DHS-II	Dakar	4.9
Small-Scale Studies [8-16]			
1963-1965	Cantrelle et al. (1980)	Niakhar	6.8
1984-1990	Projet Niakhar (1992)	Niakhar	7.8

TABLE 4-1 continued

Year	Source	Subgroup	TFR
Small-Scale Studies [8-16]			
1963-1965	Cantrelle et al. (1980)	Paos Koto	6.6
1981-1991	Pison and Desgrées du Loû (1993)	Bandafassi	6.2
1985-1992	Lagarde et al. (forthcoming)	Mlomp	5.0
Place of Residence			
1975-1978	WFS	Dakar	6.8
		Other urban	6.5
		Rural	7.5
1983-1986	DHS-I	Dakar	5.5
		Other urban	5.6
		Rural	7.3
1987-1988	Census	Dakar	4.8
		Other urban	5.6
		Rural	6.4
1989-1992	DHS-II	Dakar	4.9
		Other urban	5.4
		Rural	6.8
Ethnic Groups			
1975-1978	WFS	Wolof	7.2
		Poular	6.9
		Serer	7.9
		Mandingo	8.1
		Diola	6.3
		Other	7.0
1983-1986	DHS-I	Wolof	6.4
		Poular	6.4
		Serer	7.6
		Mandingo	6.8
		Diola	6.2
		Other	6.3
1987-1988	Census	Wolof	5.7
		Poular	6.1
		Serer	6.3
		Mandingo	6.0
		Diola	5.9
		Other	5.7
1989-1992	DHS-II	Wolof	5.6
		Poular	6.4
		Serer	7.2
		Mandingo	5.7
		Diola	5.7
		Other	6.5

continued

TABLE 4-1 continued

Year	Source	Subgroup	TFR
Level of Education			
1975-1978	WFS	None	7.4
		Primary	7.1
		Secondary+	3.6
1983-1986	DHS-I	None	7.0
		Primary	5.7
		Secondary+	3.6
1987-1988	Census	None	6.2
		Primary	5.7
		Secondary+	4.1
1989-1992	DHS-II	None	6.6
		Primary	5.7
		Secondary+	3.8

NOTES: See Appendix A for description of surveys; TFR = Total Fertility Rate, calculated for women aged 15-49.

SOURCES: Cantrelle et al. (1980); Cohen (1993); Ferry (1976); Lagarde et al. (forthcoming); Projet Niakhar (1992); Pison and Desgrées du Loû (1993); WFS, DHS-I and DHS-II data files and unpublished tabulations from the 1988 census.

adjust reported TFR, the resulting estimates are 6.0 or 5.5, depending on whether the correction coefficient is derived from the group aged 20-24 or 25-29.

The 1970-1971 NDS [2] was a multiround prospective survey. The data from this survey have been analyzed elsewhere and are thought to be of reasonably good quality (Cantrelle et al., 1986). However, the P/F ratios calculated from this survey decline steadily with age (see Figure 4-3) and average 1.27 for the age groups 20-24 and 25-29; if this factor is applied as an adjustment, the TFR estimated for 1970-1971 becomes an unrealistic 8.2.

The 1978 WFS [3], 1986 DHS-I [4], and 1992-1993 DHS-II [7] were all ad hoc fertility surveys including birth histories. As a result of using similar methodology, the estimates should be more comparable than those from the other surveys. Birth histories are usually effective at coverage of births, but fertility estimates may be distorted by errors in reports of timing. In the DHS-I, some births were undoubtedly transferred from the 5 years before the survey to an earlier period so that interviewers could avoid asking women additional questions about their children under age 5 (Arnold, 1990). Consequently, DHS-I (and DHS-II) data underestimate fertility in the last 5 years. Table 4-1 shows estimates of TFR for the period 4 years prior to the survey dates, but these also appear to be underestimates. Questions have also been raised about the quality of the WFS data (Charbit et

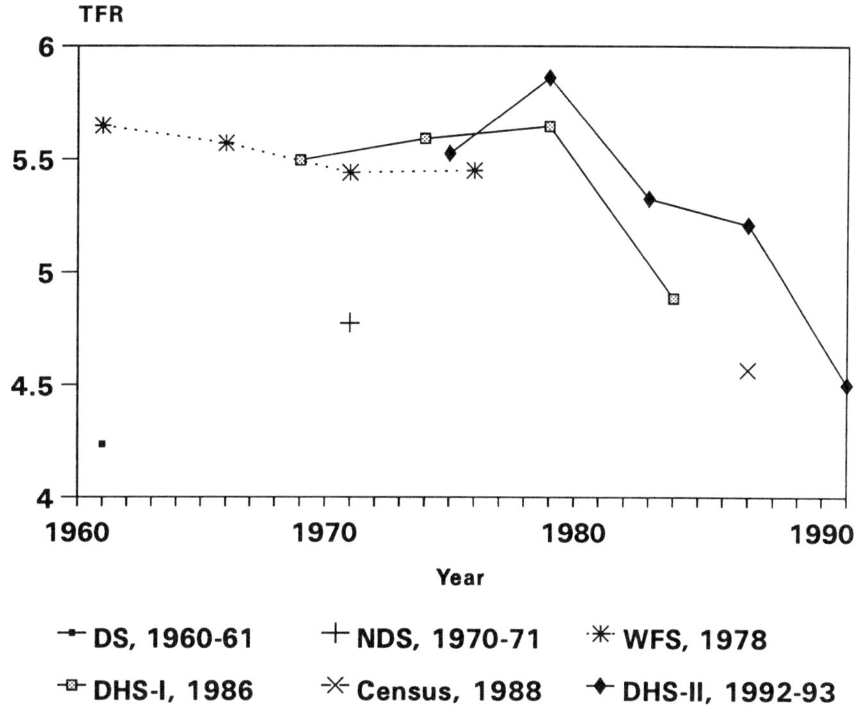

FIGURE 4-1 Total fertility rates for women aged 15-34 from national-level surveys, 1960-1993. NOTE: See Appendix A for description of surveys.

al., 1985); the complex procedure for collecting birth histories in the WFS may have resulted in fertility being overestimated, particularly among women aged 25-39.[5]

In the 1988 census, women were asked about their births in the last 12 months. This time, the problem of identifying the correct length of the period was partly resolved by taking the census exactly 1 year after an important Muslim holiday: the end of Ramadan.[6] After being adjusted (see Appendix B), the fertility estimates from the census for the period 1987-1988 are very close to those reported by the DHS-II for the period 1989-1992. On average, the ASFRs for the census are the same as those reported in the DHS-II for women under 30. On the other hand, the census estimates are slightly lower than the DHS-II estimates for women over age 30. This pattern might be explained by a relative undercount of births at all ages in the census in comparison with the DHS-II and a small fertility decline at ages under 30 during the short period between 1987-1988 and 1989-1992.

Data from the 1986 and 1992-1993 DHS surveys provide a useful con-

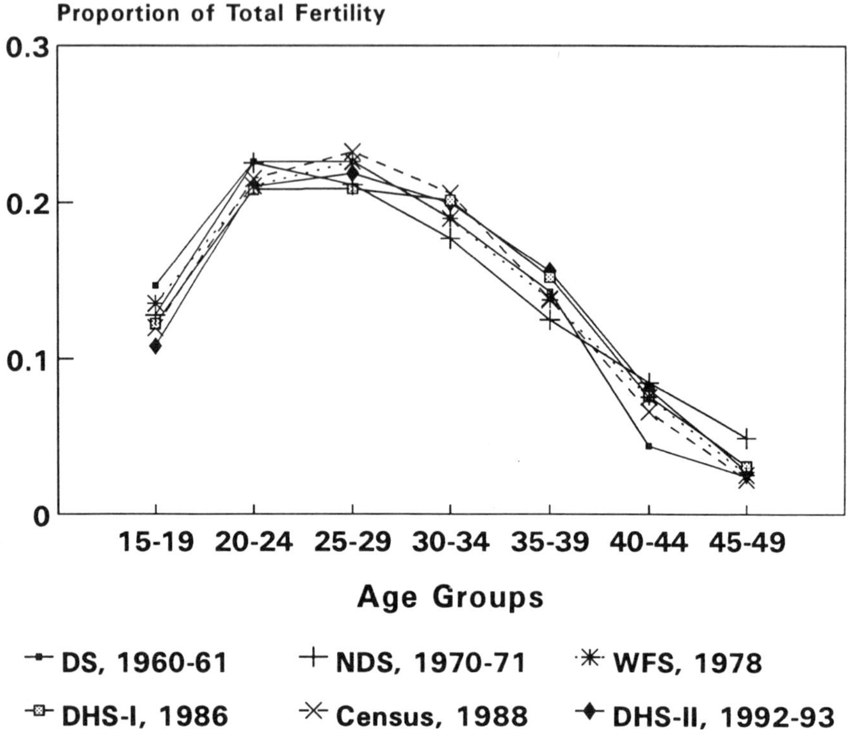

FIGURE 4-2 Proportion of the total fertility rate attributable to each age group. NOTE: See Appendix A for description of surveys.

sistency check on the accuracy of the 1988 census. Dividing all the women in the sample into 5-year cohorts, and assuming that each cohort in the 1986 DHS ages to become the next cohort in the 1992-1993 survey (i.e., those aged 15-19 in 1986 become those aged 20-24 in 1992—not exact, but good enough for present purposes), allows one to compare the cumulated ASFRs based on reported births in the year preceding the 1988 census with the change in the number of children ever born between the two DHS surveys. The denominator, commonly known as the period parity distribution, is obtained by cumulating the parity increments for different cohorts. For the age groups 20-24 and 25-29, the P/F ratios are close to 1, indicating a high degree of consistency between the census and the cohort parity changes. After age 30, the P/F ratios rise somewhat, but definitely not because fertility is falling, because the effects of falling fertility are purged by the cohort increment process. The most likely explanation for this pattern of P/F ratios is that it reflects underreporting of births by older women in the census. In summary, this analysis confirms our suspicions that there was

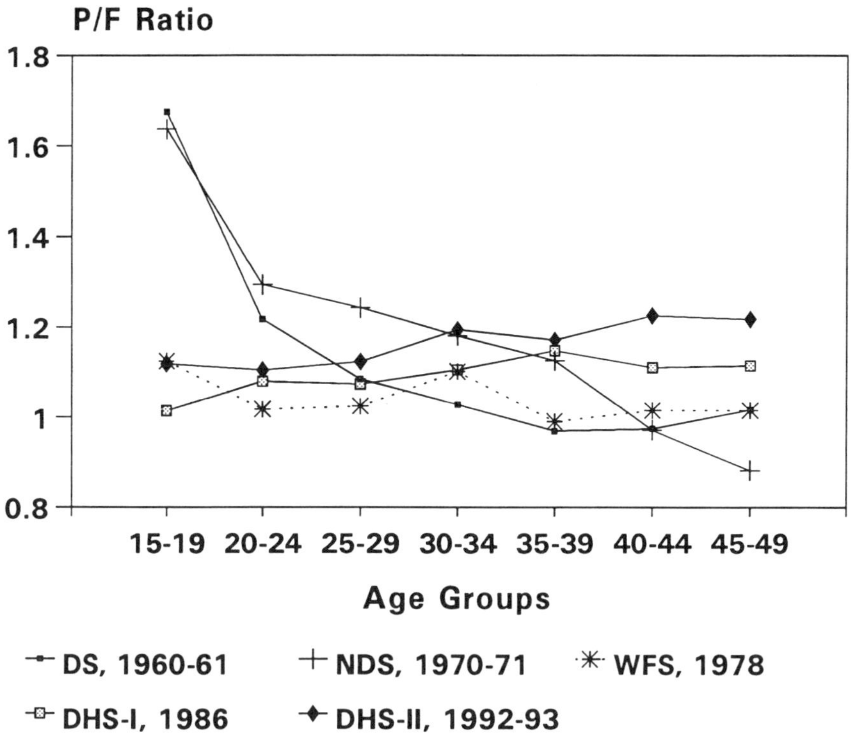

FIGURE 4-3 Brass P/F ratios. NOTE: See Appendix A for description of surveys.

differential coverage of births in the 1988 census. Specifically, the quality of reporting deteriorated for women over the age of 30. Before age 30, the fertility rates from the two DHS surveys and the 1988 census are consistent.

The fertility estimates in Table 4-1 permit different interpretations of fertility trends over the last 40 years in Senegal. The estimates for periods immediately prior to the surveys appear to show steeply rising fertility from 1960-1961 (TFR = 5.4) through 1970-1971 (TFR = 6.4) to 1975-1978 (TFR = 7.2), and then a decline from 1983-1986 (TFR = 6.6) continuing to 1989-1992 (TFR = 6.1), except for an anomalous drop to 5.9 in 1987-1988. However, when time series estimates covering the 15 years prior to the birth history surveys are considered, a different picture emerges. The estimates based on the birth history surveys show fertility (cumulated from age 15-34) declining gradually from 1960 to the late 1980s, with a few irregularities; the estimates from the 1960-1961 and 1970-1971 surveys are much lower (see Figure 4-1). The most pronounced irregularities in the birth history sequences are the points immediately preceding the DHS-I and DHS-

II; both these points are well below the general trend, and the DHS-I point is well below the corresponding time estimate from the DHS-II. These two points appear to be affected by misplacement of births in time beyond the local shifts around age 5 mentioned above.

Further analysis is required to clarify what actually happened to fertility since 1960. The P/F ratios from the 1960-1961 and 1970-1971 surveys fall smoothly with age, across all ages for 1970-1971, but to a minimum for the age group 35-39 for 1960-1961 (see Figure 4-3). The ratios from these two surveys taken together would be consistent with rising fertility affecting cohorts of women born between 1920 and 1950. However, P/F ratios from the 1978 survey show no pattern with age, showing no evidence of differences between lifetime fertility and fertility in the 5 years before the survey for cohorts born between 1930 and 1960. P/F ratios from the 1986 and 1992-1993 DHSs appear to rise with age, though not very sharply, suggesting slowly declining fertility. The 1986 and 1992-1993 series are essentially parallel, but with the 1992-1993 values slightly above the 1986 ones at all ages. Together, they suggest no major change in fertility trends between the surveys, but slightly higher overall omission of children ever born in 1992-1993.

The age pattern of P/F ratios from 1960-1961 and 1970-1971 could be explained by increasing omission of children ever born as age of mother increases, as well as by rising fertility. There are large differences in average numbers of children ever born for women at the end of their reproductive life across the surveys. Women aged 45-49 report an average of 5.4 children ever born in 1960-1961, 5.6 in 1970-1971, 7.2 in 1978, 7.3 in 1986, and 7.4 in 1992-1993. These averages would clearly be consistent with rising fertility from the cohort of women born prior to 1925 (aged 45-49 in 1970-1971) to the cohorts born after 1935. However, the age detail of the data suggests some omission from the earlier surveys. The women aged 45-49 in 1978 report an average of 7.2 births each, whereas the average number of children born reported by women aged 35-44 in 1970-1971 (of whom the 45-49 year olds in 1978 would be survivors) was only 5.7. It is unlikely that these women added on average 1.5 births in 8 years at the end of their reproductive lives; more likely is that women aged 35 and over in 1970-1971 underreported their lifetime fertility by half a child or more. A comparison of children ever born by cohort between 1960-1961 and 1970-1971 suggests the same type of error in 1960-1961 also.

The national-level data thus do not substantiate a large fertility increase in the 1960s and 1970s, though they do not rule out a moderate increase. Data from one of the population study areas, Niakhar, confirm a fertility increase (from a TFR of 6.8 in 1963-1965 to a TFR of 7.8 in 1984-1990) in one rural area of central Senegal. On balance, it seems likely that fertility did rise somewhat in the 1960s and 1970s, though not by nearly as much as the change in TFR from 1960-1961 to 1978 indicates.

It is difficult to explain what caused fertility to increase in the 1960s. It is unlikely that the increase can be attributed to a general reduction in the level of primary infertility. The proportion of women aged 50 or more with no live births in the 1960-1961 DS was already quite low, only 4-7 percent. Fargues (1989) has suggested that fertility increases in North Africa may have resulted from reduced marital disruption, particularly divorce; a similar process could underlie a fertility increase in Senegal in the 1960s and 1970s.

Figure 4-2 shows relative age patterns of fertility from the five surveys. Though there are differences between the surveys—the proportion of fertility contributed by the age group 40-44 in 1960-1961 is low, as is the contribution of the age groups 30-34 and 35-39 in 1970-1971, partially balanced in the latter case by a high contribution by women aged 45-49—these differences are probably the result of sampling or other errors, and no major trends are evident in the age pattern of fertility from 1960-1990. There is one minor trend visible, however: the percentage of total fertility contributed by the age group 15-19 does appear to be falling over time, from nearly 15 percent in 1960-1961 to 13 percent in 1978, to 11 percent by 1992-1993.

The question of whether or not there has been a recent fertility decline also requires further elucidation. Parity-specific analysis of birth history data can be a useful way to detect small changes in fertility for a country at the beginning of a transition toward lower fertility (Brass and Juarez, 1983). Recent analysis of the DHS data using censored parity progression ratios (B_{60}s)[7] revealed that the pattern of fertility decline witnessed in Kenya, Botswana, and Zimbabwe is quite unusual in comparison with the Latin American and Asian experience (Working Group on Kenya, 1993). The typical pattern of developing countries outside Africa was for initial declines to take place primarily in the middle, and sometimes in the higher, parities. The decline among low birth orders occurred more slowly. In Africa, by contrast, where fertility reductions have occurred, they have occurred across all parities (Working Group on Kenya, 1993).

The B_{60}s for women in both the DHS-I and the DHS-II are shown in Table 4-2. To simplify the table, neighboring parity progression ratios for the same cohort have been combined by multiplying consecutive indices together.[8] This procedure has the advantage of dampening fluctuations in the estimates caused by small sample size and is particularly useful because no formula exists to calculate the standard errors associated with B_{60}s: inferences about changes in fertility behavior can be drawn only by examining general patterns in the data (Brass and Juarez, 1983).

For the DHS-I data, the B_{60}s show some weak evidence of a fertility

TABLE 4-2 Censored Cohort Parity Progression Ratios, DHS-I and DHS-II

Survey and Women's Age	Censored Parity Progression Ratios (B_{60}s)			
	1-3	3-5	5-7	7-9
1986 DHS-I				
20-24	.733			
25-29	.785	.646		
30-34	.822	.771	.631	.438
35-39	.804	.753	.665	.482
40-44	.781	.755	.675	.546
45-49	.787	.797	.731	.555
1992-1993 DHS-II				
20-24	.693			
25-29	.730	.706	.554	
30-34	.779	.745	.595	
35-39	.800	.747	.641	.484
40-44	.841	.791	.690	.492
45-49	.783	.760	.736	.588

NOTE: See Appendix A for description of surveys.

SOURCE: Calculations based on data from DHS-I and DHS-II.

decline among women of middle parities, but the B_{60}s are quite erratic in the lower parities. For example, DHS-I data indicate that a little under 80 percent of women born between 1937 and 1941 (i.e., aged 45-49 in 1986) progressed from a third to a fifth birth. The comparable figure for women born between 1957 and 1961 is 65 percent. The comparable figure for women born between 1952 and 1956 is 77 percent. The proportion of women moving from a fifth to a seventh birth shows a more consistent decline across cohorts, from 73 percent among women born between 1937 and 1941 to 63 percent among women born between 1952 and 1956.

Examined by themselves, the B_{60}s from the DHS-II show clearer evidence of a fertility decline across all parities, in keeping with the pattern documented recently for other parts of sub-Saharan Africa (Working Group on Kenya, 1993). However, the results are much more ambiguous when the B_{60}s from the DHS-I and DHS-II are compared side by side. For example, consider women aged 30-34 who have had five children. According to DHS-I, 63 percent of these women progress to parity 7. As one would anticipate when analyzing a fertility decline, this is a higher progression rate than reported in DHS-II (60 percent). At the same time, however, 71 percent of women aged 25-29 at the time of the DHS-II progressed from parity 3 to parity 5, compared with only 65 percent in the DHS-I. Perhaps these findings should not come as a great surprise given that the reported use of modern contraception in Senegal is very low (see below).

Regional Variations

In 1978, the WFS reported fertility rates for four grand regions of the country:[9] west, comprising the two regions of Dakar and Thiès; center, comprising Diourbel, Fatick, Kaolack, and Louga; south, comprising Ziguinchor and Kolda; and northeast, comprising Saint-Louis and Tambacounda. Subsequently, these same regions were used in the DHS-I and DHS-II, making it straightforward to observe any regional variation in fertility over time. Fertility rates based on data from the 4 years preceding each survey are shown for each of these four regions in Table 4-1. Age-specific fertility schedules for each region for various points in time are presented in Figure 4-4.

In the late 1970s, the total level of fertility of the four grand regions was much the same (see Table 4-1); the TFR varied from 7.1 children per women in the west to 7.4 in the south. Since 1978, the level of heterogeneity has increased as fertility has started to decline. Fertility in the DHS-II ranges from 5.6 children per woman in the west to 6.6 in the northeast.

Age-specific fertility also varies by region (see Figure 4-4). Fertility among young women is lowest in the west; this region includes the cities of Dakar and Thiès, and is therefore by far the most urbanized region. On the other hand, for women over 35, fertility is lowest in the southern and central regions. These regional differences are also found in the census, in spite of its lower reliability (see Figure 4-5).

A fertility decline among women under age 25 seems to have taken place across all four regions, although the pattern of decline is quite different in each case. Comparing the WFS with the DHS-I reveals that fertility was higher in the former than in the latter in three of the four regions, although in two of the three cases the differences between surveys are slight. Only the central region exhibits no difference in the level of fertility between the two surveys. When the results of the DHS-II are added, however, the picture changes. First, the central region now exhibits lower fertility between the DHS-I and DHS-II. But the level of fertility is virtually unchanged between the two DHS surveys in the southern and northeastern regions. Only in the western region has fertility continued to decline, falling an additional 18 percent over its 1986 level and 32 percent over its 1978 level. One also observes an apparent fertility decline for women aged 25-29. The pattern is clearest in the west and northeast before 1986, less apparent in the center, and nonexistent in the south. As discussed below,

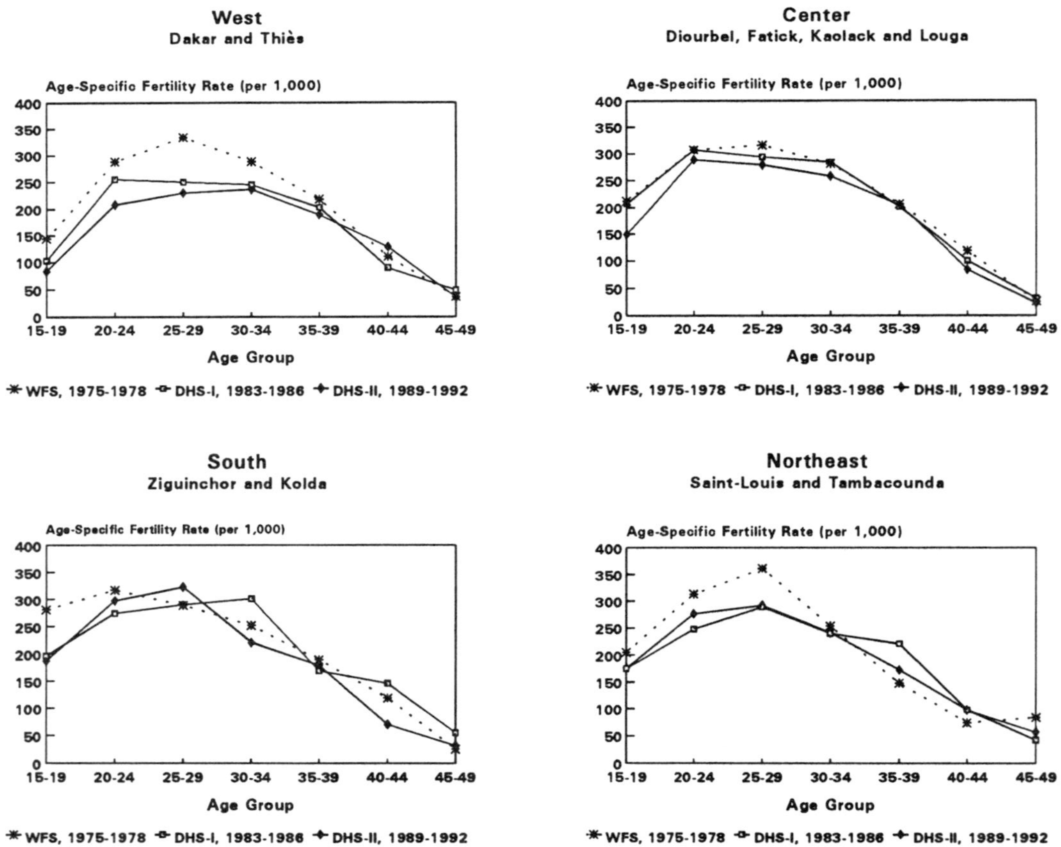

FIGURE 4-4 Changes in age-specific fertility rates, by grand region over time. NOTE: See Appendix A for description of surveys. SOURCES: Standard data files from WFS, DHS-I, and DHS-II.

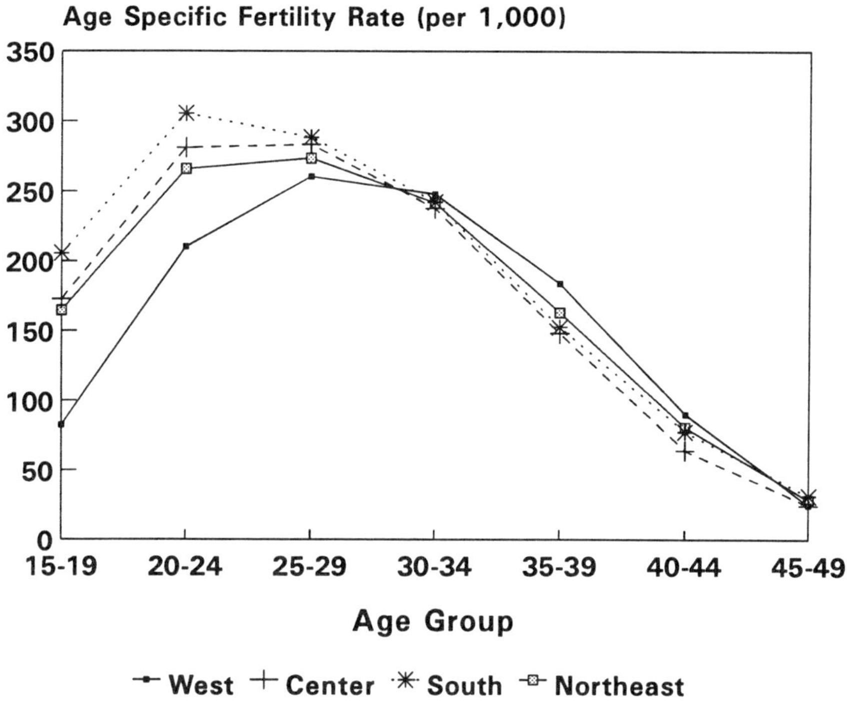

FIGURE 4-5 Age-specific fertility rates, 1987-1988, by grand region. SOURCE: 1988 census, unpublished data.

the evidence of a decline in fertility among younger women is consistent with a rise in age at first marriage.

Findings from the 1988 Census

The 1988 census allows us to investigate variations in the level of fertility by the 30 departments within Senegal. Estimates of the ASFR in each department are given in Tables B-2 to B-11 in Appendix B. The TFRs are much higher in rural than in urban areas, but they vary from department to department apparently without much of a discernible pattern, although they appear to be slightly higher in the coastal departments in the southwest of the country. Unfortunately, because the quality of reporting probably deteriorates as one moves away from the capital, it is not clear that fertility is really higher in the coastal departments.

As discussed above, women under age 30 appear to have played a central role in a fertility decline in Senegal. Consequently, it is important to examine the regional pattern of fertility among these women for whom the quality of data in the census is probably more reliable than that of the data for the older ages. Figure 4-6 shows the sum of the ASFRs for the age group 15-29. Fertility in urban areas is lowest in and around Dakar. In the south of the country, far from the influence of the capital, fertility levels in urban areas are generally higher than those elsewhere. These broad patterns of (1) lower fertility around Dakar, and (2) slightly higher fertility in the south than in the north of the country are also visible in the bottom half of the figure, which shows variations in fertility for the rural population in each department.

The geography of fertility rates before age 20 as reported by the census is comparable with that derived from the WFS, DHS-I, and DHS-II using the four grand regions defined above (see Table 4-3). But as we have seen above, this type of analysis masks considerable intraregional heterogeneity. In particular, the central region is a mix of departments, some of which are far closer to Dakar than others, and some of which are far more southerly than others—two important factors underlying fertility differentials in Senegal.

TABLE 4-3 Age-Specific Fertility Rates for Women Aged 15-19 by Grand Region, 1975-1992

Year	Source	Subgroup	Age-Specific Fertility Rate (per 1,000)
1975-1978	WFS	West	144
		Center	212
		Northeast	205
		South	281
1983-1986	DHS-I	West	103
		Center	207
		Northeast	175
		South	196
1987-1988	Census	West	82
		Center	173
		Northeast	165
		South	206
1989-1992	DHS-II	West	83
		Center	149
		Northeast	176
		South	187

NOTE: See Appendix A for description of surveys.

SOURCES: WFS, DHS-I, and DHS-II data files and unpublished tabulations from the 1988

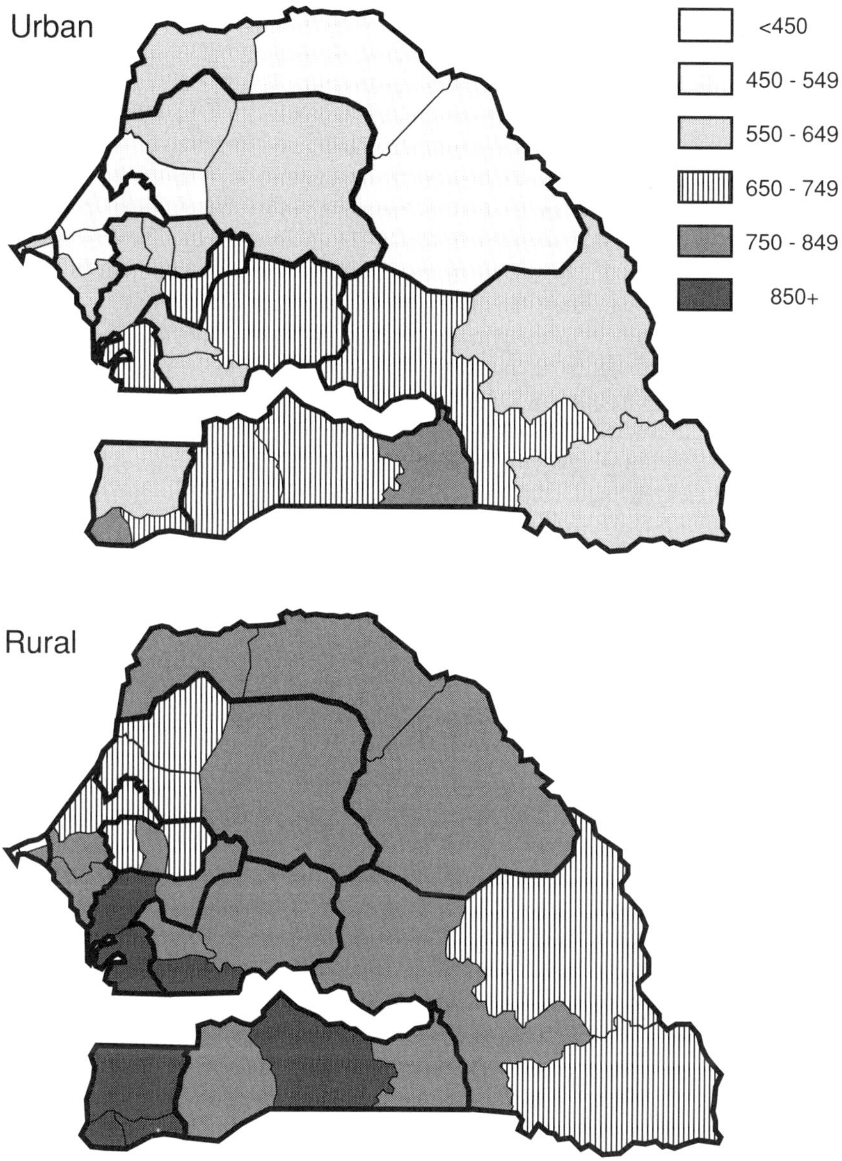

FIGURE 4-6 Map of Senegal showing variations in the fertility rates (per thousand) among women aged 15-29 in different departments, urban and rural. SOURCE: 1988 census, unpublished data.

Supplemental Information from Three Small-Scale Demographic Surveillance Systems

Apart from the information provided by national surveys and censuses described above, fertility estimates are also available for some areas from small-scale surveys [8-16]. Of course, these surveys provide information on only a small fraction of the total population, and their small populations make their estimates prone to variability. However, these drawbacks must be weighed against the fact that smaller populations enable interviewers to conduct frequent visits to the same households. Thus the enumerators can check and correct information collected during previous rounds, as well as document very carefully any events that have occurred between visits. As a result, data collected from multiround surveillance systems are often of substantially higher quality than can be achieved from a single interview, especially with regard to date and age variables.

In Senegal, the oldest and largest of these multiround surveillance systems is at Niakhar/Ngayokhème [11], where demographic data have been collected intermittently since December 1962 under the auspices of the Institut Français de Recherche Scientifique pour le Développement en Coopération (ORSTOM). Figure 4-7 shows a series of estimates derived from the ORSTOM project for various points in time.

Estimates from the Niakhar project indicate that fertility rates were extremely high over the period 1984-1990 (Projet Niakhar, 1992). The TFR was estimated to be 7.8 children per woman, approximately 2 children per woman more than the rate recorded in 1963-1965 by Cantrelle (1969). The increase in fertility occurred principally among women over the age of 25 (see Figure 4-7).[10] Although a large increase, a comparison by Garenne and van Ginneken (1994) found a satisfactory consistency between the fertility of the Serer living in the villages covered by the ORSTOM laboratory of Niakhar and the fertility of the rural Serer population measured by the WFS in 1978 and the DHS-I in 1986.

Data are also available from two other longitudinal studies, although both are of smaller size than the ORSTOM study. The Bandafassi study [8] was initiated in 1970 in the department of Kédougou, Tambacounda region and has grown steadily to include records on approximately 8,500 individuals in 1993.[11] The Mlomp study was initiated in 1984 in the department of Oussouye, Ziguinchor region, and includes information on approximately 6,500 individuals in 1990.[12]

Figure 4-8 presents fertility rates for 1981-1990 for the study area of Bandafassi. Although the reported ASFRs are rather high among teenagers, the overall level of fertility is relatively low (TFR = 6.2), invalidating the existence of a systematic association between early and high fertility in Senegal. Even within this small area, however, fertility rates vary greatly,

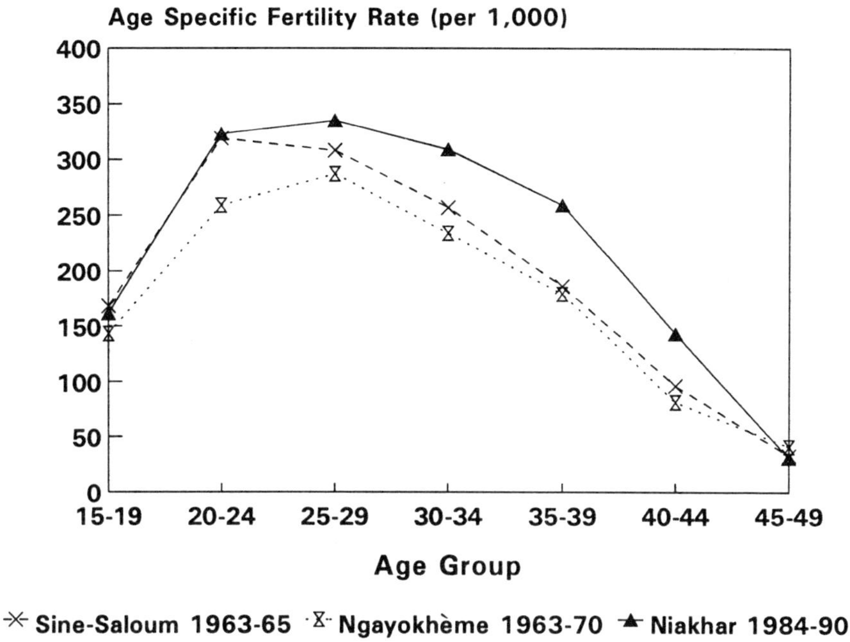

FIGURE 4-7 Changes in age-specific fertility rates, Niakhar study area, over time. NOTES: The baseline changed somewhat over the years, so the different fertility schedules are not completely comparable: the study area initially extended farther south, but not as far to the north, as the present area. See Appendix A for description of surveys. SOURCES: Cantrelle et al. (1980), Projet Niakhar (1992).

from 6.7 children per woman among the Peul to 5.5 children per woman among the Bedik (Pison and Desgrées du Loû, 1993).

The study area of Mlomp [10] is unlike any other in Senegal. It is characterized by an extremely large amount of seasonal migration, and the majority of the adult population is absent for at least half of the year (Lagarde et al., forthcoming). Eighty percent of women aged 15-24 (almost all of them unmarried) migrate to seek employment as domestic servants in the main cities of Senegal or The Gambia. Marriage takes place relatively late in Mlomp: the mean age at first marriage in the area is estimated to be 24 for women and 30 for men (Enel and Pison, 1992). Marriage probably occurred earlier one or two generations ago (Enel and Pison, 1992). Once married, women usually stop their pattern of seasonal migration and stay all year in their village. The consequences of these patterns are apparent in Figure 4-9.[13] Although Mlomp is a unique area, the rapid change in fertility shown in Figure 4-9 is an example of what might take place in Senegal in

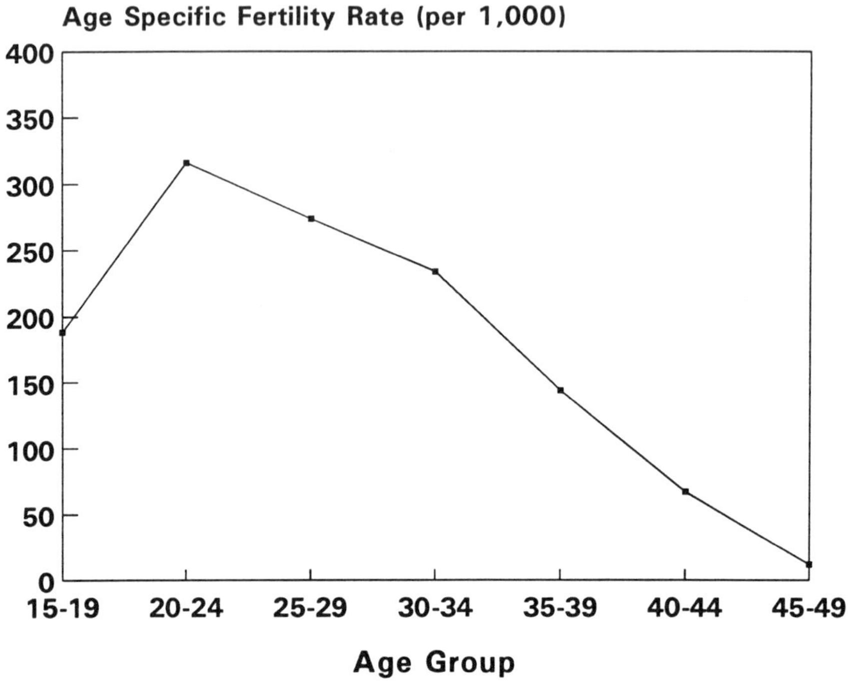

FIGURE 4-8 Age-specific fertility rates, Bandafassi study area, 1981-1990. NOTE: See Appendix A for description of survey. SOURCE: Pison and Desgrées du Loû (1993).

the years to come: a rapid decline in fertility at younger ages, following a delay in marriage.

These multiround surveillance systems provide us with an independent check on the quality of the birth data in the 1988 census. Given that the census experienced serious problems with recording of deaths of children under age 1 (see Chapter 5), it is interesting to compare the census results with ASFRs obtained from the three multiround surveillance systems. As discussed earlier, the 1988 census restricted its investigation of fertility to a single question on the number of children women had had in the last 12 months,[14] while all three multiround studies have invested considerable time and money in making repeated visits to the same households to ensure the accuracy of their data. Figure 4-10 reproduces the fertility schedules for the most recent periods for Niakhar, Bandafassi, and Mlomp. These data have been plotted with census data from the rural areas of the departments in which the surveillance systems are located.

In none of the cases is the match perfect, though encouragingly, there is

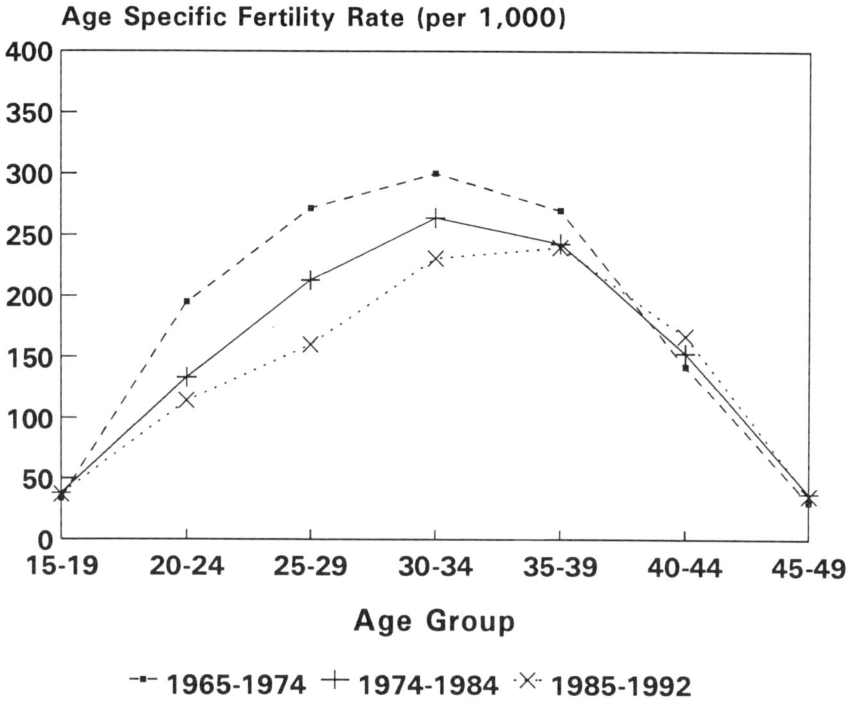

FIGURE 4-9 Changes in age-specific fertility rates, Mlomp study area, over time. NOTE: See Appendix A for description of survey. SOURCE: Lagarde et al. (forthcoming).

fairly close agreement between the Niakhar data and the census. The match is less satisfactory in the other two cases. Comparison of the ASFRs in the census with the Bandafassi data indicates that there may have been a sizable deficit of recorded births in the census in the department of Kédougou, one of the least developed parts of the country. Finally, the ASFRs for Mlomp and census data for rural Oussouye bear no resemblance to one another. However, the study area of Mlomp is considerably smaller than the department of Oussouye, has special socioeconomic characteristics, and probably should not be expected to be representative of that department.

Despite their limitations, local comparisons tend to support the hypothesis that births were underreported in the 1988 census. While fertility rates from the census for the youngest age groups, notably ages 15-19, correspond fairly well to those based on the Niakhar and Bandafassi data, the differences are greater among the older age groups, i.e., above age 20 in the census data for the department of Kédougou (compared with the Bandafassi data) and above age 30 in the census data for the department of Fatick

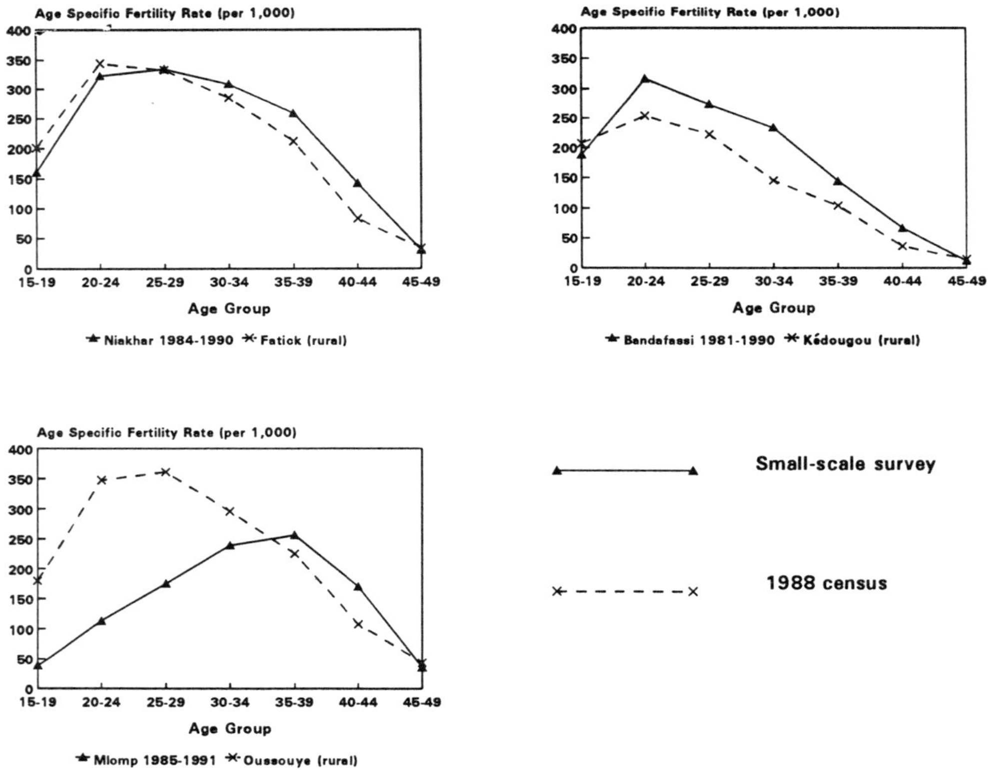

FIGURE 4-10 Comparison of age-specific fertility rates from 1988 census data with data from small-scale surveillance systems. NOTE: See Appendix A for description of surveys. SOURCES: 1988 census, unpublished data, Lagarde et al. (forthcoming), Projet Niakhar (1992), Pison and Desgrées du Loû (1993).

(compared with the Niakhar data). The extent of underreporting probably varied from one region of the country to another. This fact must be borne in mind when studying demographic variations in fertility based on census-estimated rates.

Conclusions Drawn from Regional Differences

The above discussion highlights the considerable heterogeneity among administrative regions in both the level of fertility and the timing of births. The difference in total fertility exceeds two children per woman between the small-scale studies with the highest and lowest rates. Some regions have rates of childbearing among teenagers that are three to four times higher than those in other regions. Much of the diversity among regions occurs among women under 30, suggesting that the variations may be more closely related to the timing of entry into union than to the level of fertility within unions.

Evidence for a fertility decline is strongest in Dakar and the western region of the country. Elsewhere, as in the Niakhar region, the level of fertility has increased over the past 20 years. Thus, regional differentiation has become more pronounced since the 1970s.

Fertility Differences by Socioeconomic Characteristics

A fundamental problem facing population economists attempting to explain the relationship between income and fertility is that in every major region of the world over the last two centuries, childbearing has fallen as income has risen. At first blush, this runs counter to economists' expectations because if children are desirable, one should want to acquire more of them as one accumulates more wealth. In response, economists have tended to place increasing reliance on a vast literature commonly referred to as "new home economics." This microlevel approach has been made famous over the last 30 years by Nobel Prize-winning economist Gary Becker.[15]

Within this framework, different sources of income exert differing effects on fertility. Higher male wages are assumed to increase fertility, while higher female wages are usually assumed to reduce fertility because the bearing and rearing of children competes with working in the labor force for women. Inspection of the recent empirical data appears to confirm many of the features of the neoclassical economic model (Schultz, 1994). In particular, countries with higher incomes, given their human capital resource base, were found to have higher fertility. At the same time, greater female education was found to be the dominant factor associated with a decline in fertility in both cross-sectional and longitudinal data (Schultz, 1994).

Microlevel Evidence

The 1978 WFS [3], the 1986 DHS-I [4], and the 1992-1993 DHS-II [7] allow the study of fertility differentials by some important socioeconomic characteristics, such as place of residence, ethnicity, and level of instruction. The existence of these three comparable national surveys allows us to analyze differences over time.

Figure 4-11 shows fertility differences by urban/rural residence. The vast majority of women still live in rural areas where fertility is very high. Although one small-scale study [11] indicated that fertility may have risen in Niakhar (see above), overall there appears to have been little change in fertility in rural Senegal over the past 15 years. The TFR in rural areas decreased slightly over this period, from 7.5 in the mid-1970s to 7.3 in the mid-1980s, and again to between 6.4 and 6.8 at the end of the 1980s and the beginning of the 1990s (see Table 4-1). The timing of fertility (i.e., in the total number of children ever born), like the age-specific pattern, also changed only slightly. In rural areas, childbearing still begins earlier and is ultimately higher than in the urban areas.

In urban areas, fertility has been declining since the mid-1970s. In the late 1970s, the WFS estimated fertility at 6.8 children per woman in Dakar and 6.5 children per woman in other urban areas. These levels have declined over the last 15 years. For the most recent period, 1989-1992, DHS-II data indicate that fertility is around 4.9 children per woman in Dakar and 5.4 in other cities. Some postponement of childbearing had already occurred in urban areas by the mid-1980s. In Dakar, a comparison of WFS and DHS-I data reveals that fertility decline had already occurred among women under age 35. In other cities, only women under age 30 have reduced their fertility. Overall, the changes in the timing of childbearing have led to a flatter fertility schedule that is less concentrated in the prime childbearing ages. There is virtually no indication that fertility has declined for women over the age of 30, except in Dakar. A decline in fertility among women over 30 would be significant because it would mark the beginning of a fertility decline within unions, which, when combined with the decline in fertility attributable to a delay in entry into union, can lead to a rapid change in the TFR.

Fertility was probably relatively stable in Dakar between the end of the 1960s and the mid-1970s.[16] Figure 4-12 displays the ASFR for Dakar in 1975-1978 calculated from the WFS [3] with the fertility schedule derived from the Cap-Vert (Dakar) fertility survey of 1972 [9] taken 6 years earlier. The TFR estimates are very close—6.8 and 6.6 children per woman, respectively—and we note a remarkable consistency between the two schedules.

Table 4-1 shows the variation in the TFR over time by major ethnic group. Cultural differences among ethnic groups have long been recog-

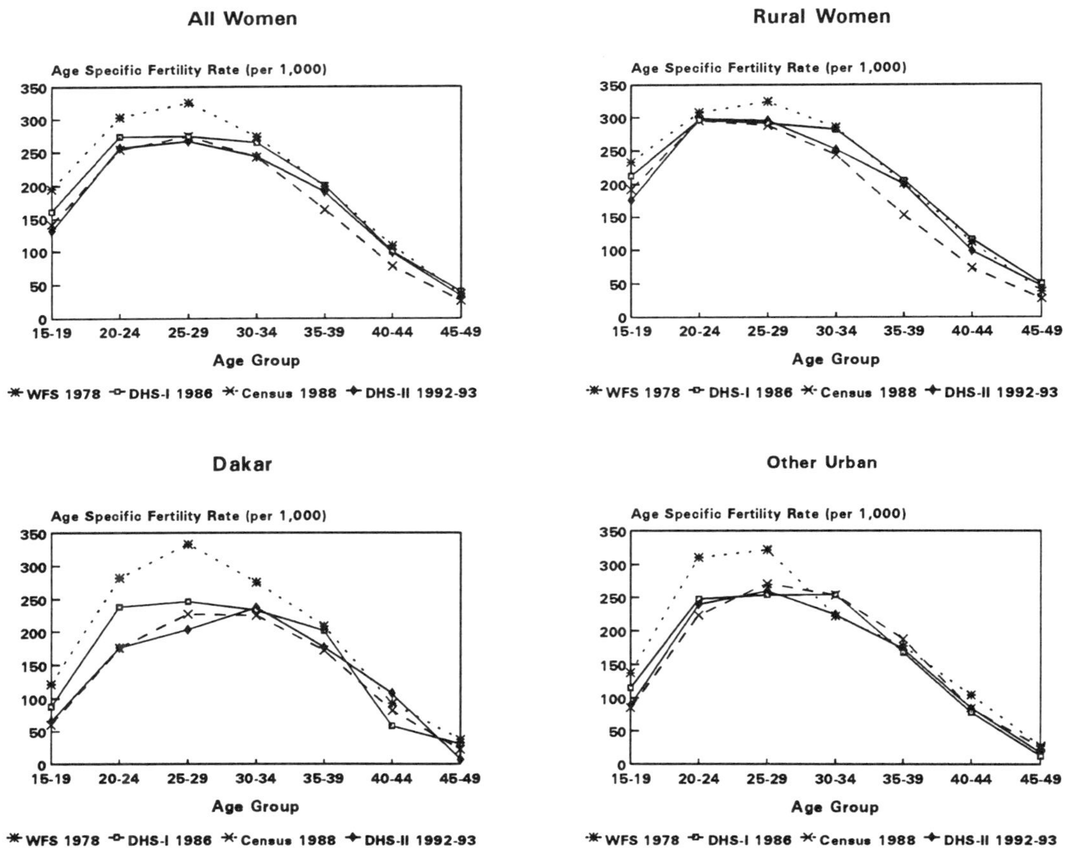

FIGURE 4-11 Age-specific fertility rates, by urban/rural residence. NOTE: See Appendix A for description of surveys. SOURCES: 1988 census, unpublished data and standard data files from WFS, DHS-I, and DHS-II.

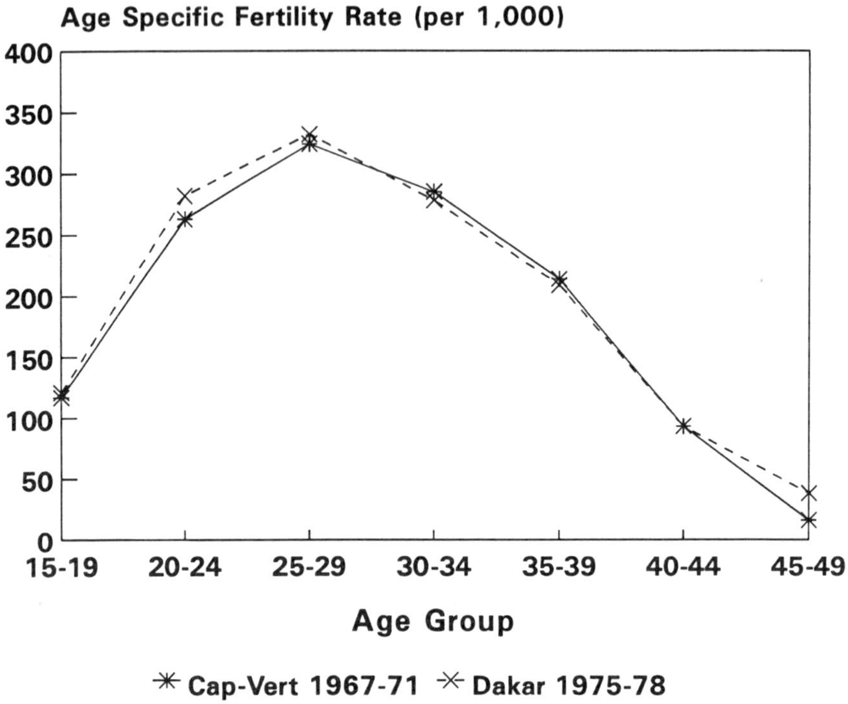

FIGURE 4-12 Changes in age-specific fertility rates, Dakar Region, over time. SOURCES: Ferry (1976) and WFS standard data tape.

nized as important determinants of the level of fertility in Senegal,[17] although the pattern of childbearing is broadly similar among the various groups. For example, fertility is considerably higher among the Serer, who live mainly in the Sine-Saloum region. The TFR for Serer women was 7.9 children per woman in 1975-1978, compared with a TFR of 7.2 for Wolof women or a TFR of 6.9 for Poular women. Although the TFR fell for all three groups between 1978 and 1986, it fell the least for the Serer. And in the DHS-II, the TFR for Serer women remains almost 1.0 child per woman higher than the TFR for the Poular and 1.6 children per woman higher than the TFR for Wolof women.[18]

The fertility schedules for the Diola, Mandingo, and other ethnic groups are based on smaller sample sizes, so they tend to be more erratic than the schedules for the Wolof, Poular, and Serer. However, Figure 4-13 shows fertility has declined significantly among young Mandingo women, who live predominantly in the south of the country. Thus, fertility variations by ethnic group partly confirm variations observed at the regional level.

Figure 4-14 shows variations in fertility over time separately for women

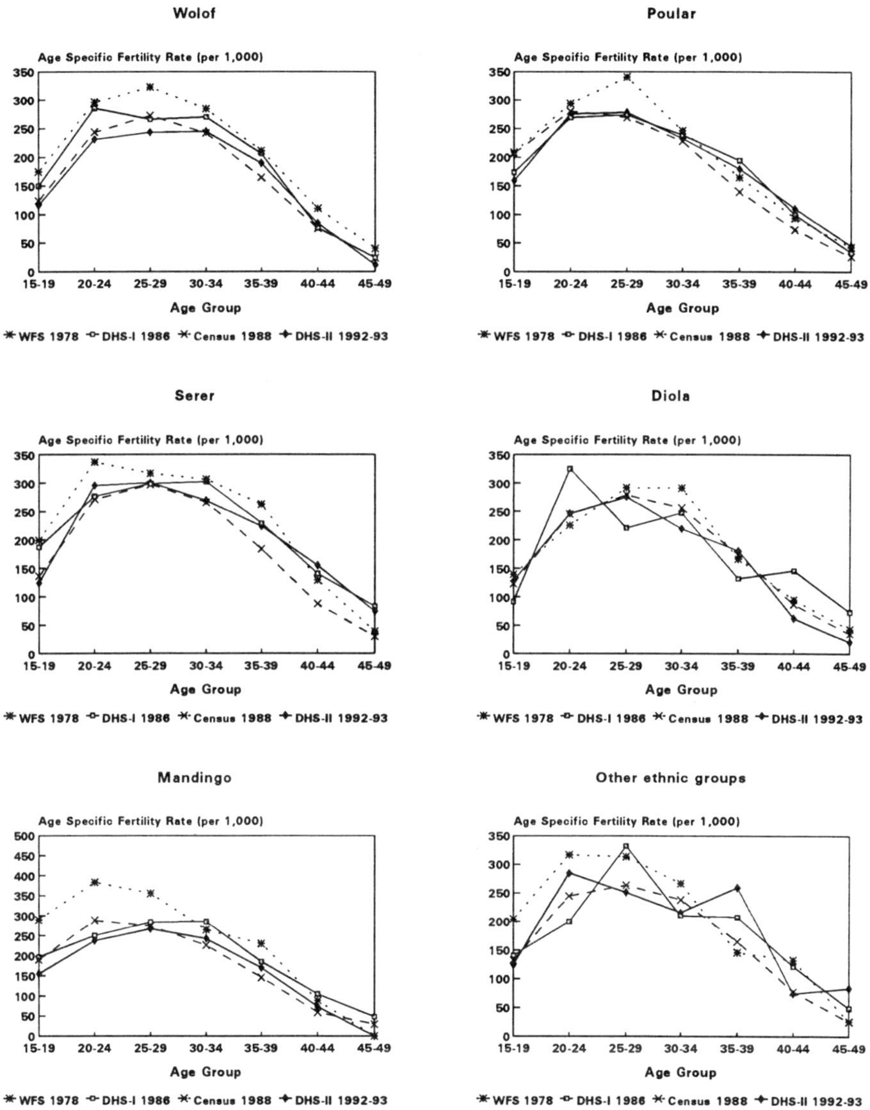

FIGURE 4-13 Age-specific fertility rates by ethnic group. NOTE: See Appendix A for description of surveys. SOURCES: 1988 census, unpublished data and standard data files from WFS, DHS-I, and DHS-II.

with different levels of education. The experiences of the three groups over time are very different. Women with no education had very high fertility in the mid-1970s. The TFR for the period 1975-1978 was 7.4 children per woman, a figure that has declined slowly over the last 15 years (see Table 4-1). On the other hand, fertility among women with only primary education fell sharply between 1975-1978 and 1983-1986; their TFR dropped from 7.1 to 5.7 children per woman over this period. Note, however, that the number of women with a primary education sampled in the WFS was quite small, so we must be careful not to read too much into small fluctuations in the shape of the fertility schedule, especially above age 35.

It is even more difficult to draw conclusions for the group of women with secondary or higher education: the fertility schedule estimated from the WFS is quite erratic, reflecting the small sample size. There is, however, little doubt that women in this group have lower fertility than women with less education. The TFR among the former group has changed little over the period—the TFR has remained around 3.6 children per woman—but the peak of the fertility schedule may have moved from ages 25-29 to ages 30-34.[19]

Macrolevel Evidence

The cross-sectional relationships among various socioeconomic, fertility, and marriage indicators can be analyzed using data from the 1988 census.[20] Three fertility indicators are used in this analysis: the period TFR for women aged 10-54 (TFR_{10-54}), the period TFR for women aged 15-29 (TFR_{15-29}), and the period ASFR for women aged 15-19 ($ASFR_{15-19}$). The marriage indicators used are the singulate mean age at first marriage for men and women ($SMAM_m$, $SMAM_f$), the proportion of men aged 20-24 who have ever been married, and the proportion of women aged 15-19 who have ever been married.

The correlation coefficient is a useful statistic that provides a measure of the association between two random variables. Correlation coefficients between selected socioeconomic and demographic indices at the department level ($N = 30$) are provided in Table 4-4.

Until recently, there was little evidence of any parity-specific fertility control among married women in Senegal, so it is not surprising to find a low correlation between the TFRs and the various measures of socioeconomic development displayed in Table 4-4. When these indicators are correlated with the fertility rate of females aged 15-29, the associations become more pronounced. Fertility among women aged 15-19 is even more strongly associated with socioeconomic status, so that a department's level of socioeconomic development becomes a good predictor of the level of adolescent childbearing. Figure 4-15 is illustrative of the departmental

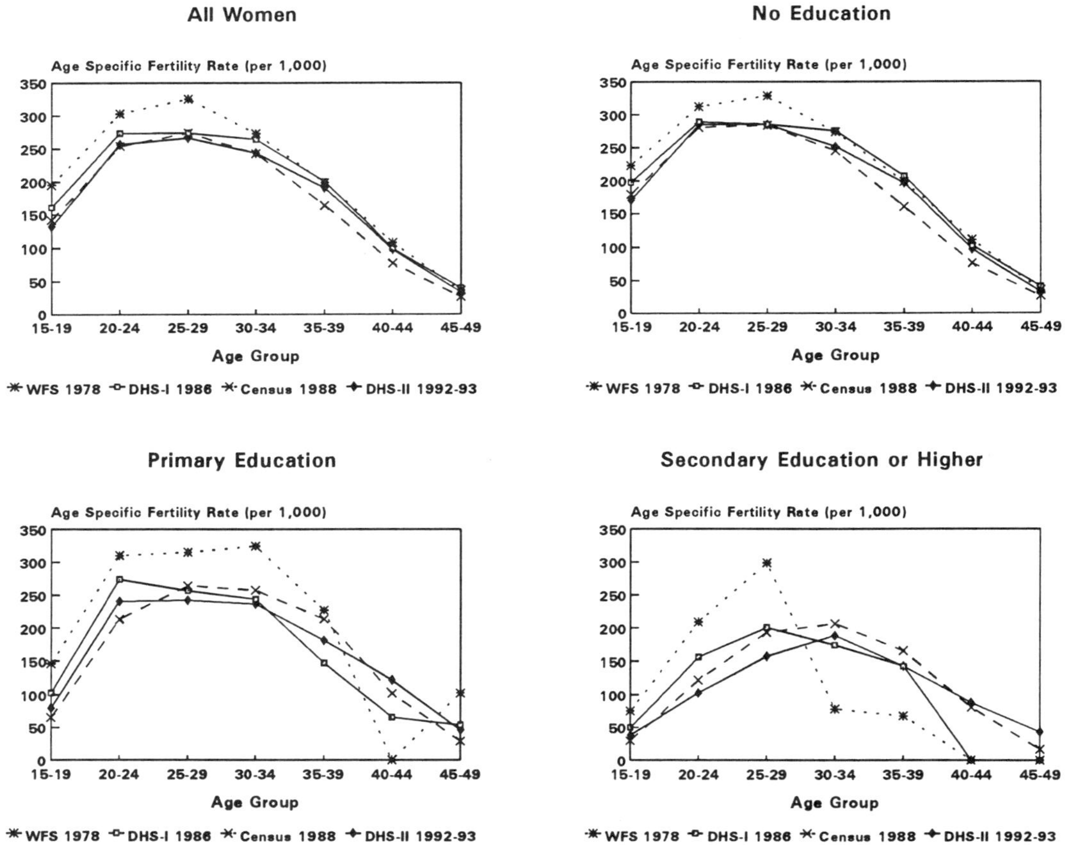

FIGURE 4-14 Age-specific fertility rates by level of education. NOTE: See Appendix A for description of surveys. SOURCE: 1988 census, unpublished data and standard data files from WFS, DHS-I, and DHS-II.

TABLE 4-4 Correlation Coefficients Between Socioeconomic and Demographic Indicators

	Fertility Indicators			Nuptiality Indicators			
Socio-economic Indicator	TFR	TFR_{15-29}	$ASFR_{15-19}$	% Males Married, 20-24	% Females Married, 15-19	$SMAM_m$	$SMAM_f$
Housing	–.365	–.754	–.879	–.703	–.818	.744	.812
Electricity	–.551	–.833	–.799	–.548	–.656	.584	.673
Latrine	–.502	–.709	–.682	–.416	–.488	.434	.511
Water	–.544	–.812	–.846	–.462	–.598	.476	.579
Composite	–.516	–.822	–.843	–.557	–.673	.585	.674
Urban	–.440	–.747	–.780	–.671	–.766	.695	.781
Ever school	–.225	–.606	–.727	–.852	–.898	.890	.920
School enrollment rate (male)	–.028	–.435	–.639	–.882	–.916	.925	.933
School enrollment rate (female)	.008	–.416	–.628	–.871	–.909	.936	.933

NOTE: See Chapter 2 for details on how the socioeconomic indicators were constructed.

SOURCE: Unpublished tables, 1988 census.

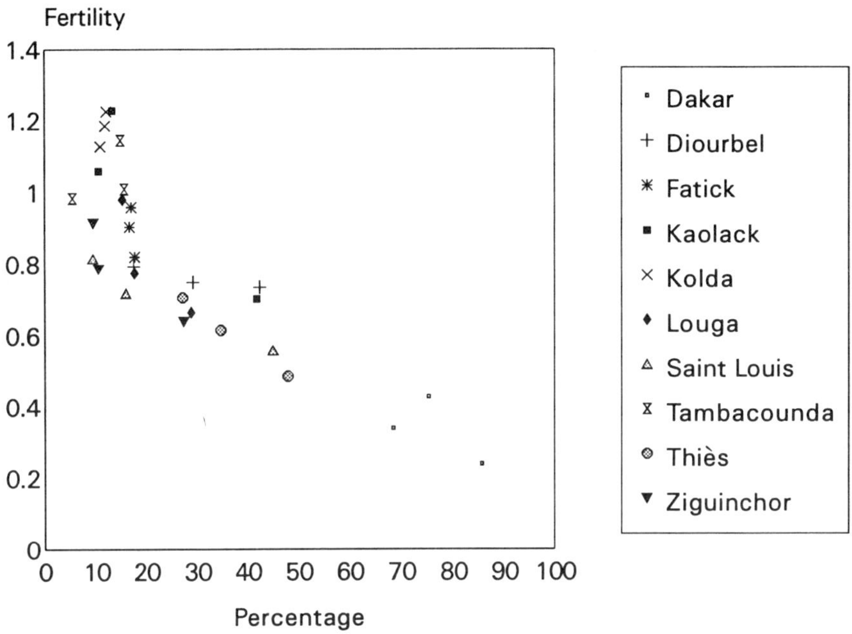

FIGURE 4-15 Departmental variations in fertility by the composite facilities indicator, women aged 15-19. NOTE: The composite facilities indicator is the arithmetic mean of (1) the percentage of households obtaining their water supply from a faucet or standpipe, whether placed inside or outside the home; (2) the percentage of households with electricity; (3) the percentage of households with toilets or latrines; and (4) the percentage of households whose houses have been built using good construction techniques. See Chapter 2 for more details. SOURCE: 1988 census, unpublished tables.

relationship between age-specific fertility of women aged 15-19 and the level of socioeconomic development.

As seen later, age at first marriage is an important proximate determinant of fertility among women aged 15-19. The correlations between various indicators of marriage and socioeconomic status reported in Table 4-4 are rather large. Figure 4-16 is illustrative of this relationship at the department level. One region is a notable outlier on the figure: Ziguinchor. Given the department's socioeconomic status, fewer young women in Ziguinchor are married than would be expected, probably because a high proportion of Diola women (the major ethnic group in the area) tend to spend their early adult years working in urban areas, and consequently tend to marry relatively late.

In summary, fertility rates and socioeconomic indicators tend to be

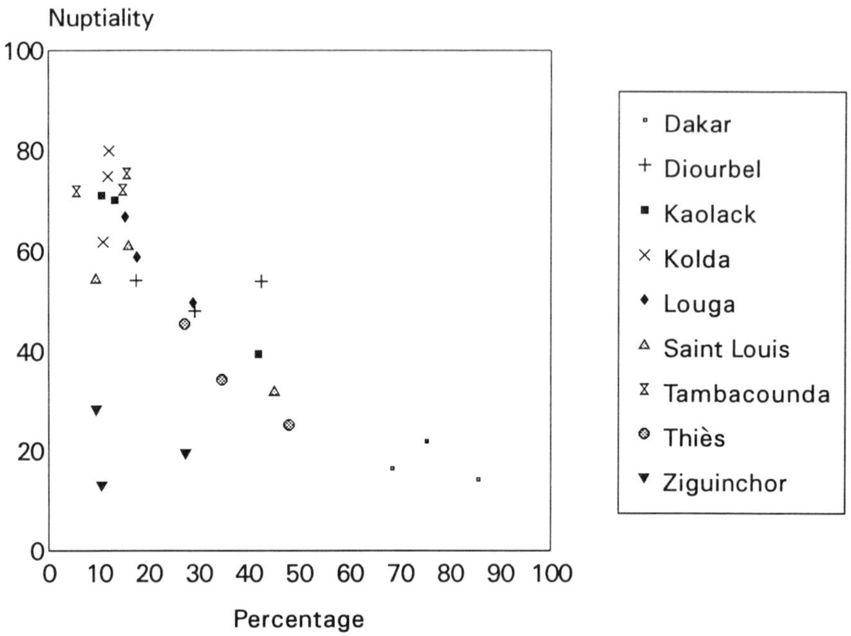

FIGURE 4-16 Departmental variations in nuptiality by the composite facilities indicator, women aged 15-19. NOTE: See note for Figure 4-15. SOURCE: 1988 census, unpublished tables.

inversely related. Fertility for younger women tends to be more strongly related to socioeconomic status than does fertility for older women. The percentage of males and females married is also inversely related to socioeconomic status, the relationships being stronger for females than for males. With one notable exception, Ziguinchor, mean age at marriage tends to increase with socioeconomic status.

Summary of Fertility Levels and Trends

Senegalese women have high fertility. On average, each woman has about 6 children over the course of her reproductive life. Although a substantial number, this figure actually represents a decline of approximately 1 child per woman from the fertility level observed at the end of the 1970s. It is possible that this decline was preceded by an increase in fertility during an earlier period. Until recently, there was a general reluctance to accept any signs of recent fertility decline in Senegal, but it now appears that such a decline has in fact occurred. This decline started first in the capital and extended progressively, although slowly, to other regions of the country. Until now, this decline has affected only the urban population.

Examination of differentials by region, place of residence, education, and ethnicity reveals that the western region, which is the most educated and urbanized, is the one with the lowest fertility. Variations in reproductive behavior by ethnicity may also explain some regional differences.

What other variables might help explain these changing patterns of fertility? The decline in ASFRs among women aged 15-19 and 20-24 indicates that the fertility decline may be linked to a delay in the entry into union (Sadio, 1985). However, some of the other observed fertility differentials, such as those between women with secondary education and women with no education, are very large and cannot be explained solely by differences in the timing of marriage. Other proximate determinants, such as contraceptive use, abortion, and sterility, also play a role in limiting total fertility. The relative importance of these factors is quantified below using the proximate determinants framework of Bongaarts and Potter (1983).

PROXIMATE DETERMINANTS OF FERTILITY

Overview

Regardless of the survey examined, ASFRs in Senegal remain high over a woman's entire reproductive period. However, as noted above, fertility rates have fallen over the last 15 years, particularly among the young. Why have these changes taken place? It is analytically convenient to differentiate factors influencing fertility into two distinct classes: (1) a set of biological "proximate" determinants that exert a direct influence on fertility, and (2) all social, cultural, and economic factors that can influence fertility only through these proximate determinants. Originally specified by Davis and Blake (1956) as "intermediate variables," the major proximate determinants were identified by Bongaarts (1978) and adopted into a straightforward framework so that the relative importance of each could be easily assessed. The following is a complete list of the quantitatively important proximate determinants:

- the proportion of women married (or more strictly the proportion of women in sexual unions);
- the contraceptive prevalence and effectiveness rate;
- the induced abortion rate;
- the length of the postpartum infecund interval (primarily the result of breastfeeding patterns);
- the frequency of coitus;
- the level of spontaneous intrauterine mortality; and
- the prevalence of primary or secondary sterility.

Each proximate determinant has a different degree of importance in explaining variations in fertility. It has been shown, however, that differences in fertility rates among populations are due predominantly to variations in only four of the determinants: the proportion married, the level and effectiveness of contraceptive use, the incidence of induced abortion, and the length of the postpartum infecund interval (Bongaarts and Potter, 1983). In sub-Saharan Africa, high levels of pathological sterility may also lead to important variations in fertility among certain ethnic groups (Frank, 1983; Bongaarts et al., 1984). The respective effects of the main proximate determinants on fertility can be quantified using the following model:

$$TFR = C_m * C_c * C_i * C_a * I_p * TF,$$

where:

TFR = total fertility rate,
C_m = index of marriage,
C_c = index of contraception,
C_i = index of postpartum infecundability,
C_a = index of induced abortion,
I_p = index of sterility, and
TF = potential fertility.[21]

The effect of each of the proximate determinants is quantified by an index that varies between 0 and 1. The model has been constructed in such a way that when an index is close to 1, the proximate determinant will have a negligible inhibiting effect on total fertility, whereas when the index is close to 0, the proximate determinant will have a large inhibiting effect.

Table 4-5 shows the Bongaarts indices, estimated using data from the WFS [3], DHS-I [4], and DHS-II [7]. The level of fertility is scarcely reduced by contraceptive use (C_c), or pathological sterility (I_p). Both these indices are close to 1, and together reduced potential fertility by less than 2 percent in 1978 and 5 percent in 1986 and 1992. The 4-percent increase in fertility reduction can be attributed to a recent increase in the use of modern contraception. On the other hand, the inhibiting effect of postpartum infecundability (C_i) is very large. This index alone reduced potential fertility by 37 percent in 1978, 42 percent in 1986, and 41 percent in 1992.[22] The importance of postpartum infecundability to the reduction of fertility is typical in Africa and is mainly due to extended periods of breastfeeding (see Jolly and Gribble, 1993).

The second smallest index—the second largest fertility-inhibiting index—is C_m, the index of marriage. It is calculated as the ratio of the TFR

TABLE 4-5 Indexes of the Effect of Proximate Determinants on Fertility in Senegal, WFS, DHS-I, and DHS-II

Year and Survey	TFR	C_m	C_c	C_i	C_a	I_p
1978 WFS	7.2	.935	.992	.625[a]	1.000	.992
1986 DHS-I	6.6	.898	.973	.576	1.000	.976
1992 DHS-II	6.1	.843	.951	.595	1.000	1.000

NOTES: See Appendix A for description of surveys; TFR, C_m, C_c, C_i, C_a, and I_p are defined in the section Proximate Determinants of Fertility and in endnote 21.

[a]The WFS did not ask women whether they were currently amenorrheic, so i was imputed using the formula $i = 1.753\exp(.1396B - .001872B^2)$, where B is the duration of breastfeeding (Bongaarts and Potter, 1983).

SOURCES: République du Sénégal (1981), Ndiaye et al. (1988) and unpublished tabulations of DHS-II data.

to the TMFR, the total marital fertility rate. As Table 4-5 demonstrates, this index fell from .935 in 1978 to .898 in 1986 to .843 in 1992. Thus, the decline in the TFR, which fell from 7.2 in 1978 to 6.1 in 1993, was the result mainly of a change in marriage patterns. As we shall see below, the major change was a trend towards later age at first marriage for women.

For all three surveys, the index C_a has been set to 1.000. Owing to the sensitivity of the issue, no data were collected on abortions in any of the three surveys. However, Coeytaux (1988) and others have suggested that the incidence of induced abortion in sub-Saharan Africa is nontrivial and higher than generally realized. Given that age at first marriage in Senegal is rising, the likelihood of conceptions occurring before marriage and being aborted has probably also risen, so research into the prevalence of abortion and its impact on fertility in Senegal should be a priority.

In the following subsections, the effects of each index are discussed in greater detail.

Marriage and Fertility

Bongaarts' index of marriage (C_m) takes into account the global effect of marriage on fertility, including age at first marriage, marital stability, and the proportion of women ever married. These elements are discussed separately below, along with the relationship between the age at first marriage and age at first birth, and the role of polygyny.

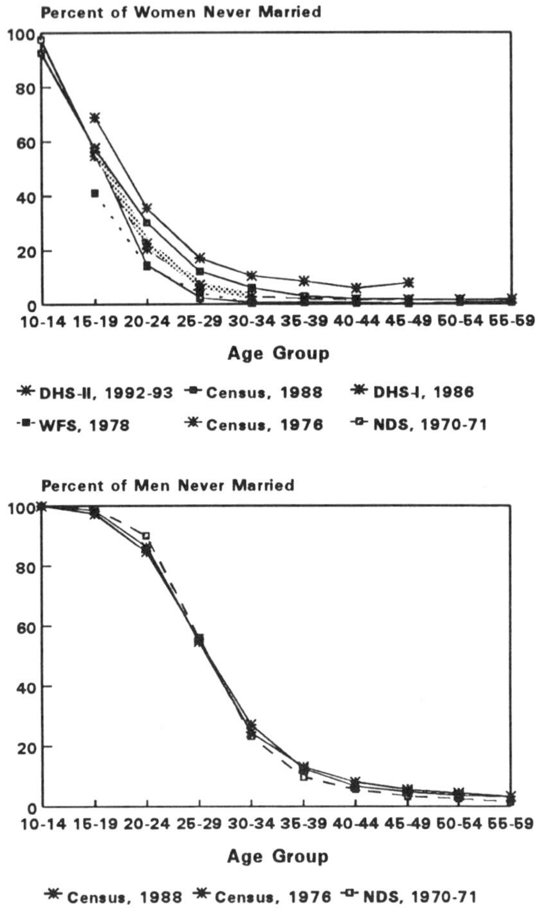

FIGURE 4-17 Percent never married, by age.
NOTE: See Appendix A for description of surveys.
SOURCES: République du Sénégal (1974, no date, and 1988 census, unpublished tables) and standard data files from WFS, DHS-I, and DHS-II.

Age at First Marriage

To examine changes in marriage patterns over time, we observe the proportion of men and women never married by age at various points in time. Figure 4-17 plots the percent of women (top half of the figure) and men (bottom half of the figure) never married, by age, for different census and survey dates. Table 4-6 provides more detailed information on the percent of women who have never married by ages 15-19 and 20-24 for various subgroups of the population.

Little is known about the marital lives of men. Many of the national demographic surveys in the country have been restricted to women, reflecting a long tradition of research on nuptiality, primarily as a determinant of a woman's fertility. The bottom half of Figure 4-17 provides information on

TABLE 4-6 Percent of Women Never Married, Aged 15-19 and 20-24, 1978-1992

Year	Source	Subgroup	% Never Married 15-19	20-24
National Level				
1970-1971	NDS	n.a.	57	15
1976	Census	n.a.	55	21
1978	WFS	n.a.	41	14
1986	DHS-I	n.a.	57	23
1988	Census	n.a.	57	30
1992-1993	DHS-II	n.a.	69	36
WFS and DHS Regions				
1978	WFS	West	64	26
		Center	30	10
		Northeast	28	4
		South	29	6
1986	DHS-I	West	77	40
		Center	44	8
		Northeast	38	12
		South	50	20
1992-1993	DHS-II	West	85	52
		Center	62	25
		Northeast	54	21
		South	58	28
Administrative Regions				
1988	Census	Dakar	83	52
		Thiès	66	33
		Saint-Louis	52	25
		Tambacounda	27	9
		Louga	43	18
		Diourbel	48	18
		Fatick	52	22
		Kaolack	41	19
		Ziguinchor	78	45
		Kolda	30	10
Small-Scale Studies				
1963	Cantrelle (1969)	Sine	40	9
1963	Cantrelle (1969)	Saloum	27	5
1984	Enel et al. (1994)	Mlomp	99	89
1984	Delaunay (1994)	Niakhar	50	11
1991	Delaunay (1994)	Niakhar	62	13

continued

TABLE 4-6 continued

Year	Source	Subgroup	% Never Married	
			15-19	20-24
Small-Scale Studies				
1992	Pison and Desgrées du Loû (forthcoming)	Bandafassi		
		Peul	35	4
		Malinké	74	7
		Bedik	88	21
Place of Residence				
1978	WFS	Dakar	73	31
		Other urban	62	24
		Rural	29	5
1986	DHS-I	Dakar	81	44
		Other urban	79	38
		Rural	37	8
1988	Census	Dakar	85	57
		Other urban	79	44
		Rural	40	16
1992-1993	DHS-II	Dakar	91	58
		Other urban	82	56
		Rural	53	19
Ethnic Groups				
1978	WFS	Wolof	48	18
		Poular	29	8
		Serer	45	11
		Mandingo	24	14
		Diola	77	21
		Other	40	11
1986	DHS-I	Wolof	64	26
		Poular	43	11
		Serer	60	22
		Mandingo	53	21
		Diola	89	49
		Other	54	27
1992-1993	DHS-II	Wolof	73	40
		Poular	55	25
		Serer	74	31
		Mandingo	66	41
		Diola	91	62
		Other	72	27
Level of Education				
1978	WFS	None	29	8
		Primary	63	24

TABLE 4-6 continued

Year	Source	Subgroup	% Never Married	
			15-19	20-24
Level of Education				
		Secondary+	90	47
1986	DHS-I	None	41	11
		Primary	85	40
		Secondary+	95	68
1988	Census	None	44	19
		Primary	87	55
		Secondary+	95	73
1992-1993	DHS-II	None	56	22
		Primary	86	52
		Secondary+	96	82

NOTE: See Appendix A for description of surveys.

SOURCES: Cantrelle (1969); Delaunay (1994); Enel et al. (1994); Pison and Desgrées du Loû (forthcoming); WFS, DHS-I, and DHS-II data files and unpublished tabulations from the 1988 census.

men's marital status by age from three independent sources. Entry into marriage occurs at a much slower rate for men than for women, so that the mean age at first marriage for men is quite high—27.6 years. By age 24, only about 30 percent of men have married. Figure 4-17 demonstrates that there has been virtually no change in the age at first marriage for men.

The top half of Figure 4-17 presents similar information for women. Despite the potential ambiguities surrounding the definition of marriage,[23] the data show a clear trend towards later age at first marriage. In 1978, the WFS found that 14 percent of women aged 20-24 and 41 percent of women aged 15-19 had not been married. In 1986, the DHS-I found that the percentage of women who had never married had risen to 23 percent for women aged 20-24 and 57 percent for women aged 15-19. In the DHS-II, these percentages had increased again, to 36 and 69 percent, respectively. Figure 4-18 shows that there is considerable heterogeneity in marriage patterns among the four grand regions: women marry much later in the west than in the three other regions. These differences reflect important differences in education attainment and urban/rural residence, as explained below, as well as differences in the accepted age at first marriage among the various ethnic groups. The Poular, for example, marry relatively early, while the Serer and the Diola marry somewhat later, in part because women from these two latter ethnic groups often migrate to urban areas for a short period to accumulate goods before they marry (Ndiaye, 1992:18).

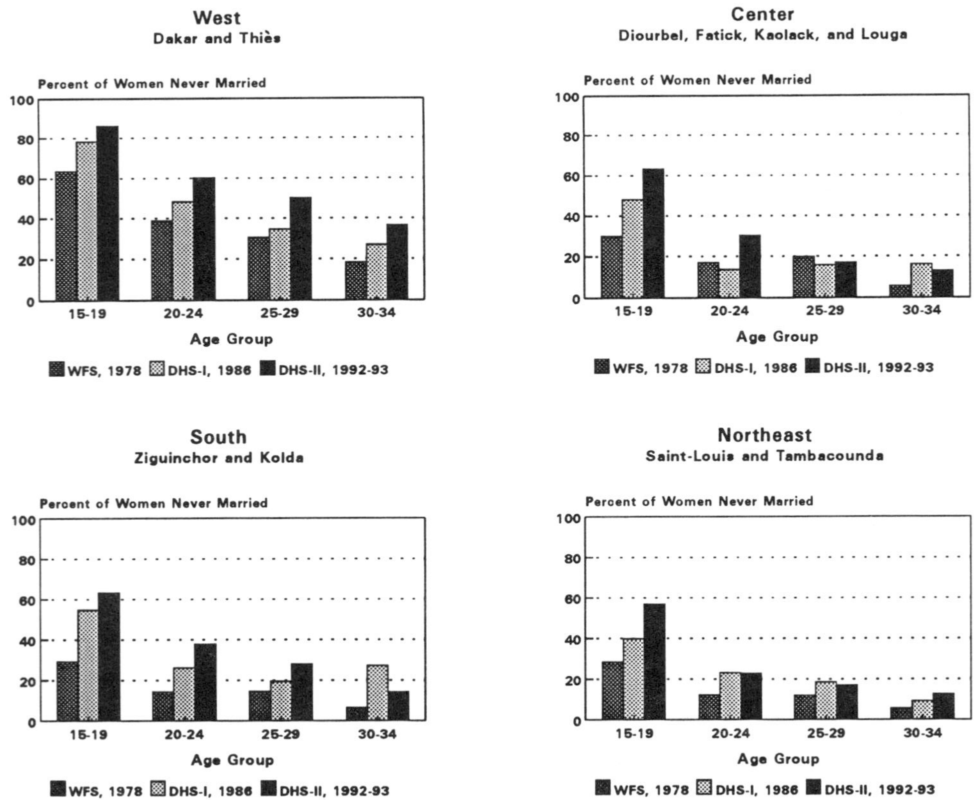

FIGURE 4-18 Percent of women never married, by age and region. NOTE: See Appendix A for description of surveys. SOURCES: Standard data files from WFS, DHS-I, and DHS-II.

A comparison of the findings of the WFS, DHS-I, and DHS-II demonstrates that signs of changing marriage patterns are appearing in all four grand regions of the country. The changes are partly attributable to increasing levels of education and urbanization. Figures 4-19 and 4-20 show the percent of women who have never married for various socioeconomic groups. Marriage occurs earliest among women with little or no education and among women living in rural areas. However, there is a perceptible increase in the age at marriage within each educational level and within both urban and rural areas. Antoine and Nanitelamio (1991) recently documented a rise in the number of single women in Dakar, but Figure 4-20 demonstrates that the phenomenon is not restricted to the capital. Further, one of the largest rises in age at first marriage has been for women with primary school education. Even among women with no education, there are still signs of a pattern towards later marriage. The immediate demographic consequence of these changes is an increase in the period of adolescence for females. In the past, early marriage meant the abrupt end of a woman's childhood and a transition into being a wife and a mother. Now, with later marriage, women can experience a period of adolescence before they marry (Working Group on the Social Dynamics of Adolescent Fertility, 1993).

Marital Stability

Information on divorce and remarriage comes principally from the WFS because it was the only national-level demographic study that collected complete information on marital histories. The DHS-I, DHS-II, and census questions on marriage were rather limited and concerned current marital status and age at first marriage. Because of the high quality and uniqueness of the WFS data, they have been analyzed in considerable detail (République du Sénégal, 1981; United Nations, 1983b; Smith et al., 1984; Ndiaye, 1985). These analyses revealed the following findings:

- In 1978, 71 percent of married women were in their first marriage. For those who were not, the principal reason for the dissolution of their marriage was divorce or separation: 20 percent of the married women had been divorced or separated. The remaining 9 percent of married women had been widowed.
- The survivorship rate of marriages in Senegal is low compared with that in Kenya and Lesotho (two other sub-Saharan African countries where a WFS was conducted). On average, women are married 1.32 times over the course of their life, and 5 percent of women are married 3 or more times.
- Senegal's relatively high (by African standards) marital instability is

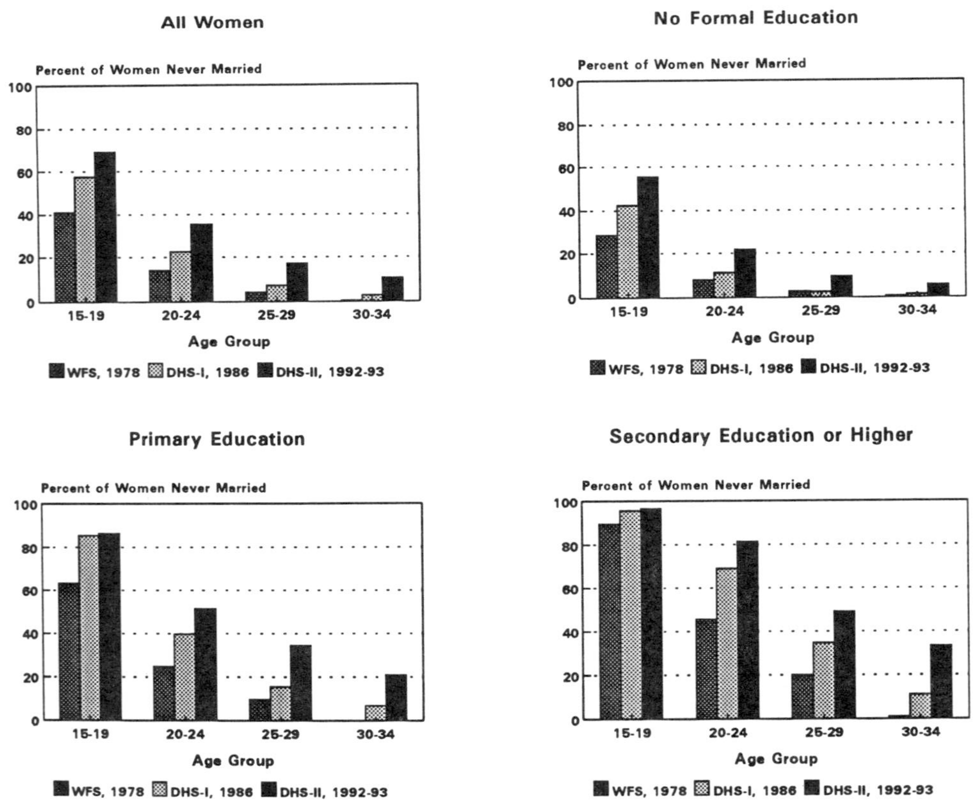

FIGURE 4-19 Percent of women never married by age and education. NOTE: See Appendix A for description of surveys. SOURCES: Standard data files from WFS, DHS-I, and DHS-II.

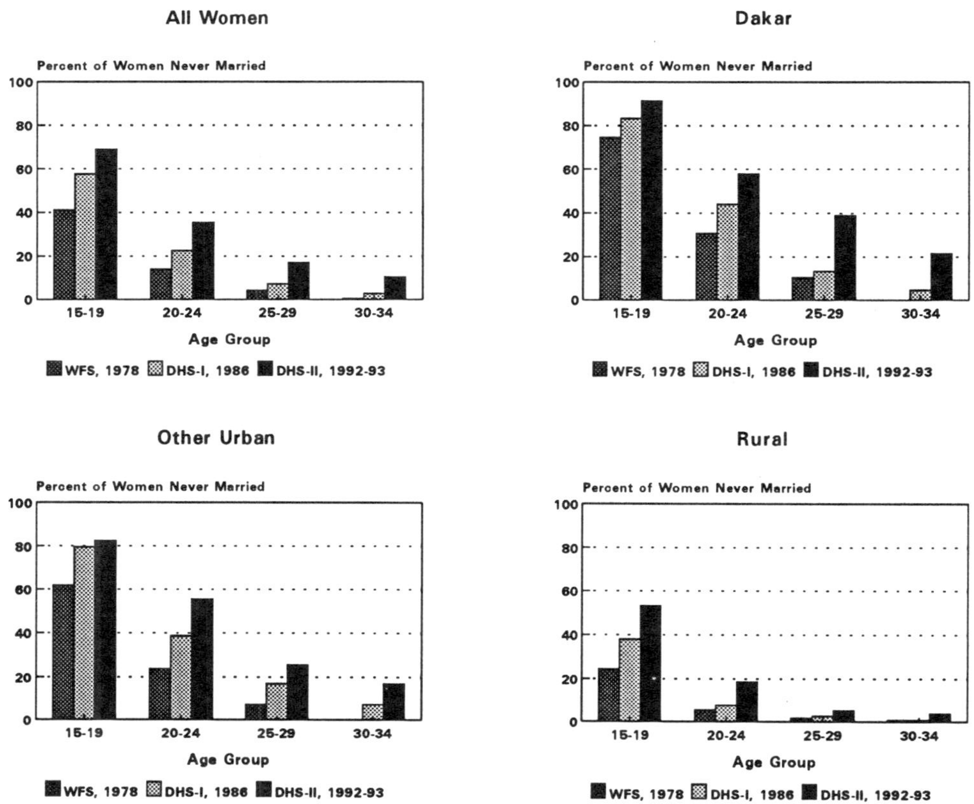

FIGURE 4-20 Percent of women never married, by age and urban/rural residence. NOTE: See Appendix A for description of surveys. SOURCES: Standard data files from WFS, DHS-I, and DHS-II.

largely compensated for by rapid and high rates of remarriage. Among women who are widowed or divorced, 90 percent remarry within 5 years.

• Marriages are generally more stable in rural areas, among women who have never attended school, and among women who have given birth to at least one child within the first 5 years of the marriage (Ndiaye, 1985). Marriages are less stable among urban women, literate women, and the Poular, who have the youngest average age at first marriage of any ethnic group. The high divorce rate among the Poular is probably the result of the high percentage of arranged marriages. Why should urbanization and literacy affect the probability of divorce? Both increase the probability that the woman has paid employment in the wage sector, thus increasing a woman's independence. Women in urban areas may also be less stigmatized by a separation or a divorce than women in rural areas.

In summary, the percentage of women who are single between marriages at any time is low, and the average length of time women spend married is high. Consequently, divorce and remarriage have little role to play in explaining fertility differentials in Senegal, either over time or among various socioeconomic groups.

Proportion of Women Ever Married

In the case of Senegal, the ultimate proportion of women ever married has not varied significantly over time: the proportion of never-married women aged 45-49 was less than 1 percent in all three surveys and was estimated to be 1.8 percent based on the 1988 census. Thus, the index C_m has not been affected by a change in the proportion of women ever married.

Age at First Marriage and Age at First Birth

Marriage is the legal and cultural institution that sanctions childbearing, and the Bongaarts formula assumes that all fertility occurs within marriage. How good is this assumption in Senegal? Illegitimate fertility in the late 1970s was relatively low in Senegal: 6 percent of first births took place outside of marriage according to the WFS (Guèye and Ferry, 1985). Has the delay in marriage brought about a delay in the age at first birth, and if so, is it responsible for the decline in fertility among young women noted above?

One simple measure of the extent of early childbearing is the proportion of women of a given age having had their first birth before the age of 20. To minimize biases due to the omissions and errors of dating that are frequent for older women (Arnold and Blanc, 1990), we consider only women aged 20-29 at the time of the survey. In 1978, 65 percent of all women aged 20-29 had had their first birth before the age of 20. These percentages fell only slightly in the 1986 DHS-I: 61 percent of women aged 25-29 and 60 percent of women aged 20-24 had had their first birth by age 20. In the 1992-1993 DHS-II, these proportions fell by about 10 percent, so that 57 percent of women aged 25-29 and only 52 percent of women aged 20-24 had had their first birth by age 20. This represents a more substantial decline than the one that took place between 1978 and 1986, but is it more or less than what one might expect from an increase in the age at marriage?

The trends in teenage marriage and teenage childbearing are displayed in Figure 4-21, which shows the percentage of women marrying by age 20, the percentage giving birth by age 20, and the percentage having a premarital birth before age 20. There are two points for each survey: one represents women aged 20-24 at the time of the survey, while the other represents women aged 25-29. These women were aged 20-24 5 years before the survey, so their information has been plotted 5 years to the left of the survey date. Hence the three surveys have been combined to show the experiences of women aged 20-24 at various points in time. The observations from different age groups and surveys fit together closely over time, arguing for the general quality of the data. The solid downward-sloping line at the top of the figure represents the proportion of women aged 20-24 marrying by age 20. The downward slope of this line means a decline in early marriage. The downward-sloping line below the early marriage line represents the percentage of women giving birth by age 20. Again, a downward-sloping line represents a decline in early childbearing. However, the gap between the two lines narrows over time, indicating that early childbearing has declined more slowly than early marriage. These changes could be the result of an increase in the frequency of premarital conception, or a shortening of the interval between marriage and first birth.[24] We return to this topic below.

As noted above, there are few reported cases of premarital births in Senegal. There are two reasons for this. First, the young age at first marriage implies that a large proportion of unmarried women are young and still infecund. Second, older women often misreport age at first birth if they were unmarried at that time. However, Figure 4-21 suggests that there has been a slight increase in premarital childbearing. The triangles scattered across the bottom of the figure represent the percentage of women who reported having a premarital birth before age 20. (Note that these triangles have been plotted on the second scale displayed on the right of the figure.) The upward-sloping dotted line fitted to these points shows, though it does not fit tightly, the upward trend in premarital births. Thus, the figure indicates that there has been a slight weakening of the link between marriage and childbearing.[25]

The observation of a certain weakening of the relation between age at

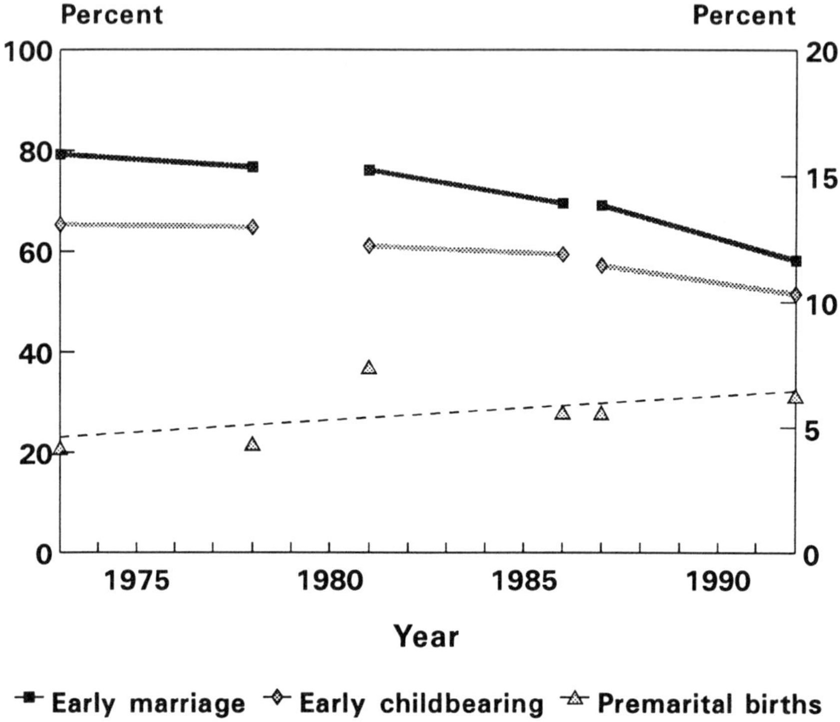

FIGURE 4-21 Early marriage, early childbearing, and premarital births over time. NOTE: See Appendix A for description of surveys. SOURCE: Standard data files from WFS, DHS-I, and DHS-II.

marriage and age at first birth is confirmed using local data sets. For example, marriage occurs very late in Mlomp, especially by rural standards, and many young women have their first—and sometimes even their second—child while still unmarried (Enel et al., 1994; Lagarde et al., forthcoming).

The Bandafassi survey [8] reveals that the relationship between age at first marriage and age at first birth can be quite complex. This survey covers three ethnic groups (Peul, Malinké, and Bedik), each of which lives in a different village.[26] Age at first marriage and age at first birth differ among the groups, and the correlation between the two is weaker than one would have expected. According to the survey, women in the Peul ethnic group marry, on average, at age 16.6 and have their first child at age 17.9, or 13 months later. On average, Malinké women marry at age 19.4, but often they have already had their first child; their average age at first birth is 4 months earlier than their age at first marriage. Finally, among the

Bedik, premarital births are even more common: for these women, the average age at first marriage is 20.6 years, compared with an average age at first birth of 19.2 years, or 14 months earlier (Pison and Desgrées du Loû, 1993).

The Niakhar data [11] allow us to observe the change in the timing of first marriage since the beginning of the 1960s. Comparing the estimates reported by Cantrelle (1969) with those of Delaunay (personal communication, 1993), it is clear that the proportion of women aged 15-19 and 20-24 who are single has increased over the last 30 years. But over the same period, the fertility of women aged less than 25 has remained unchanged (see above and Figure 4-7).

Although the relationship between age at first marriage and age at first birth may be complex locally, it should not overshadow the main point: age at first marriage has increased, and, whether as a result or not, age at first birth has increased and fertility fallen. The general relationship between early marriage and early childbearing at the regional level in Senegal is shown in Figure 4-22. The figure plots the percentage of women aged 15-19 who are single and the ASFR for women aged 15-19. The data are from the 1988 census. Each of the ten administrative regions of the country is represented by two data points, one for rural women and one for urban women. The figure demonstrates the strong negative relationship between the proportion of women single and the extent of teenage childbearing.

The relationship between delayed marriage and fertility is particularly clear in Dakar. Table 4-6 shows that the percentage of women aged 15-19 who are unmarried has increased over time from 73 percent in 1978 to 91 percent in 1992-1993. Over the same period, the percentage of women having their first child before age 20 has fallen, and the fertility rate for this age group has decreased significantly (see above and Figure 4-11).

The Role of Polygyny

Polygyny is perhaps the most distinctive feature of African marriage, and any discussion of the effect of marriage on fertility would be incomplete without a brief examination of the relationship between polygyny and fertility. This relationship has been described often, so we only summarize the more important elements here. When discussing the influence of polygyny on fertility, it is important to distinguish between micro- and macrolevel effects (Pison, 1986). At the micro- or individual level, women in polygynous unions are usually thought to have lower fertility than those in monogamous unions for a number of reasons. First, coital frequency is likely to be lower because the husband's attention is divided among several competing wives. Second, coital frequency and fecundity tend to decline with age, and for the practice of polygyny to be sustainable, there must be a

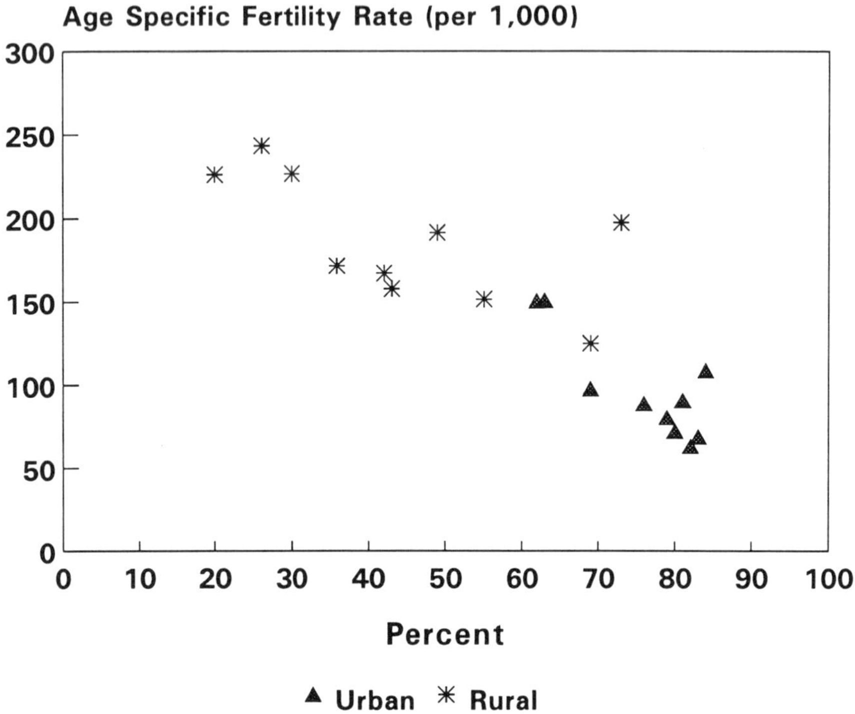

FIGURE 4-22 Urban/rural variation in percentage of women aged 15-19 never married and age-specific fertility rates. SOURCE: 1988 census, unpublished tables.

large difference in the average age of spouses. Polygynous wives thus tend to have older-than-average husbands whose fecundity is lower. Third, polygyny makes it easier to maintain traditional birth-spacing practices, such as a postpartum taboo on sexual relations until the child is weaned. Fourth, African society places high premiums on childbearing. Consequently, if, as the result of male or female infertility, a monogamous marriage does not produce any children, that may be sufficient incentive for a man to look for a second wife. This can introduce a selection bias, so that a disproportionate number of subfecund men and women are in polygynous relationships.

At the macro- or societal level, polygyny is often associated with a number of lifestyle factors (early marriage and almost universal remarriage for widows and divorcees) that tend to raise the total length of time a woman spends in marriage. These factors tend to raise fertility.

A number of studies based on Senegalese data have contributed to the debate on the relationship between polygyny and fertility (United Nations, 1983b; Ndiaye, 1985; Pison, 1986; Garenne and van de Walle, 1989). Garenne and van de Walle (1989: 282) studied the relationship between polygyny and fertility among the Serer using time-series data collected from the Ngayokhème study [11] during 1962-1981. The authors found that fertility of monogamous wives exceeds that of polygynous wives, and the fertility of the latter decreases as their rank in the union increases. They attribute this finding to two factors: first, polygynous wives spend more time separated from their husbands; second, older men probably have lower fecundity and coital frequency.

Using WFS data, Ndiaye (1985) found few differences in fertility over the first 5 years of marriage between women in monogamous and polygynous marriages. Furthermore, the author concludes that failure to have children in the first 5 years of a marriage is not associated with the probability that a husband takes a second wife.

Table 4-7 shows the percentage of currently married women in polygynous unions, by age, in the three most recent national-level demographic surveys, WFS, DHS-I, and DHS-II. Senegal has one of the highest rates of polygyny in western Africa: in 1992-1993, 49.2 percent of women aged 30-34 and 68.4 percent of women aged 40-44 were in polygynous unions. One-quarter of all currently married women aged 15-19 are also in polygynous unions, and the vast majority of these young women must have married directly into a polygynous relationship. The increasing occurrence of polygynous unions with age reflects the fact that husbands may marry a second or third wife after a few years, so that even if women enter a monogamous marriage they are likely to lead some part of their married life in a polygynous relationship.

The incidence of polygyny differs across socioeconomic and ethnic boundaries (Table 4-8). Polygyny is usually more common among women that have no formal education and those who live in rural areas. For example, 51 percent of currently married women who have not had any formal education are in polygynous unions, compared with only 29 percent of those with secondary education or higher. Similarly, 51 percent of currently married women in rural areas are in polygynous unions, compared with only 40 percent in urban areas. Women with more education are less likely to accept being in a polygynous union.[27]

The incidence of polygyny is dwindling, at least in part because of increasing urbanization and female education. Table 4-7 lends some support to this hypothesis among women aged less than 35. The percentage of these women reporting that they are in polygynous unions tends to be generally smaller in the DHS-II than it was in the DHS-I, and smaller in the DHS-I than in the WFS. If correct, this represents a very recent trend in marriage, because both the WFS and Garenne and van de Walle (1989) suggest that polygyny was rising during the 1960s and 1970s. However, while polygyny may be declining, other forms of union that closely re-

TABLE 4-7 Percentage of Currently Married Women in Polygynous Unions by Age, 1978-1993

National Survey	15-19	20-24	25-29	30-34	35-39	40-44	45-49	Total
1978 WFS	30.6	35.5	46.5	57.7	56.5	65.5	64.8	48.5
1986 DHS-I	27.1	33.2	40.9	56.0	63.7	59.7	62.0	46.5
1992-1993 DHS-II	25.0	32.9	42.5	49.2	58.1	68.4	59.6	47.3

NOTE: See Appendix A for description of surveys.

SOURCE: Ndiaye et al. (1988:16) and unpublished DHS-II tables.

TABLE 4-8 Percentage of Currently Married Women in Polygynous Unions, by Age and Various Socioeconomic Variables, 1992-1993

Variable	15-19	20-24	25-29	30-34	35-39	40-44	45-49	Total
Level of Education								
None	24.7	35.0	46.3	55.3	61.2	69.7	61.9	50.5
Primary	27.8	25.6	24.5	28.3	45.9	55.8	27.3	32.1
Secondary+	16.7	17.2	26.8	20.0	35.1	65.4	12.5	28.8
Place of Residence								
Urban	24.7	26.3	31.6	33.7	51.8	64.4	55.3	40.2
Rural	25.1	35.6	48.2	58.7	61.5	70.3	61.8	50.7
Ethnic Group								
Wolof	27.7	33.4	46.8	54.0	59.9	74.7	67.8	51.4
Poular	22.3	38.3	43.6	48.2	61.3	69.8	52.8	46.6
Serer	17.6	27.6	35.5	38.6	54.5	56.7	57.1	41.1
Mandingo	22.2	28.6	56.5	58.5	63.5	68.5	44.4	50.3
Diola	66.7	32.0	17.1	28.2	36.4	51.6	43.8	34.6
Other	30.8	26.9	31.0	56.9	52.4	69.4	58.3	44.4

NOTE: See Appendix A for description of survey.

SOURCE: Derived from unpublished DHS-II tables.

semble polygyny (for example, outside wives) may be increasing. It is improbable, therefore, that a change in polygynous behavior would have influenced fertility significantly.

Summary of the Effect of Marriage Patterns on Fertility

Analysis of the influence of marriage on fertility shows that the current trend for women to delay first marriage is associated with lower fertility in the younger ages. These changes are occurring predominantly in Dakar and, to a lesser extent, in other urban centers. At the same time, the slight rise in premarital births indicates that these changes in marriage patterns do not necessarily reflect an increase in the age at first sexual encounter.

Breastfeeding and the Length of Birth Intervals

In a population where contraception is scarcely used, the average length of time between births is determined primarily by the duration of postpartum infecundity and the duration of postpartum abstinence. The duration of infecundity (i.e., the length of the anovulatory interval) is determined primarily by the duration and intensity of breastfeeding, which tends to delay the normal resumption of menses.[28] It is analytically convenient to distinguish between factors that are designed to restrict the total number of children, and those that are not parity-specific which are adopted after each birth regardless of parity to protect the health of the mother and child, rather than to limit family size. One example of a nonparity-specific practice is postpartum abstinence. Consequently, it is factored into the index of postpartum infecundability (C_i), rather than the index of contraception (C_c).

In Senegal, as in many other sub-Saharan African countries, people have a clear idea of what length of time constitutes an appropriate birth interval. A quick pregnancy following a birth is viewed as overly burdensome and fatiguing for the woman. It also leads to premature weaning for the most recent child, which is viewed as particularly harmful to the child's health (Ferry, 1981). Consequently, traditional practices have been established to ensure that birth intervals remain relatively long.

Table 4-9 provides various estimates of the median length of birth intervals and the median duration of breastfeeding, postamenorrhea, and abstinence both for the whole country and for various subgroups and specific areas. Women in Senegal maintain long birth intervals—around 30 months, on average—with birth intervals being slightly shorter in urban than in rural areas.

In Senegal, breastfeeding is essentially universal and lasts a long time. The median duration of breastfeeding is around 19-20 months, with little change over time (see Table 4-9). This is the primary reason why birth intervals in Senegal are rather long (Cantrelle and Léridon, 1971; Ferry, 1977, 1981; Cantrelle and Ferry, 1979; Guèye and Ferry, 1985; Sow, 1994a,b). Postpartum abstinence overlaps the period of breastfeeding and so has little additional effect on fertility. As shown in Table 4-9, the length of postpartum abstinence is relatively short. Averaging over the various surveys indicates that the median duration of postpartum abstinence is around 6 months. This is longer than the prescribed 40 days under Islamic code, but is still too short to have a great influence on the length of the subsequent birth interval.

Fertility behavior in the region of Sine-Saloum has been studied in depth over the past 30 years. Table 4-9 provides various estimates of the length of birth intervals made by different authors at different times on the various subpopulations of the region. There is a general consistency among the sources, despite the methodological differences among the various surveys. Breastfeeding and amenorrhea are particularly long in this region, but postpartum abstinence is usually short. Thus these sources support the hypothesis that the length of time a woman breastfeeds is the most important determinant of long birth intervals.

In a population where lengthy breastfeeding is the norm, the main determinant of the length of breastfeeding is usually the survival of the child. If the child dies, breastfeeding ceases, and the mother quickly regains her fecundity. The difference in the length of the subsequent birth interval between women whose children die at 3 months and women whose children die at 18 months can exceed 12 months (Cantrelle and Léridon, 1971; Ferry, 1976; Lagarde et al., forthcoming). Because child mortality decreased notably in the 1970s and 1980s, one may expect a slight increase in the median duration of breastfeeding and consequently in birth intervals. At the national level, the length of breastfeeding has risen, on average, since 1978, but this has not translated into a significant change in the length of birth intervals. The implication is that changes in breastfeeding practices have occurred, such as reduced breastfeeding intensity, that have changed the relationship between breastfeeding duration and amenorrhea duration.

Closely related to the long duration of breastfeeding, the duration of postpartum amenorrhea in Senegal is also relatively long, though there are large differences between urban and rural areas. The median duration of postpartum amenorrhea varies from 16-18 months in rural areas to around 12 months in urban areas. Note that factors other than breastfeeding may also influence the postpartum period, particularly in rural areas. Chronic malnutrition associated with physical activity can contribute to long periods of amenorrhea, especially among rural women (Rosetta, 1989). However, the duration of postpartum amenorrhea decreased by approximately 2 months between the two DHS surveys, even though the length of breastfeeding appears to have risen. Again, this is consistent with a decline in the intensity of breastfeeding—which is partly a determinant of the duration of infecundity—accompanying the earlier introduction of solid food.[29]

In summary, birth intervals have remained relatively long, primarily as a result of extended breastfeeding. The length of postpartum amenorrhea is shorter in urban than in rural areas, although one might expect the reverse to be true on the basis of child mortality differentials alone (child mortality is lower in urban areas). The explanation lies in differences in the length and intensity of breastfeeding between rural and urban areas. On average, breastfeeding is shorter in urban than in rural areas by about 2 months. However, the difference in amenorrhea between urban and rural areas is even greater—3-5 months—suggesting either better nutrition or less intense breastfeeding in the urban areas. Finally, postpartum abstinence may be declining, although the reported decline between the DHS-I and DHS-II is too rapid to be convincing.

TABLE 4-9 Median Length of Birth Intervals and Duration of Breastfeeding, Amenorrhea and Postpartum Abstinence (in months)

Year	Source	Subgroup	Birth Interval	Breast-feeding	Amenorrhea	Abstinence
National Level						
1978	WFS	National	33.4	18.5	—	—
1986	DHS-I	National	31.5	18.8	16.2	7.9
1992-1993	DHS-II	National	32.4	20.1	14.3	3.5
1978	WFS	Urban	32.3	17.6	—	—
1986	DHS-I	Urban	31.2	16.2	12.4	6.7
1992-1993	DHS-II	Urban	32.1	18.4	11.8	3.6
1978	WFS	Rural	33.8	19.1	—	—
1986	DHS-I	Rural	31.7	20.2	18.1	8.4
1992-1993	DHS-II	Rural	32.6	20.9	15.8	3.4
Local Studies in the Sine-Saloum Region						
1973	Lacombe (1973)	Fakao	33.8	—	—	—
1973	Lacombe (1973)	Diahanor	34.5	—	—	—
1963-1968	Cantrelle and Léridon (1971)	Niakhar	30.9	24.3[a]	—	2.3[a]
1963-1968	Cantrelle and Léridon (1971)	Paos-Koto	30.9	24.0	—	2.3[a]
1968-1969	Cantrelle and Ferry (1979)	Thiénaba	32.6[a]	23.7	17.9	2.3[a]
1981-1982	Mbacké (p.c.)	Thiénaba	—	21.0	17.0	2.0
1981-1982	Mbacké (p.c.)	Fissel	—	22.0	17.0	3.0
1981-1982	Rosetta (1989)	Ndiaganio	—	22.8	19.0	—
1991	Projet Niakhar (1992)	Niakhar	31.0	26.0	—	—

Other Rural Studies						
1980-1992	Pison and Desgrées du Loû (forthcoming)	Bandafassi	32.9	—	—	—
1985-1992	Lagarde et al. (forthcoming)	Mlomp	29.6	—	—	5.0
Semi-rural Studies						
1968-1969	Ferry (1981)	Khombole	32.3[a]	19.7[a]	15.4[a]	2.4[a]

NOTES: —, not available; p.c., personal communication; see Appendix A for description of surveys.

[a]Mean duration used instead of median.

SOURCES: Cantrelle and Ferry (1979), Cantrelle and Léridon (1971), Ferry (1981), Lacombe (1973), Lagarde et al. (forthcoming), Projet Niakhar (1992), Pison and Desgrées du Loû (forthcoming), Rosetta (1989) and WFS, DHS-I, and DHS-II data files.

Contraception

Though prolonged breastfeeding and postpartum abstinence result in avoidance of pregnancy and so may be considered a form of contraception, the traditional intention was not to restrict family size but rather to ensure adequate spacing between births as a way of maximizing the number of surviving children. Despite (or because of) effective traditional birth-spacing practices, use of modern contraception had a relatively late start in Senegal. Although efforts to promote use began before 1980 (Osmanski et al., 1991; République du Sénégal, 1990), it was not until that year that a 1920 French law outlawing the use of modern contraceptives was repealed (République du Sénégal, 1991). Since 1980, political support for family planning has increased within the government, and international donor agencies have played a substantial role in building the country's family planning effort (République du Sénégal, 1990). Both the number of family planning clinics and the number of family planning acceptors increased substantially between 1985 and 1990 (Osmanski et al., 1991). (See the appendix to Chapter 5 for a general description of the expansion of health services, of which family planning has been a part.)

Not surprisingly, knowledge of contraceptives has increased over the last 15 years. As can be seen in Table 4-10, knowledge of modern methods of contraception increased more than threefold in the 15 years between 1978 and 1992-1993. By 1992-1993, over 70 percent of currently married women knew of a modern method. This increase in knowledge has taken place in both rural and urban areas and at all educational levels.

Table 4-10 also shows the increases that have taken place in contraceptive use. Modern contraceptive use is still very low (less than 5 percent of currently married women reported that they were current users in 1992-1993), but the proportion of users has increased over the recent past. Predictably, contraceptive use is much more frequent in cities (where 12 percent of women use modern contraception, according to DHS-II data) than in rural areas (1 percent), and among women with secondary or higher (29 percent) or primary (13 percent) schooling than among those with no formal education (2 percent). The most popular modern method of contraception is the pill; almost half of the currently married women who were current users of modern methods in 1992-1993 reported using the pill. Other methods of contraception reported include intrauterine devices (IUDs) (1 percent), female sterilization (0.4 percent), and condoms (0.4 percent).

The relatively frequent use of contraception in urban areas, especially among women who have attended school, partly explains why marital fertility has decreased among that population. Elsewhere, for the great majority of the population, contraception is not yet sufficiently widespread to have had a noticeable influence on the total fertility rate.

TABLE 4-10 Percentage of Currently Married Women Aged 15-49 Who Know of Modern Contraception and Who Use Contraception

Year	Source	Subgroup	Knowledge of Modern Methods	Contraceptive Users: Traditional Method	Contraceptive Users: Modern Method
National Level					
1978	WFS	n.a.	20.4	3.3	0.6
1986	DHS-I	n.a.	67.6	9.0	2.4
1992-1993	DHS-II	n.a.	70.3	2.7	4.8
Place of Residence					
1986	DHS-I	Urban	87.5	7.5	6.7
		Rural	58.1	9.6	0.3
1992-1993	DHS-II	Urban	88.4	4.3	11.8
		Rural	61.6	1.9	1.4
Level of Instruction					
1986	DHS-I	None	64.0	8.8	1.0
		Primary	86.9	9.0	5.9
		Secondary+	97.3	10.7	22.2
1992-1993	DHS-II	None	65.5	1.9	2.2
		Primary	93.7	6.3	12.8
		Secondary+	98.6	7.2	29.3

NOTE: Injection and sterilization were included as modern methods in 1986 and 1992-1993, but not in 1978; see Appendix A for description of surveys.

SOURCES: République du Sénégal (1981:Table 4.2.1B, p. 265); DHS-I: Ndiaye et al. (1988:Tables 4.1, 4.3, 4.7, and 4.8, pp. 43, 45-46, 52, 54-55); DHS-II: unpublished tables supplied by Macro International, Inc.

Additional information about the potential demand for family planning can be obtained by examining women's responses to questions relating to (1) their desire for (and timing of) more children, and (2) their reported ideal family size. Differences in women's responses to such questions have been observed between the DHS-I in 1986 and the DHS-II in 1992-1993, suggesting that the potential demand for family planning may be increasing. For example, the percentage of currently married women who want to have another child decreased from 79 percent in the DHS-I to 70 percent in the DHS-II (Table 4-11). At the same time, the proportion stating they wanted no more children changed little, from 19 to 20 percent, but those undecided increased from 2 to 7 percent. Although this change in preferences may be

TABLE 4-11 Percent Distribution of Currently Married Women by Desire for Children, According to Number of Living Children

Preference	Number of Living Children 0	1	2	3	4	5	6+	Total
Wants to have another child								
1986 DHS-I	97.0	97.2	94.7	88.6	80.1	66.3	34.4	79.3
1992-1993 DHS-II	89.3	91.5	89.1	80.4	74.8	58.8	34.8	69.9
Wants no more children								
1986 DHS-I	1.9	2.1	4.2	10.9	18.8	31.0	61.6	19.0
1992-1993[a] DHS-II	1.0	1.4	4.2	9.1	16.6	28.3	52.6	20.1
Undecided								
1986 DHS-I	0.9	0.7	1.1	0.5	0.9	2.7	3.8	1.6
1992-1993 DHS-II	2.8	3.0	4.3	8.2	6.1	9.6	9.5	6.6
Declared infecund								
1986 DHS-I	—	—	—	—	—	—	—	—
1992-1993 DHS-II	6.6	4.0	2.3	2.3	2.5	3.4	3.0	3.2

NOTE: See Appendix A for description of surveys.

[a]Includes women who have been sterilized.

SOURCES: DHS-I: Ndiaye et al. (1988:Table 5.1, p. 68); DHS-II: unpublished tables supplied by Macro International, Inc.

partly the function of a change in the wording of the questionnaire, it appears to have occurred across almost all parities and all age groups (see Tables 4-11 and 4-12).

Another indicator suggesting that the demand for family planning may increase in the future is the decline, since 1978, in the number of children women reported as "ideal." The ideal number of children for all women fell from 8.5 in 1978 to 6.8 in 1986, and then to 5.9 in 1992-1993. As can be seen in Figure 4-23, this trend is apparent for all age groups. However, 5.9 children per woman is still very close to the potential supply of children, so that with the trend towards later age at first marriage, the small decline in ideal family size can be realized without resorting to contraception.

Abortion

As in most developing countries, there are few firm statistics on the extent of abortion in Senegal. Although reliable statistics are unavailable,

TABLE 4-12 Proportion of Currently Married Women Aged 15-49 by Desire for Another Child, According to Age of Woman

Preferences	Age of Woman 15-19	20-24	25-29	30-34	35-39	40-44	45-49	Total
Wants to have another child								
1986 DHS-I	98.5	98.2	91.8	78.1	61.7	45.8	33.9	79.3
1992-1993 DHS-II	94.2	93.7	86.1	72.7	57.6	34.8	20.2	69.9
Wants no more children								
1986 DHS-I	1.2	1.7	7.6	19.4	36.5	50.5	59.0	19.0
1992-1993[a] DHS-II	1.8	1.7	7.3	17.6	33.0	47.8	52.1	20.1
Undecided								
1986 DHS-I	—	0.1	0.6	2.3	1.6	3.7	7.1	1.6
1992-1993 DHS-II	3.8	4.0	5.4	8.5	7.2	8.5	10.8	6.6
Declared infecund								
1986 DHS-I	—	—	—	—	—	—	—	—
1992-1993 DHS-II	0.2	0.4	1.2	1.3	2.0	8.8	17.0	3.2

NOTES: Totals by age for each year may not equal 100; in both years, 0.1 percent of cases were missing. See Appendix A for description of surveys.

[a]Includes women who have been sterilized.

SOURCES: DHS-I: Ndiaye et al. (1988:Table 5.2, p. 68); DHS-II: unpublished tables supplied by Macro International, Inc.

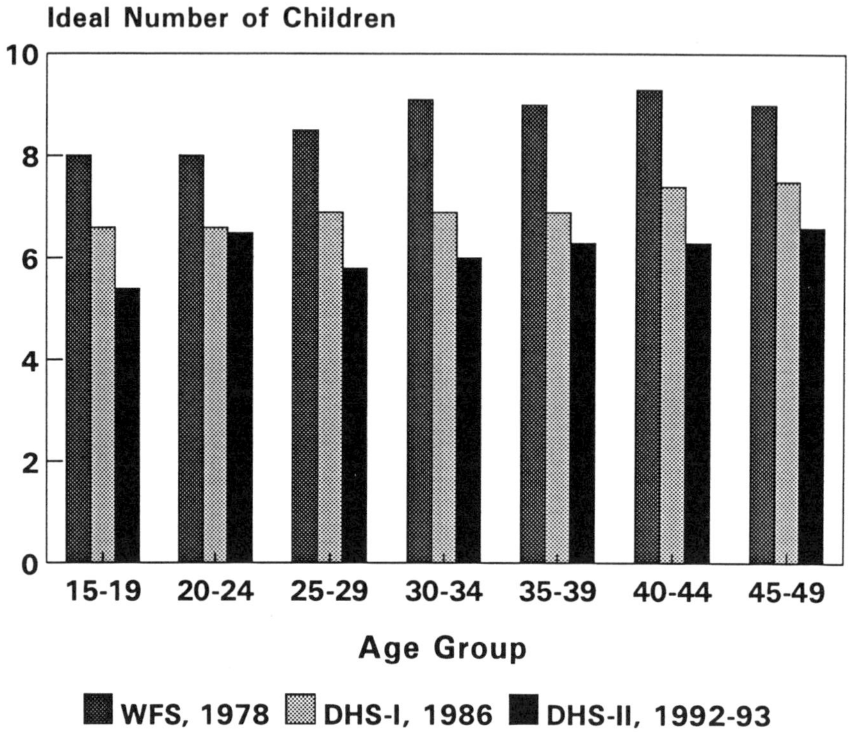

FIGURE 4-23 Variations in ideal family size over time. NOTE: See Appendix A for description of surveys. SOURCES: Standard data files from WFS, DHS-I, and DHS-II.

illegal abortion is generally considered to be an increasingly serious problem, especially in urban areas (Ferry, 1981; Pillsbury, 1990; Diouf, 1994). Because abortion can carry a fine that ranges from 20,000-50,000 CFA (US$40 to US$100) and 6-10 months in prison, both for the woman undergoing the abortion and for the performer, abortions are often carried out clandestinely. Botched abortions are a major cause of all hospital admissions for women of reproductive age. In 1988, abortion complications were one of the two major reasons for the emergency transfer of women from Pikine to Dakar (Guèye et al., 1989, cited in Pillsbury, 1990).

Limited data on abortions are available from several sources. Information on abortion from the WFS is limited because the relevant questions did not distinguish between spontaneous and induced abortions, but it appears that between 10-12 percent of women reported having had an abortion (Diouf, 1994). Sow (1985) estimates that at the time of the WFS, women had, on average, 0.3 abortions over their lives, although the basis for this estimate is unclear.

Because of the moral and religious sensitivity surrounding the issue, no questions on abortion were asked in the 1986 DHS-I, but there was a rather roundabout attempt to measure the abortion experience of women in Senegal in the 1992-1993 DHS-II. In DHS-II, women were asked whether they had ever had an unwanted pregnancy, and, if so, what they had done about this pregnancy. Out of 6,299 women, 1,131 admitted that they had had an unwanted pregnancy. Of these women, 1,058 carried the pregnancy to term and 37 were currently pregnant. Only 19 women admitted that the pregnancy was terminated, either spontaneously or by induced abortion, although a further 15 women admitted that they had attempted to induce an abortion but had failed.*

The prevalence of abortion in the WFS survey appears to be in reasonably close agreement with a survey undertaken in 1986 in Pikine. Out of 9,196 pregnancies, 804 or 8.7 percent of them resulted in spontaneous or induced abortions (Antoine and Diouf, 1989:507). The frequency of abortion varied by age of women, marital status, ethnic group, level of instruction, and number of children ever born. Abortion in Pikine appeared to be particularly frequent among 15-19 year olds and among unmarried women (Diouf, 1994). However, abortions were also fairly common among women over age 30 and among married women.

In the Bongaarts model presented above, the index measuring the effect of abortion on fertility is set to 1 for the WFS and the DHS-I. The assumption is that, given the general high demand for children, deliberate abortion is not important in determining final fertility outcomes. This assumption almost certainly leads to a serious underestimation of the extent of abortion among adolescent schoolgirls. Taking the DHS-II figures at face value implies an index of C_a of .999, an unsatisfactory result and no improvement over the basic (poor) assumption of zero abortion. Clearly, much more research on abortion is needed, especially among young women, although the effect of abortion on total fertility is probably of little importance.[30]

Sterility

For pathological or other reasons, some couples will never bear children (primary infertility). Others lose the ability to bear children following an earlier birth (secondary infertility). Sterility can occur either naturally, primarily by aging, or pathologically, primarily by complications resulting

*Two women failed to answer the follow-up part of the question.

from infection with a sexually transmitted disease, which in Africa is most frequently gonorrhea.

In the absence of fertility regulation, a reasonable estimate of the level of infertility is given by the proportion of women aged 40-49 who have never had a live birth. In a population with a "normal" level of sterility, one would expect around 5 percent of women to be nulliparous (Frank, 1983), although the level depends strongly on the age pattern of first births. In Senegal, the figure ranges from 2.7 to 4.6 percent across the last three national-level surveys, WFS, DHS-I, and DHS-II. The small number of nulliparous women in each sample does not permit us to establish a trend between surveys. Other local studies confirm the general level of sterility (Ferry, 1981) or indicate slightly higher levels, possibly reaching 8 percent, as in Bandafassi (Pison and Desgrées du Loû, forthcoming). In summary, the prevalence of primary sterility in Senegal appears rather normal, and sterility scarcely diminishes the reproductive potential of Senegalese women.

SUMMARY AND CONCLUSIONS

The 1978 WFS established that fertility in Senegal was very high in the mid-1970s—7.2 children per woman. There are some indications that fertility may have been lower two or three decades earlier and increased in the preceding years. Fertility declined by around one child per woman between the mid-1970s and the beginning of the 1980s, and the differences in the fertility levels among various regions and sociocultural subgroups have increased.

The decline has occurred almost exclusively among women under age 30. A comparison of ASFRs between 1975-1978 and 1989-1992 reveals that the decline in fertility among women aged 15-19 is approximately twice as large as that among women aged 20-29, which, in turn, is almost twice as large as that among women over age 30. After age 30, fertility has remained much the same.

The driving force behind these changes has been a trend towards later marriage. In some areas of Senegal, for example in Casamance, women have always married relatively late. However, the larger trend towards later marriage probably began in Dakar in the early 1980s and has been spreading to other urban areas ever since. The pattern of later marriage is closely linked to formal education, although signs of change are emerging even among women who have never attended school. Little of the fertility decline appears to be attributable to either a decrease in ideal family size or an increase in the use of modern contraception. Nationally, use of modern contraception has enjoyed only modest success. Contraceptive use among currently married women increased from 1 percent in 1978 to 5 percent in

1992-1993. However only certain subgroups of the population use modern contraception, so that the absolute number of users is still very low.

In summary, these features indicate that Senegal's small fertility decline is unlike those that have occurred recently in other sub-Saharan African countries. In Botswana, Kenya, and Zimbabwe—usually considered the three countries in the vanguard of an African fertility transition—fertility declines are associated with increased use of modern contraception. In Senegal, the decline is associated with a trend toward later marriage. In addition, although Botswana, Kenya, and, to a lesser extent, Senegal and Zimbabwe have all experienced a decline in teenage marriages, Senegal has not experienced such a dramatic separation of teenage marriage and teenage fertility. Consequently, Senegal has not seen the same increase in premarital fertility as these other countries.

The Senegalese pattern matches more closely, but not exactly, the pattern found in certain Northern African countries during the first phase of their fertility declines. For example, most of the first decreases in fertility observed in countries such as Algeria, Egypt, and Tunisia can be attributed to later age at first marriage (Fargues, 1989; National Research Council, 1982). It is interesting to note that in these countries, the initial phase of fertility decline was followed immediately by a second phase linked to a substantial decline in the demand for children and a corresponding increase in modern contraceptive use among married women. Whether Senegal follows this pattern and experiences a second phase of fertility decline immediately following the first remains to be seen.[31] Much will depend on what happens to the demand for children. There has been a trend towards wanting fewer children that extends across all parities and all age groups of women. However, current preferences still lie very close to the physiological maximum, assuming a continued regime of delayed marriage and long birth intervals.

If the education sector can overcome its fiscal constraint and continue to make advances in primary and secondary school enrollment for women, further declines in fertility can be expected in the near future. In rural areas, a further reduction in fertility can be achieved solely by later marriage. Urban areas, particularly Dakar, have already experienced most of the decline in actual fertility that is achievable solely by an increase in the age at marriage. Future fertility reductions will have to await greater coverage of modern contraception.

If the government of Senegal wishes to influence the timing and shape of the fertility decline, it must implement strong policies that target both girls and women of reproductive age. For girls, policy should be aimed at increasing formal education. For women, action should be taken to promote the availability of contraception while increasing women's functional literacy and reducing their domestic burden. When combined with interventions aimed at improving maternal and child health, such policies should have a good chance of making women more receptive to the use of modern contraception.

NOTES

1. The TFR expresses the total number of children a woman would have if she experienced the same level and pattern of fertility throughout her reproductive life as those in effect at the time of the survey. An advantage of using the TFR over other measures of fertility, such as the crude birth rate, is that it is independent of the age structure of the population.

2. See Appendix A for a complete list and brief description of all the major surveys used in this report.

3. Apart from not reporting children that died, respondents frequently are unable to identify the beginning of the reference period, and this can also lead to systematic bias. Fortunately, this was probably not a serious problem in the 1988 census (see endnote 6).

4. For example, the infant mortality rate based on data for deaths occurring during the preceding 12 months was estimated to be 93 deaths per 1,000 live births, or approximately half the presumed actual rate.

5. There was also a tendency in the WFS to shift the dates of births towards the survey date, and there were a number of omissions of births for more remote time periods (Guèye, 1984; van de Walle and Foster, 1990).

6. The 1988 census was conducted between May 20 and June 3, but May 27, 1988, was adopted as the official reference date. The holiday of "Korité," which marks the end of Ramadan and is widely celebrated in Senegal, fell on May 29 the year before, nearly 12 months to the day before the census reference date. Consequently, the holiday was used as a reference point to identify any births and deaths that occurred in the 12 months preceding the census.

7. B_{60}s measure the proportion of women in an age cohort (a group of women defined by 5-year age groups at the time of the survey) who, having attained an nth birth, go on to an $(n + 1)$th birth within 60 months. Thus B_{60}s are a form of censored parity progression ratios (CPPRs). B_{60}s have been designed to correct for an inherent bias in the usual calculation of CPPR suggested by Rodriguez and Hobcraft (1980) that results from systematically excluding women with long birth intervals (see Brass and Juarez, 1983).

8. That is, we report the probabilities that a woman in a particular cohort who has had her nth birth goes on to have an $(n + 1)$th birth within 60 months of her nth birth, *and* subsequently goes on to have an $(n + 2)$th birth within 60 months of her $(n + 1)$th birth.

9. The term "grand region" is used throughout this report in reference to the four WFS and DHS regions, as opposed to the ten administrative regions.

10. Other data from local studies in the Sine-Saloum region are not presented here because of the small population size from which they are taken, their poor quality that is acknowledged by those responsible for their collection, and the lack of published data.

11. See Pison et al. (1991), Pison and Desgrées du Loû (forthcoming), and Appendix A for additional information.

12. See Pison et al. (1991), Lagarde et al. (forthcoming), and Appendix A for additional information.

13. Note that given the longitudinal nature of the survey, the omission of births in recent periods is probably not a large problem. For the most recent period, 1985-1992, the estimates of the fertility rate are based on the number of recorded events between multiple rounds of the survey. Thus the most recent estimates take advantage of the longitudinal nature of the survey. Fertility estimates for the earlier periods are from retrospective biographical data.

14. The census did not include an additional question on the number of children a women had ever borne, which would have enabled us to use indirect estimation techniques to correct for underreporting of births, nor did it ask one further question, on the number of children that had died, which would have provided information for the estimation of child mortality.

15. Briefly, this neoclassical model holds that households decide on the number of children to have by attempting to maximize household utility subject to time and income constraints. Children, both in quantity and quality, enter the problem in exactly the same way as other goods. Together with other competing sources of satisfaction, they create household demand, which can be satisfied by a combination of (1) income from either a household's wealth or the labor-force participation of its members, and (2) time. Because the bearing and rearing of children is an extremely time-intensive activity, especially for women, having children competes with other activities, such as working in the labor force. Hence, women are forced to trade off their time among (1) working in the labor force so that they can purchase additional goods and services, (2) bearing and raising children, and (3) doing other things. The problem is further complicated by the fact that the wages and opportunities for women are likely to be functions of previous labor-market experience, which in turn depends on the timing and frequency of earlier children in a woman's early working life (Willis, 1973; Becker, 1981; Schultz, 1981). Note, however, that this demand-side approach is often viewed as being overly simplistic in developing countries because it largely ignores the economic contribution of children through farm work and child-minding activities—which can be considerable—and the role of children as care providers for their parents in old age (Anker and Knowles, 1982). These factors provide an important incentive for high fertility. Finally, the neoclassical model assumes that individual households act alone and ignores the role extended families play as decision makers and, in some cases, as child rearers.

16. Ferry (1981) observes that fertility rates in Dakar were at least as high as, if not higher than, those in rural areas in the late 1960s.

17. See, for example, Lacombe (1972) who provides estimates of fertility rates by ethnic group from as early as 1957.

18. Comparisons among ethnic groups, and in particular between the Serer and the other groups, are made difficult because of a tendency for Serer women to declare themselves to be Wolof in surveys. This practice, which has been termed "Wolofization" (Ferry, 1977), is more prevalent in urban than in rural areas. Thus the Serer ethnic group disproportionately comprises women who remain in rural areas, which introduces an important selection bias into the data.

19. Secondary education of women is also likely to be correlated to the probability that the husband works in the formal sector, which itself can have an independent effect on fertility outcomes (see Mboup, 1993).

20. See Chapter 2 for a description of each of the socioeconomic indicators.

21. TFR = total fertility rate; C_m = index of marital fertility calculated using the formula C_m = TFR/TMFR, where TMFR is the total marital fertility rate. (Both rates are estimated for the 4 years prior to the survey.) C_c = index of contraception, calculated as $C_c = 1\text{-}1.08ue$, where u is the current contraceptive use prevalence rate among women in sexual unions, and e is the average effectiveness of the chosen contraceptive methods, calculated as the weighted average of the proportion of women using each method times the effectiveness of the method. Following Jolly and Gribble (1993), we have divided other methods into other traditional methods and other modern methods. The following effectiveness levels have been assigned to specific methods: sterilization = 1.0; IUD, Depo-Provera, Norplant = .95; pill = .90; other modern methods = .70; traditional methods = .30. Breastfeeding and postpartum abstinence are not included in contraception, since they are not parity-specific practices and are adopted to protect maternal and child health, rather than as a means to limit family size. Furthermore, there is substantial variation among surveys in the proportion of women practicing abstinence as a method of contraception, which probably has more to do with differences in definitions and interviewers' instructions than with changes in women's behavior. Finally, traditional methods, such as the use of ritual charms or potions (*gris-gris*), have been excluded; in essence, these methods are equated with using no contraception. C_i = index of postpartum infecund interval, calculated using the formula $C_i = 20/(18.5 + i)$, where i is the mean number of months of postpartum infecundability (estimated as the mean number of months of postpartum amenorrhea or abstinence, whichever is longer) for women in union. C_a = index of induced abortion, taken to be 1.00 in the absence of additional information; and I_p = index of sterility, calculated as $I_p = (7.63 - .11s)/7.3$, where s is the proportion of women aged 40-49 who have never had any children.

22. It would be a mistake to read too much into the differences in the C_i index among surveys. The WFS did not ask women whether they were currently amenorrheic, so the C_i index for the WFS was imputed using a formula provided by Bongaarts and Potter (1983), based on the duration of breastfeeding.

23. When examining age at first marriage in any African setting, it is important to remember that marriage in Africa may be better described as a process than an event (van de Walle, 1968, 1993; Lesthaeghe et al., 1989; Pison, 1989; Meekers, 1992; Working Group on the Social Dynamics of Adolescent Fertility, 1993). Unlike births or deaths, entry into marriage may take place over an extended period of time. Consequently, the date on which a marriage occurs is subject to several interpretations.

First, marriages are usually marked by a ceremony and the transfer of a bridewealth that can range from symbolic tokens to large transfers of cash or goods spanning several years. However, the payment of bridewealth, the ceremony, the cohabitation of spouses, and the consummation of the marriage often occur several months apart and not necessarily in the same order (Meekers, 1992). Among the Poular, for example, consummation of marriage may occur several years after a marriage ceremony. This traditional waiting period (known as "le jebalé") is often decided mutually among the parents of the newly married couple and helps explain the paradoxically low levels of fertility in the first years of marriage among the Poular (République du Sénégal, 1981:97). Different members of society may also give full recognition to the union at different stages of the process, perhaps depending on the ethnic group(s) involved, the degree of personal involvement, or simply individual interpretation. The practice of dating marriage by date of cohabitation was abandoned in the DHS-I for Senegal and was replaced with date of consummation.

Furthermore, there are multiple forms of marriage in Senegal, so that as an institution, marriage is not always easy to measure. Customary marriage practices in Senegal include monogamy, polygyny, and a wide range of consensual unions such as "sugar daddies" and "outside wives." Unfortunately, the need for survey and census takers to categorize and reduce the various forms of marriage into a small number of discrete units means that much of this diversity in marriage patterns is lost. In the 1988 census, information on marriage was collected for all persons aged 6 and over. Marriage was defined to include both civic and traditional marriages, but excluded conjugal unions (i.e., unsanctioned unions), a more restrictive definition than that used in either the DHS-I or the DHS-II. Marriage was defined quite loosely in both the DHS surveys, and a series of questions was used to identify such possibilities as a couple living together but not in a sanctioned union and a "visiting relationship." In the 1988 census, these variants of marriage were probably captured in the category "autres cas," which was left suitably ambiguous. Confusion surrounding the definition of marriage extends far beyond researchers in their efforts to categorize people as being either married or unmarried in the Western tradition. Couples in apparently identical situations may describe their condition in quite different ways, and in some instances, even the partners in the same union may not agree on their marital status (Locoh, 1988, cited in Working Group on the Social Dynamics of Adolescent Fertility, 1993).

Van de Walle (1993) suggests that the processional nature of marriage in Africa presents an inherent ambiguity to respondents that could introduce systematic biases into their responses. For example, some unions that have only partially completed the process of marriage may be reported as marriages at the time of a survey, but may appear never to have taken place if the union dissolves. At the same time, other partial unions that prove successful may not have been reported as "marriages" in their earlier stages, but with the benefit of hindsight appear to have started at a time when their status was actually quite uncertain (van de Walle, 1993). This ambiguity also makes it difficult to define what constitutes a premarital birth, since in some instances the birth of a child is actually part of a longer marriage process (Working Group on the Social Dynamics of Adolescent Fertility, 1993).

24. In fact, Guèye and Ferry (1985) and Ndiaye (1985) note that there is an inverse relation between age at marriage and the length of the interval between marriage and first birth in Senegal.

25. A similar finding has emerged from many other DHS studies in Africa (see Working Group on the Social Dynamics of Adolescent Fertility, 1993; Diop, 1993), but the extent of the rise in premarital adolescent childbearing in Senegal is relatively small in comparison with the experience of several other sub-Saharan Africa countries (e.g., Kenya and Botswana).

26. The Malinké belong to the Mandingo group, and the Bedik, a small group also called the Tenda, are close to the Bassari.

27. "Polygyny is often perceived by more educated women as being a type of union that is incompatible with their social aspirations" (République du Sénégal, 1981:81).

28. The calculation of C_i can be done directly on the basis of the duration of postpartum amenorrhea or indirectly on the basis of a model linking the duration of amenorrhea to that of breastfeeding. On the basis of data from the DHS-I, comparison of direct and indirect results shows that the period of infecundability is longer if one considers declarations of postpartum amenorrhea than if one infers the length of amenorrhea indirectly from the duration of breastfeeding (Jolly and Gribble, 1993).

29. We have no data on the intensity of breastfeeding over time.

30. An alternative approach is to calculate C_a indirectly from Table 4-5. Assuming a level of total fecundity of 15.3 children per woman (Bongaarts and Potter, 1983) and applying the formula $TFR = C_m \times C_c \times C_i \times C_a \times I_p \times 15.3$, implies levels of C_a between .82 and .88 across the three surveys.

31. An important element in these other countries' fertility decline is that as women's educational status has improved, the gain due to more widespread contraception and the loss due to shorter breastfeeding—the most important determinant of amenorrhea—have practically canceled each other out (Fargues, 1989). In contrast, recent data from the DHS-II do not indicate that the average length of breastfeeding is decreasing in Senegal.

5

Mortality

INTRODUCTION

Throughout the world, wherever data are available, we know that mortality has declined over the last century. In regions where long time-series data are unavailable, our knowledge of mortality trends over the recent past is drawn from sources such as ad hoc surveys of women's birth histories. In sub-Saharan Africa, available information shows that mortality was very high in the middle of the twentieth century and that it has declined substantially since. In the 1950s, 30-40 percent of newborn children died before reaching age 5 (Hill, 1992, 1993). In the 1970s, the proportion was much lower—10-25 percent. Adult mortality has probably also decreased substantially over this period, though the data to document the decline are scanty (Timæus, 1993).

Both health programs and economic development have probably contributed to the mortality decline in African countries. In the past, the development of health services in Senegal mirrored the development in industrialized countries: most individual services were provided through hospitals, supplemented by disease-control public health measures. Specific programs were organized to control infectious diseases, such as those for the eradication of smallpox or the control of leprosy. Some of these programs reached into rural areas, but most health care services were located in urban settings. The reorientation of health policy towards primary health care is one of the great changes of the modern era. As was decided at the World Health

Assembly in 1978 at Alma-Ata, primary health care aims to provide limited but affordable services at the community level in an integrated manner using community health workers.

Following the 1978 conference, Senegal reformulated its health care policy, placing greater emphasis on primary health care in rural areas. The number of hospitals, health posts, community health workers, and pharmacies increased throughout Senegal, particularly in areas outside of Dakar. In 1981, the Expanded Programme on Immunization (EPI) was established, with the purpose of increasing vaccination coverage in rural as well as in urban areas. The results of the EPI efforts have been notable. Vaccination coverage has increased substantially over the past couple of decades, particularly in rural areas, narrowing the inequalities in vaccination coverage between urban and rural areas (see the appendix to this chapter for more detail on health programs in Senegal). From the early 1980s, efforts toward the provision of better health services have taken place against a background of economic crises and more recently of the HIV/AIDS epidemic.

This chapter reviews the levels and trends in mortality in Senegal. The next two sections address data sources and national levels, trends, and geographical variations in child mortality and adult mortality, respectively. The final section presents conclusions.

CHILD MORTALITY

Sources and Quality of Data

Five surveys and one census supply data that permit estimation of the national level of child mortality: the 1960-1961 Demographic Survey (DS) [1], the 1970-1971 National Demographic Survey (NDS) [2], the 1978 World Fertility Survey (WFS) [3], the 1986 Demographic and Health Survey (DHS-I) [4], the 1988 census[18], and the 1992-1993 Demographic and Health Survey (DHS-II) [7] (see Appendix A).

The type and quality of data gathered vary among surveys, as do the methodologies used. Accordingly, it is preferable to focus initially on a simple, robust indicator of child mortality, such as the probability that a newborn will die before the age of five (${}_5q_0$), also called the under-5 mortality rate. The advantage of this indicator is that it is less sensitive to age-reporting errors (for ages of surviving children or ages at time of death) than is the infant mortality rate or the probability of death prior to 1 year, ${}_1q_0$, which is more often used. Moreover, ${}_5q_0$ is less sensitive to biases linked to the estimation method (Cantrelle et al., 1986; Fargues and Khlat, 1989).

The 1960-1961 DS [1] gathered information on the number of births and surviving children of each woman interviewed. These data allow the indirect estimation of the risk of death between 0 and 5 years of age. The method applied here is that of Brass, as adapted by Trussell and described in United Nations (1983a).

The 1970-1971 NDS [2] gathered prospective data on births and deaths occurring during a 12-month period in a sample of households. Three visits were made to each household at 6-month intervals. This method of data collection reduces the risk of omitting childhood deaths, so the data are of fairly good quality. The probability of dying by age 5 was calculated directly by relating deaths to person-years of exposure to risk.

The WFS [3], DHS-I [4], and DHS-II [7] collected birth histories for all sampled women, providing information for each live-born child on date of birth and, if the child had died, age at the time of death. These data permit direct calculation of the risks of death for different periods preceding the survey. A bias that often affects this kind of information is that some children who die young are omitted, thereby causing underestimation of mortality. In general, the risk of omission is greater for older than for younger women and for events further in the past. Another kind of error concerns the identification of the correct date of birth, which is often known only approximately, particularly in environments where illiteracy is prevalent. It appears that, in the WFS, births tended to be shifted toward the survey date, a phenomenon that leads to slight overestimation of the mortality rate at a given date if mortality is declining. This bias is not apparent in the other surveys. In fact, in the DHS-I, some births were probably moved from the most recent 5-year period to an earlier period, which could, conversely, lead to an underestimation of mortality. A third common type of error is in the reporting of age at death, both rounding to numbers of years (such as "1 year") and exaggerating age at death. This error may reduce the infant mortality rate relative to young child mortality, but has little effect on our chosen indicator, ${}_5q_0$.

The 1988 census [18] provided data about deaths occurring during the preceding 12 months. This type of data is normally of poor quality, because of respondents' difficulty in situating the beginning of the previous 12 months. Respondents tend either to over- or (more typically) underestimate mortality, depending on whether the beginning of the period is mistakenly placed before or after the true beginning of the reference period. Low reliability also results from the omission of certain deaths, especially those occurring shortly after birth, as in all retrospective surveys.

With respect to the 1988 census, it is possible that the first bias, tied to the difficulty in accurately situating the beginning of the preceding 12 months, was less important than usual because the major Muslim holiday, the Korité, took place exactly 1 year prior to the census and was thus used as point of reference (see Chapter 4, footnote 6 for details).

The census data on child mortality can be evaluated by comparison with other sources, namely the ongoing small-scale surveys conducted in three rural areas, Niakhar/Ngayokhème [11] (Projet Niakhar, 1992), Bandafassi [8] (Pison and Desgrées du Loû, 1993), and Mlomp [10] (Lagarde et al., forthcoming). Because the census data and data from the small-scale surveys do not exactly coincide in terms of area, comparisons can be made only between each study area and the rural part of the department in which that area is located. Comparisons were focused on the probability of dying before age 1 and the probability of dying between age 1 and 5 (${}_1q_0$ and ${}_4q_1$, respectively). The results appear in Table 5-1.

In each case, the census estimate of ${}_1q_0$ for the rural area of the department falls substantially below the estimate of the corresponding local study. The census estimates amount to 30 percent, 38 percent, and 41 percent of the local study estimates, respectively, for rural Fatick as compared with Niakhar/Ngayokhème, rural Oussouye as compared with Mlomp, and rural Kédougou as compared with Bandafassi. On the other hand, census estimates of ${}_4q_1$ differ little from those of the local studies: 141 per 1,000 in rural Fatick as compared with 152 in Niakhar, 90 per 1,000 in rural Oussouye as compared with 71 in the Mlomp study area, and 117 per 1,000 in rural Kédougou as compared with 121 in Bandafassi. Local comparisons thus indicate underreporting by as much as two-thirds of the deaths of children below the age of 1 year recorded in the census. Conversely, the local comparisons indicate a relatively high level of recording of deaths among those aged 1-4.

These conclusions are supported by national-level data. Table 5-2 gives the national estimates from the 1988 census and the national surveys, DHS-I and DHS-II. The infant mortality rate reportedly fell from 86 per 1,000 in 1981-1986 (DHS-I estimate) to 34 per 1,000 in 1987-1988 (census estimate), or a decline of more than one-half (60 percent) within 4 years, before rising thereafter to 68 per 1,000 (or 100 percent) in 1988-1992 (DHS-II estimate). These short-term fluctuations are highly implausible. Differentials among the various estimates most likely result from a pronounced underreporting in the census of deaths of children less than 1 year of age. On the other hand, mortality of children aged 1-4 reportedly fell from 114 per 1,000 in 1981-1986 to 83 per 1,000 in 1987-1988, and to 68 per 1,000 in 1988-1992, which is a plausible decline.

Thus, the usual bias of retrospective studies—the omission of early deaths—is encountered in the census. On the other hand, the omission of deaths does not seem to be a problem above 1 year of age. Moreover, as noted above, the bias arising from the difficulty in temporally situating the beginning of the preceding 12 months was probably less of a factor than usual because of the Korité.

Comparison of deaths registered in vital records in the city of Saint-

TABLE 5-1 Comparison of Mortality Estimates from the 1988 Census and Selected Local Studies

Region	Source	Date	$_1q_0$ (per 1,000)	$_4q_1$ (per 1,000)
Department of Fatick (rural)	1988 census	1987-1988	36	141
Portion of the Niakhar and Tataguine arrondissements	Niakhar study	1987-1988	122	152
Department of Oussouye (rural)	1988 census	1987-1988	19	90
Portion of the Loudia Wolof arrondissement	Mlomp study	1985-1991	50	71
Department of Kédougou (rural)	1988 census	1987-1988	58	117
Portion of the Bandafassi arrondissement	Bandafassi study	1986-1991	140	121

NOTES: Method of calculation for the 1988 census: annual mortality rates were calculated as the ratio of the number of deaths in the last 12 months to the average population in the last 12 months. The latter was estimated from the census adjusted downward by 1.5 percent, the annual growth rate of the population being around 3 percent. The mortality rates were then converted into the corresponding probabilities of dying. See Appendix A for description of surveys.

SOURCES: Bandafassi study: Pison and Desgrées du Loû (1993); Mlomp study: Lagarde et al. (forthcoming); Niakhar study: Projet Niakhar (1992); 1988 census: 1988 census (unpublished data)

Louis between May 1987 and May 1988 with those reported in the census yields the same conclusions: deaths occurring before 1 year of age are less than half as numerous in the census as in vital records, that is, 99 as compared with 210. For ages 1-4, however, the two sources are much closer: 109 deaths according to the census and 84 according to the vital records (Diop, 1990).

This analysis of the quality of data from the 1988 census thus gives an unexpected result: aside from deaths of children under 1 year of age, the data gathered concerning deaths during the last 12 months seem relatively complete.

At the national level, if one discards the census estimate for $_1q_0$ and combines the census estimate for $_4q_1$ with $_1q_0$ from another source, esti-

TABLE 5-2 Comparison of National-Level Mortality Estimates from the 1988 Census (data on deaths in the last 12 months) and Estimates from DHS-I and DHS-II

Source	Period	$_1q_0$ (per 1,000)	$_4q_1$ (per 1,000)
1986 DHS-I	1981-1986	86	114
1988 census	1987-1988	34	83
1992-1993 DHS-II	1988-1992	68	68

NOTE: See Appendix A for description of surveys.

SOURCES: 1986 DHS-I: Ndiaye et al. (1988); 1992-1993 DHS-II: Ndiaye et al. (1994); 1988 census (unpublished data)

mates for $_5q_0$ can be calculated. For example, combining the midpoint between the $_1q_0$ indicated by the DHS-I for the period 1981-1986 and that of the DHS-II for 1988-1992, or 77 per 1,000, with the $_4q_1$ estimate of 83 per 1,000 from the census gives an estimate of $_5q_0$ for the period June 1987-May 1988 of 154 per 1,000, as seen in Table 5-3.

Mortality Levels and Trends Among Children Under Age 5

National Level

Table 5-3, illustrated in Figure 5-1, shows $_5q_0$ estimates for all of Senegal obtained from the five national surveys and the census for different dates and periods. The table also summarizes the type of data gathered and the method of estimation employed. Although these measurements result from different surveys and estimation techniques, they are fairly consistent.

Broadly speaking, in the 45 years following the end of World War II, child mortality ($_5q_0$) declined by two-thirds, falling from an estimated level of 373 in 1946 to 131 in the years 1988-1992. The decline appears to have occurred rather slowly until the early 1970s, with $_5q_0$ falling only to 281 per 1,000 by 1970, a 25 percent decline in 25 years. The reduction seems to have accelerated thereafter, with $_5q_0$ falling by more than 50 percent in the next 20 years, from 281 per 1,000 in 1970 to 131 in 1988-1992.

The Case of Dakar

Multiple sources of information make it possible to track the trend in $_5q_0$ in Dakar over time (see Figure 5-2). The estimates from the various

TABLE 5-3 Proportion of Children Dying Before Age 5 in Senegal, 1945-1990

Source	Period	Reference Date	$_5q_0$ (per 1,000)
1960 DS	—	1946.2	373[a]
		1951.6	343[a]
1970-1971 NDS	1970-1971	1970.5	281[b]
1978 WFS	1964-1968	1966.1	293[c]
	1969-1973	1971.1	283[c]
	1974-1978	1976.1	262[c]
1986 DHS-I	1971-1975	1973.5	287[c]
	1976-1980	1978.5	236[c]
	1981-1986	1983.0	191[c]
1988 census	1987-1988	1987.9	154[d]
1992-1993 DHS-II	1978-1982	1980.6	199[c]
	1983-1987	1985.6	185[c]
	1988-1992	1990.6	131[c]

[a]Estimate calculated using an indirect method with data on number of children born and number of children surviving (Hill, 1992).

[b]Estimate calculated using a direct method with data on deaths collected by multiround survey.

[c]Estimate calculated using a direct method with data on women's birth histories (status of each child—living or dead—and age at death, if deceased).

[d]Estimate calculated using a direct method with data on deaths within the last 12 months (with a correction due to underreporting of deaths under 1 year of age). (See the discussion earlier in this section.)

SOURCES: 1960: DS (Hill, 1992); 1970-1971: NDS (République du Sénégal, 1974) 1978: WFS (Rutstein, 1983); 1986: DHS-I (Ndiaye et al., 1988); 1992-1993: DHS-II (Ndiaye et al., 1994); 1988: 1988 census (unpublished data)

sources are broadly consistent, and differences among them are due primarily to variations in methodology and data quality, as well as to differences in the populations of children studied.

Garenne et al. (1992) analyzed the birth histories of women from the WFS and DHS-I in the region of Dakar who had lived in the city since childhood. These series are shown on Figure 5-2 as WFS-Dakar and DHS-I-Dakar. The DHS-I-Dakar series seems more plausible than that of the WFS-Dakar. For the period 1975-1979, the former matches almost perfectly the estimate from vital registration (Dakar-2), while the WFS-Dakar

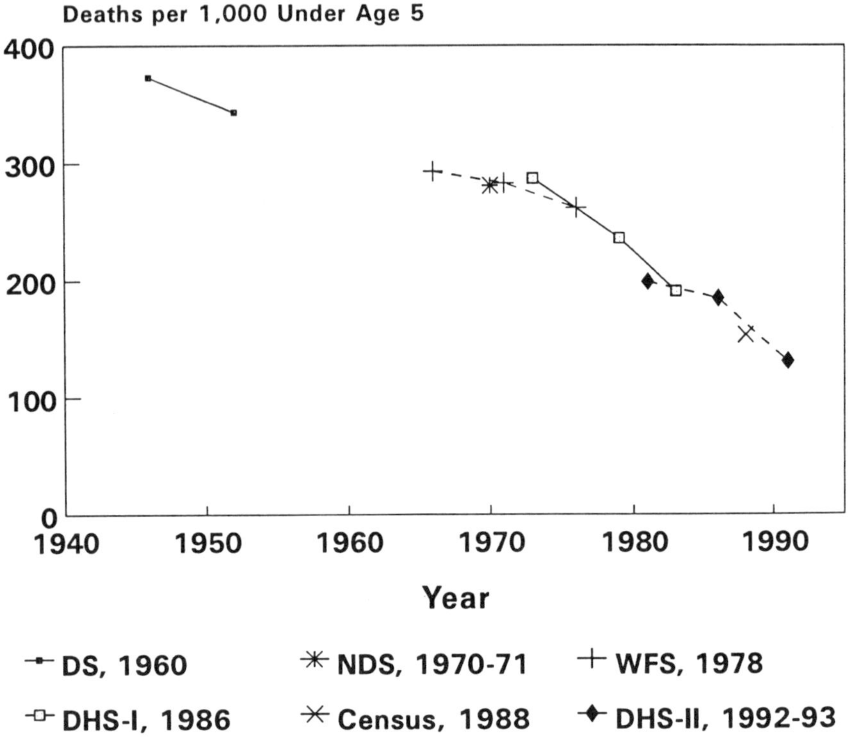

FIGURE 5-1 Trends in child mortality ($_5q_0$ per 1,000), Senegal, 1945-1992. SOURCES: Hill (1992); Ndiaye et al. (1988, 1994); Rutstein (1983); Antoine and Mbodji (1991); and unpublished data from the 1988 census.

series shows a pronounced, and not very plausible, increase of mortality around 1960, probably reflecting poorer-quality data for earlier periods. Note that taken together the WFS-Dakar and DHS-I-Dakar sequences indicate a stagnation of $_5q_0$ during the period 1965-1983 at a level of approximately 100-150 per 1,000. This stagnation is also found in the birth history data collected in Pikine in the 1986 Dakar-Pikine Survey [15] if one considers only children born in Pikine to mothers native to the Dakar urban area (Antoine and Diouf, 1992). The level of $_5q_0$ for the same period from this survey was also about 100 per 1,000 (data not shown).

Restricting the analysis to children whose mothers have lived in Dakar since childhood excludes children born in Dakar to migrant mothers from rural areas. The mortality of the latter group is higher (Antoine and Diouf, 1992; Garenne et al., 1992). However, the differential between the level of child mortality for *all* children from Dakar and the estimated level for the

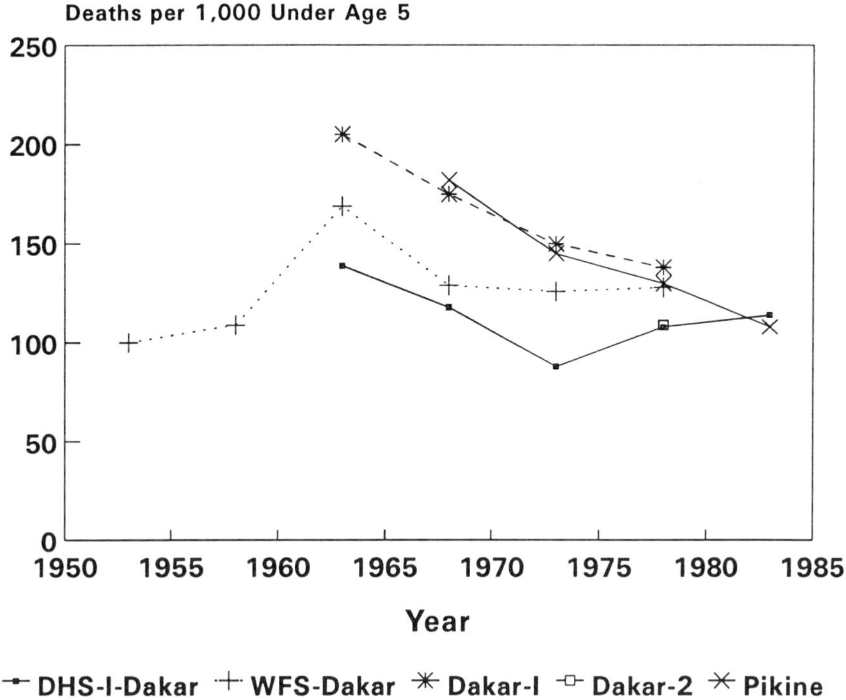

FIGURE 5-2 Child mortality trends in Dakar ($_5q_0$ per 1,000), multiple sources. NOTES: DHS-I-Dakar: Direct estimates of the risk of death by period, based on data from the 1986 DHS-I [4] conducted solely among women residing in Dakar since childhood. WFS-Dakar: Direct estimates of the risk of death by period, based on data from the 1978 WFS [3] conducted solely among women residing in Dakar since childhood. Dakar-1: Direct estimates of the risk of death by period, based on data from the 1986 Dakar-Pikine Survey [15]. Estimates include only children born in Dakar to women residing in Pikine at the time of the survey. Dakar-2: Mean 1975-1979 estimate from vital records. Pikine: Direct estimates of the risk of death by period, based on data from the 1986 Dakar-Pikine Survey [15]. Estimates included only children born in Pikine to women residing in Pikine at the time of the survey. SOURCES: Antoine and Mbodji (1991); Garenne et al. (1992:Table 5, p. 24, Table 7, p. 26); Cantrelle et al. (1986:Table 76, p. 112).

subgroup of children whose mothers have lived in Dakar since childhood may have changed over time. Data from the Pikine survey allow us to analyze these changes (see Figure 5-2). The estimates from the Pikine survey encompass all of the children covered by this survey and born in either Dakar (Dakar-1 in Figure 5-2) or Pikine (Pikine in Figure 5-2), regardless of their mothers' origin. These estimates show a mortality level that (1) was apparently higher during the 1960s than the mortality level of children whose mothers had lived in Dakar since childhood, and (2) declined during the two decades between the early 1960s and the early 1980s ($_5q_0$ fell from 200 per 1,000 at the beginning of the 1960s to less than 150 per 1,000 in the early 1980s).

Overall mortality was probably not as high as that of children born to women residing in Pikine (a relatively low socioeconomic section of Dakar) regardless of their origin, and not as low as that of children born to women who had resided in Dakar since childhood. The most plausible scenario is that during the period 1960-1985, mortality declined at a relatively slow pace, especially at the end of the period.

Rural Areas

Figure 5-3 shows the trend of $_5q_0$ in all rural areas in Senegal, according to the WFS, DHS-I, and DHS-II. These measurements were obtained using a method similar to the preceding one, that is, by selecting rural women who had lived in rural areas since childhood (Garenne et al., 1992, and unpublished tables from DHS-II). For the region of Dakar, the WFS series seems less plausible than either of the DHS series, especially before 1965. If only DHS estimates are considered, the trend shows stagnation at a level between 350 and 400 per 1,000 until the early 1970s, followed by a rapid decline beginning in the late 1970s: according to the DHS-I, $_5q_0$ reportedly fell from 369 per 1,000 in 1970-1974 to 231 per 1,000 in 1980-1984, a reduction of 37 percent in 10 years. The DHS-II shows a similarly rapid decline, but with consistently lower mortality than in the DHS-I: according to the DHS-II, $_5q_0$ fell from 303 per 1,000 in 1968-1972 to 133 per 1,000 in 1988-1992.

Figure 5-4 compares the trends of $_5q_0$ in rural areas, those discussed earlier in the region of Dakar, and the Saint-Louis series estimated from that city's vital records (Diop, 1990). The contrast between the mortality levels in the cities (Dakar, Pikine, and Saint-Louis) and those in rural areas is enormous during the period 1960-1975. The Saint-Louis series shows that the differentials are long-standing, resulting from the early, sizable decline in mortality in the cities beginning during the first half of the century. At the end of the 1970s, the situation changed. Because of the pronounced decline in mortality in rural areas and a slowing of the decline in the Dakar region, the gap between Dakar and rural areas narrowed to a factor of around two at the beginning of the 1980s.

The rural areas did not evolve as a homogenous entity. Figure 5-5 shows some localized differences recorded by reliable surveys. In the various regions studied, we find, more or less, the pattern observed for the

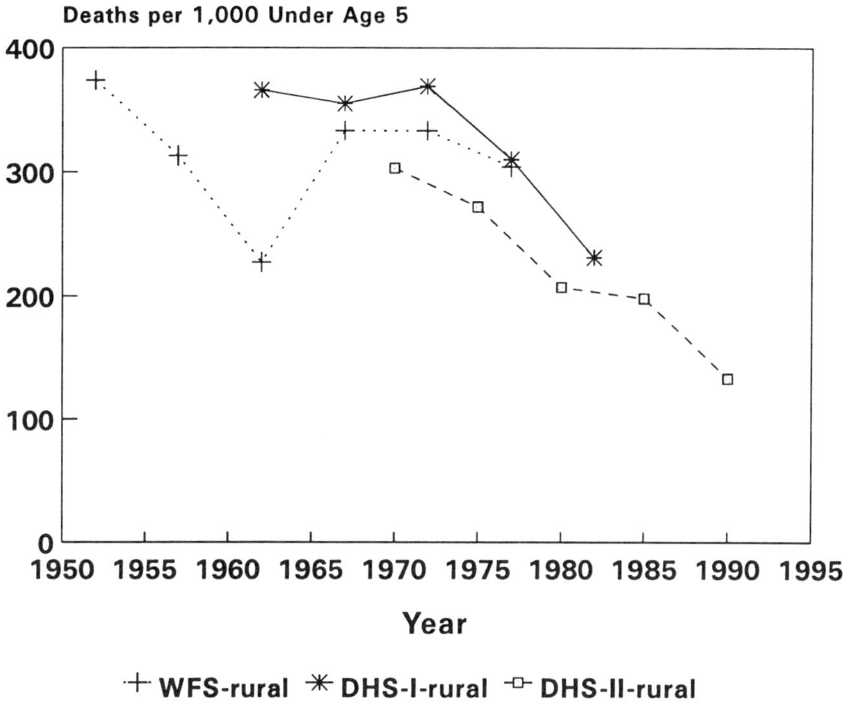

FIGURE 5-3 Trends in child mortality ($_5q_0$ per 1,000) in rural areas, 1978 WFS, 1986 DHS-I, and 1993 DHS-II. NOTE: Only children whose mothers lived in rural areas since childhood are included. SOURCE: Garenne et al. (1992).

whole of rural areas in Senegal: a plateau, followed by a rapid decline. Differences among regions appear mainly with respect to timing.

In Bandafassi, the study area furthest from Dakar (700 km), the decline in child mortality began only in the mid-1980s, coincident with the accelerated 1986-1987 EPI (Pison and Desgrées du Loû, 1993) (see the appendix to this chapter for discussion of the EPI). In Niakhar/Ngayokhème, 150 km from Dakar, the decline began earlier, in the early 1970s. The decline during that period is attributed mainly to reduced rainfall, leading to reduced incidence of malaria (Cantrelle et al., 1986); however, the decline persisted at the same pace after the dry years ended, so that other factors undoubtedly already at work must have continued the trend. The rural areas of Fissel and Thiénaba are somewhat closer to Dakar (120 and 90 km, respectively). Thiénaba is 15 km from the major city of Thiès and only 10 km from Khombole, the only rural maternal-child health center in Senegal, which began operation in 1957. Earlier measurements are not available for

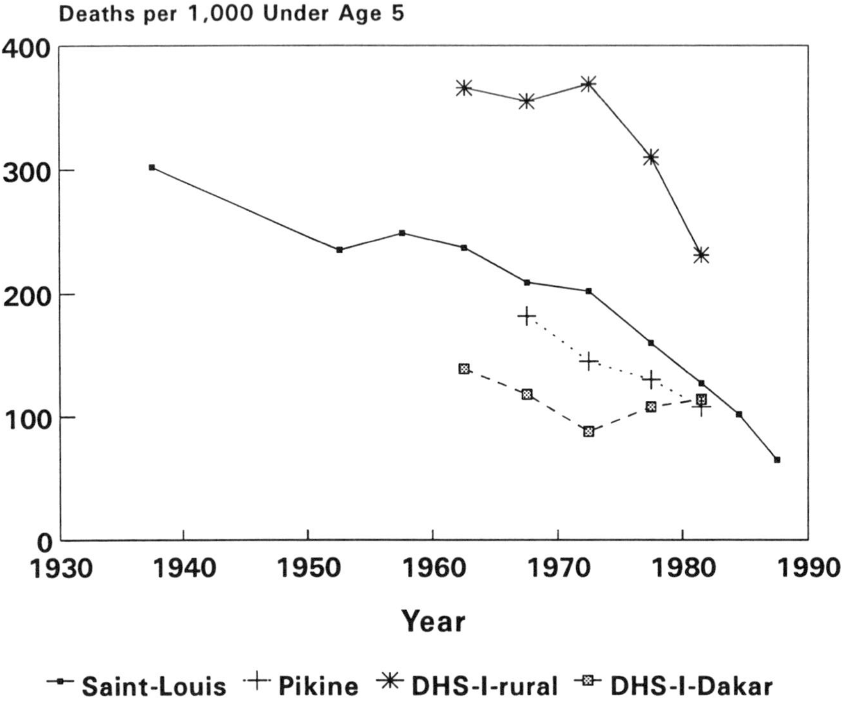

FIGURE 5-4 Trends in child mortality ($_5q_0$ per 1,000), comparison between two large cities—Dakar-Pikine and Saint-Louis—and rural areas in Senegal. NOTES: DHS-I-rural: Direct estimates of the risk of death by period, based on data from the 1986 DHS-I [4] conducted solely among rural women residing in rural areas since childhood. DHS-I-Dakar: Direct estimates of the risk of death by period, based on data from the 1986 DHS-I conducted solely among women residing in the Dakar region at the time of the survey and those residing in urban areas since childhood. Pikine: Direct estimates of the risk of death by period, based on data from the 1986 Dakar-Pikine Survey [15]. Estimates include only children born in Pikine to women residing in Pikine at the time of the survey. Saint-Louis: Saint-Louis vital records. SOURCES: Antoine and Mbodji (1991); Diop (1990); Garenne et al. (1992:Table 5, p. 24).

dating the start of the child mortality decline for the entire Fissel-Thiénaba region covered by the Survey on Child Mortality in the Sahel of 1981-1984 [16]. However, this decline probably began still earlier than in Niakhar/ Ngayokhème and apparently progressed very rapidly during the 1970s. During the period 1981-1984, child mortality in Thiénaba was 25 percent lower than that in Fissel ($_2q_0$ was 202 per 1,000 in Fissel, as compared with 149

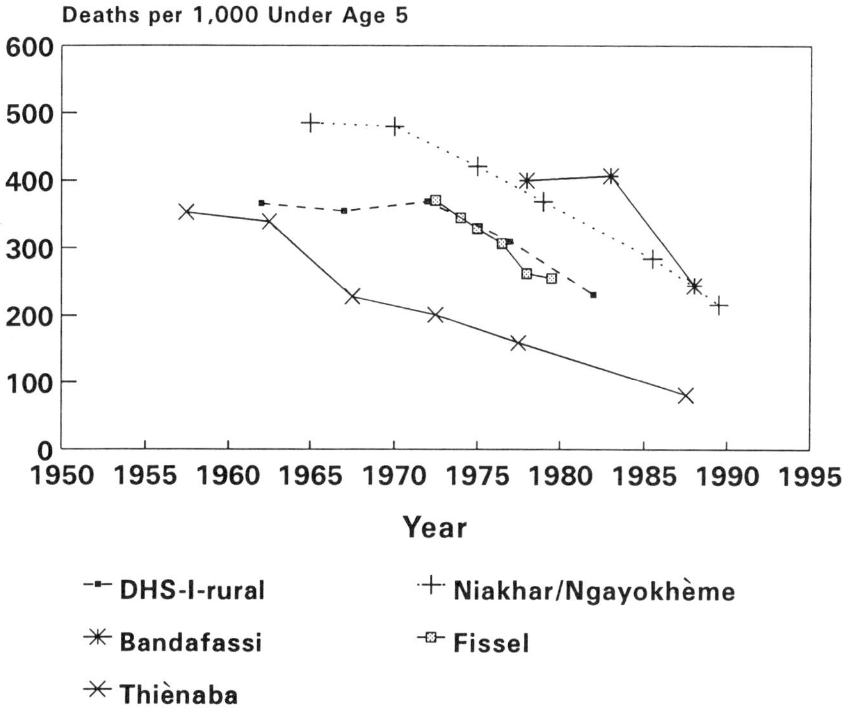

FIGURE 5-5 Trends in child mortality ($_5q_0$ per 1,000), rural areas, Senegal. SOURCES: Antoine and Mbodji (1991); Diop (1990); Garenne et al. (1992:Table 5, p. 24).

per 1,000 in Thiénaba); this is attributable to an improved health infrastructure and more frequent use of health services in Thiénaba (Mbodji, 1988).

Mlomp presents a special case. This rural area, about 500 km from Dakar, is 50 km from Ziguinchor, the regional capital. In Mlomp, the population benefited from the establishment of a private dispensary and a maternity clinic in 1961, which soon after their establishment were providing high-quality health services to a large majority of the area's residents (Pison et al., 1993). An early and very rapid decline in child mortality occurred in this area in the mid-1960s; the risk of dying before age 5 was cut fourfold in 20 years.

With the exception of Mlomp, the onset of child mortality decline appears to be correlated with distance from Dakar, a factor that is, in turn, correlated with the availability of health services. The educational level of women and household income level were uniformly low in all of these areas during this time, so these factors cannot explain the observed differences in timing. The relatively rapid trend toward declining child mortality in rural areas beginning in the late 1970s can, however, be linked in large part to infrastructure decentralization and to the new health policy implemented during that period (see the appendix to this chapter for a discussion of these issues).

Geographic Variations

Regional Differences

Table 5-4 shows that the western grand region, encompassing the Dakar and Thiès administrative regions, is clearly different from the other grand regions—the center (including the administrative regions of Louga, Diourbel, Kaolack, and Fatick), the northeast (Saint-Louis and Tambacounda), and the south (Ziguinchor and Kolda)—where child mortality is 1.5 times greater.[1] Despite the overall decline in mortality, the ranking of these three grand regions remained approximately the same between 1968 and 1988—an appreciably lower mortality in the northeast and a higher mortality in the south, with the center remaining in the middle.

TABLE 5-4 Variations in Child Mortality (${}_5q_0$ or ${}_4q_1$) by Grand Regions, 1968-1992

	1968-1972		1976-1985		1987-1988		1988-1992	
Grand Region	${}_5q_0$	Ratio[a]	${}_5q_0$ or ${}_4q_1$	Ratio	${}_4q_1$	Ratio	${}_5q_0$ or ${}_4q_1$	Ratio
${}_5q_0$								
West	183		156		—		111	
Northeast	253	1.4	200	1.3	—		183	1.6
Center	304	1.7	244	1.6	—		170	1.5
South	335	1.8	262	1.7	—		195	1.8
${}_4q_1$								
West	—		89		50		60	
Northeast	—		109	1.2	83	1.7	84	1.4
Center	—		166	1.9	101	2.0	106	1.8
South	—		164	1.8	103	2.1	108	1.8

NOTE: Results are from univariate analysis of data from national surveys (1978 WFS, 1986 DHS-I, 1992-1993 DHS-II, and 1988 census).

[a]Ratio between regional ${}_5q_0$ and ${}_5q_0$ from the first category (west).

SOURCES: 1968-1972: Guèye and Sarr (1985); 1976-1985: Ndiaye et al. (1988); 1987-1988: 1988 census (unpublished tables); 1988-1992: Ndiaye et al. (1994)

Departmental Differences

Since the mortality data for children aged 1-4 from the 1988 census appear to be fairly reliable, we have used them to study variations in child mortality on a more discriminating scale—departmental.

Table 5-5 shows mortality rates for children aged 1-4 in 1987-1988 by department and rural or urban area, based on the 1988 census. Excluding the region of Dakar, mortality in this age group varies by a factor of two. At one extreme are the departments experiencing low rural mortality—Kébémer, Louga, and Tivaouane—in which the annual mortality rate for this age group is 19 per 1,000; at the other extreme are departments having high rural mortality—Fatick (37), Bambey (38), Mbacké (33), and Sédhiou (33). On average, rural mortality is lower in the north and higher in the south (see Figure 5-6). This distinction is particularly clear in the western half of Senegal, where the vast majority of the population resides. If, leaving Saint-Louis in the north, one travels southward keeping to the city of Saint-Louis' longitude, one passes in turn through the departments of Dagana (annual mortality rate for children aged 1-4 of 20 per 1,000), Louga (19), Kébémer (19), Tivaouane (19), Bambey (38), Fatick (37), and Foundiougne (29). Mortality abruptly doubles when one goes from Tivaouane to Bambey. The gradient still exists on a north-south line closer to Dakar, such as from Tivaouane through Thiès to Mbour, but the pattern is complicated by an additional low-mortality effect associated with proximity to Dakar.

Several departments constitute exceptions to this north-south division. Bakel has a mortality rate lower than that of Matam, the neighboring department farther to the north, and the departments of Kaolack and Oussouye, where mortality is lower than the average for the south.

This north-south contrast in rural mortality among children aged 1-4 in 1987-1988 could be explained by a more marked underreporting of deaths in the northern departments during the census. The lower mortality rate in the north is, however, confirmed by earlier surveys. We found this especially in the DHS-I survey, in which the northeastern grand region has a mortality rate one-third lower than that of the central and southern grand regions (see Table 5-4). The northeastern grand region in the WFS and the two DHS surveys corresponds approximately to the northern portion of the country we are describing here.

The line separating the north (lower mortality) and the south (higher mortality) lies parallel to the isohyet (equal average annual rainfall) lines. The lower rainfall and shorter rainy season in the north may explain the contrast: they may be the underlying factors associated with diarrhea—more frequent during the rainy season—and malaria. Malaria is a major cause of death among children aged 1-4, as discussed below. The role of this disease in child mortality differentials may have been particularly high

TABLE 5-5 Annual Mortality Rates for Children Aged 1-4 (per 1,000) by Department and Rural/Urban Residence: Deaths in Last 12 Months According to 1988 Census

Region and Department	Rural	Urban
Dakar		
Dakar	—	7.6
Pikine	—	9.2
Rufisque	14	10
Diourbel		
Bambey	38	22
Diourbel	30	19
Mbacké	33	17
Fatick		
Fatick	37	20
Foundiougne	29	20
Gossas	27	20
Kaolack		
Kaffrine	29	12
Kaolack	23	11
Nioro du Rip	30	28
Kolda		
Kolda	31	14
Sédhiou	33	24
Vélingara	24	12
Louga		
Kébémer	19	1.4
Linguère	20	18
Louga	19	7.3
Saint-Louis		
Dagana	20	10
Matam	25	30
Podor	26	2.9
Tambacounda		
Bakel	20	19
Kédougou	31	23
Tambacounda	27	8.7
Thiès		
Mbour	24	13
Thiès	23	9.2
Tivaouane	19	7.5
Ziguinchor		
Bignona	27	15
Oussouye	23	24
Ziguinchor	28	17

SOURCE: 1988 census (unpublished tables)

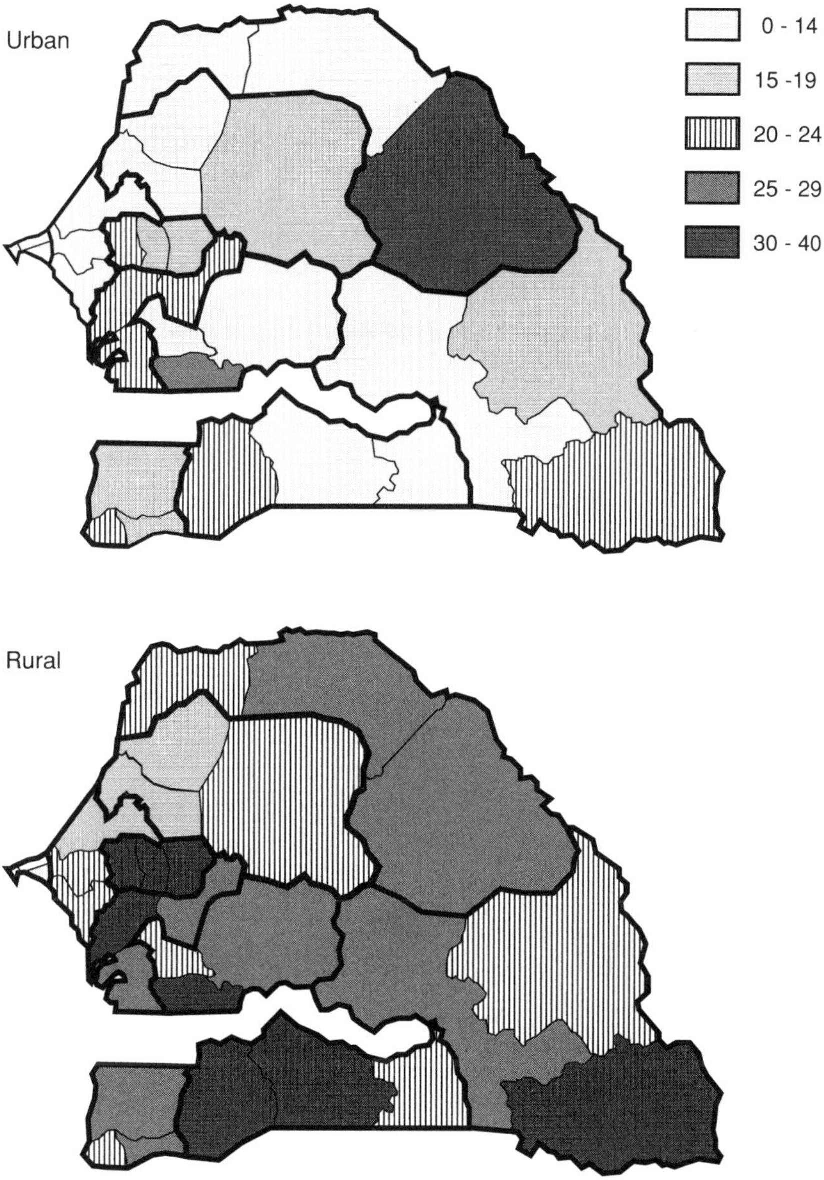

FIGURE 5-6 Departmental variations in annual mortality rate (per thousand) of children aged 1-4 years in rural and urban areas, 1987-1988. SOURCE: Unpublished tables, 1988 census.

in 1987 and 1988 because of the probable decrease in mortality from a number of infectious diseases due to increases in the proportion of children vaccinated. For example, measles must have diminished throughout Senegal during these years, following the accelerated EPI in 1986-1987.

The relatively low rural mortality rate in the department of Bakel, which stands out as an exception in the south, may be the result of the relative wealth of Soninke villages, which make up a major part of the department's population and which receive earnings from migrant workers abroad. A portion of such remittances is invested in dispensaries and medicines (Condé and Diagne, 1986).

The low rural mortality in the department of Oussouye, again an exception in the south, is corroborated by the Mlomp study [10], which showed in particular a very low level of malaria-caused mortality linked to the antimalaria program implemented by the private dispensary in this rural area (Pison et al., 1993). The abundance of dispensaries in this department probably contributes to its low child mortality as well. The department of Kaolack, although located in the south, also enjoys low rural mortality, which is associated with its proximity to a major town, Kaolack, and thus with better-than-average access to health care, despite its high incidence of mosquitos and its relatively poor sanitation.

Age and Sex Patterns in Child Mortality

Age Patterns

Senegal has been noted for having an unusual age pattern of child mortality, with very high mortality for the ages 1-5 and comparatively low mortality before age 1. This pattern was noted by Cantrelle (1969) on the basis of data from the Niakhar/Ngayokhème population study [11], and has been confirmed by national-level surveys since.[2] In the 1960s and 1970s, the probability of dying between the ages of 1 and 5 (${}_4q_1$) was 50 percent higher than the probability of dying in the first year of life, though in the 1980s, ${}_4q_1$ declined more rapidly than ${}_1q_0$, so that the two rates were equal around 1990. Table 5-6 shows estimates of ${}_1q_0$ and ${}_4q_1$ for Senegal as a whole and from a variety of subnational studies. Figure 5-7 compares the infant and child mortality patterns with the historical patterns embodied in the Coale-Demeny (1983) model life tables, plotting ${}_4q_1$ against ${}_1q_0$. The unusual nature of the Senegalese age pattern of child mortality is immediately evident, as is the recent convergence toward the historical norms.

The tendency of ${}_4q_1$ to fall more rapidly than ${}_1q_0$ is encountered everywhere. For example, in Dakar, which had experienced a pronounced decrease in mortality since the beginning of the century, ${}_1q_0$ and ${}_4q_1$ were already low during the 1960s: ${}_1q_0$ was 58 per 1,000 in 1973, while ${}_4q_1$ was

75 per 1,000. Thereafter, ${}_1q_0$ stagnated, at least until 1980, while ${}_4q_1$ continued its decline by falling almost 50 percent between 1973 and 1988 (see Table 5-6). The same type of change occurred in Saint-Louis (Table 5-6 and Figure 5-7). The period 1955-1988 saw a steady decline in both ${}_1q_0$ and ${}_4q_1$, but the pace of the decline was more rapid for ${}_4q_1$ than for ${}_1q_0$. As a result, from being higher than ${}_1q_0$, ${}_4q_1$ became lower. The decline in ${}_4q_1$ accelerated in the middle of the 1980s.

Niakhar/Ngayokhème and Bandafassi (Table 5-6 and Figure 5-7) show the same type of change over time in rural areas. The decline of ${}_4q_1$ in the mid-1980s was particularly rapid, especially in Bandafassi. The Mlomp rural area is an exception to the general pattern (see Table 5-6 and Figure 5-7). There, the reduction of ${}_1q_0$ preceded and occurred more rapidly than that of ${}_4q_1$.

Table 5-7 shows the changes in age-specific mortality rates over time for several rural areas with greater age detail. Until the mid-1980s, mortality rates were higher between ages 6 months and 1 year than between ages 1 and 5 months and remained high until age 24 months. This increase in risk, especially well-defined in Niakhar/Ngayokhème, but present virtually everywhere else, decreased or disappeared altogether beginning in the mid-1980s.

High mortality for ages 1-4 has been attributed to a combination of three factors: a relatively high incidence of infectious diseases, poor climate, and widespread malnutrition. Because of their seasonal or epidemic character in this country, malaria and measles are particularly problematic.

The epidemiological patterns of measles are unique, especially in rural areas. First, the transmission of measles is seasonal; transmission is highest at the end of the dry season, when most of the migrations occur and when the climate favors transmission. Second, because the density of the population is low in rural areas, the population is grouped in villages distant from one another, so the disease is epidemic. For several years, there may be no measles cases, and then an epidemic occurs and affects many children, nearly all those born since the last epidemic. As a result, children tend to get measles when they are rather old. Third, the average family size is large, which favors secondary transmission of the disease (between siblings or children living in the same family). Such transmissions are associated with increased severity and higher case fatality ratios.

Child mortality (for ages 1-4) is also high due to malaria. Due to the climate, its transmission is also seasonal. A short rainy season, during which malaria is transmitted, alternates with a long dry season, during which the transmission is interrupted. Children tend to be infected for the first time at a higher age than if the rate of transmission was the same throughout the year.

The disappearance of this pattern of relatively high mortality for ages

1-4 in the late 1980s is related to health programs that focused on these diseases, including, in particular, measles immunization and antimalaria chemoprophylaxis. These programs were instituted earlier and were more effective than programs focused on improved pregnancy follow-up and delivery conditions, which affect primarily early mortality before 6 months of age. This fact explains the more rapid decline in $_4q_1$ than in $_1q_0$. The particular situation of Mlomp, where pregnancy monitoring and delivery in

TABLE 5-6 Age Pattern of Child Mortality: National- and Regional-Level Variation and Change, 1955-1992

Level and Year or Period	$_1q_0$ per 1,000	$_4q_1$ per 1,000	$_5q_0$ per 1,000
National Level			
1963-1967[a]	119	198	293
1968-1972[a]	123	183	283
1970[b]	102	199	281
1971-1975[c]	120	189	287
1973-1977[a]	112	170	262
1976-1980[c]	96	155	236
1978[d]	94	149	229
1978-1982[e]	90	119	199
1981-1985[c]	86	114	191
1983-1987[e]	84	109	185
1987-1988[f]	—	83	—
1988-1992[e]	68	68	131
Dakar			
1973	58	75	128
1980	60	43	101
1987-1988	—	36	—
Saint-Louis			
1955-1959	124	142	249
1960-1964	117	136	237
1965-1969	109	112	209
1970-1974	101	112	202
1975-1979	82	85	160
1980-1985	73	65	133
1986-1988	42	24	66
Ngayokhème			
1963-1967	223	340	485
1968-1972	214	342	480
1973-1977	182	291	421
1978-1980	167	242	369
1984-1986	101	202	282
1987-1991	104	142	230

TABLE 5-6 continued

Level and Year or Period	$_1q_0$ per 1,000	$_4q_1$ per 1,000	$_5q_0$ per 1,000
Bandafassi			
1970-1985	197	202	360
1986-1992	140	131	253
Mlomp			
1930-1964	168	225	355
1965-1974	86	141	215
1975-1984	56	97	148
1985-1991	50	71	112

NOTE: See Appendix A for description of surveys.

[a]WFS
[b]1970-1971 NDS
[c]DHS-I
[d]1978-1979 survey
[e]DHS-II
[f]1988 census

SOURCES: National level: 1970-1971 NDS (Cantrelle et al., 1986); 1978-1979 survey (Cantrelle et al., 1986); 1988 census (unpublished tables); WFS (Rutstein, 1983); DHS-I (Ndiaye et al., 1988); DHS-II (Ndiaye et al., 1994). Sub-National level: Dakar: Cantrelle et al. (1986); Saint-Louis: Diop (1990); Ngayokhème: 1963-1980: Cantrelle et al. (1986); 1984-1991: Projet Niakhar (1992); Bandafassi: Pison and Desgrées du Loû (1993); Mlomp: Pison et al. (1993)

maternity units was expanded relatively early, before the other health programs were expanded, shows the reverse effect—a reduction in $_1q_0$ that occurred earlier and more rapidly than that in $_4q_1$. A portion of early deaths was thus eliminated well before the other health programs had the time to produce an effect on later deaths.

Sex-Related Differences in Mortality

The national surveys, the 1978 WFS, 1986 DHS-I, and 1992-1993 DHS-II, and the 1988 census reveal an excess mortality among boys as compared with girls, which appears to increase as mortality declines (see Table 5-8).[3]

This excess mortality of boys could be tied to an underreporting of the mortality of girls in the surveys. However, with the exception of the 1989-1991 population in Niakhar/Ngayokhème, excess male mortality is found in all three of the population studies where we do not expect such underreporting

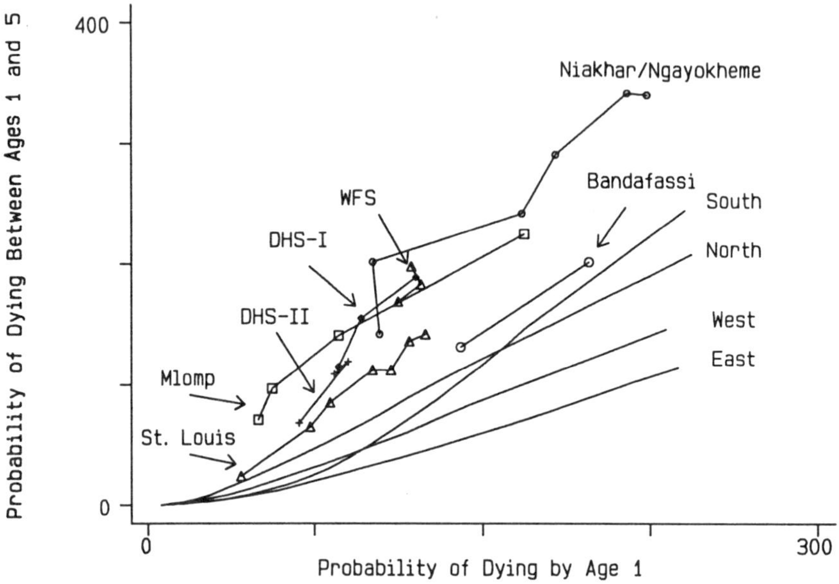

FIGURE 5-7 Comparison of the pattern of infant and child mortality versus historical patterns embodied in the Coale-Demeny model life tables.

to be a problem (Niakhar/Ngayokhème [11], Bandafassi [8], and Mlomp [10]). Moreover, again with the exception of the 1989-1991 population in Niakhar/Ngayokhème, data from Niakhar/Ngayokhème and Bandafassi show a trend toward a widening of the gap between the sexes over time (see Table 5-8).

Several mechanisms probably play a role in the widening of the boy-girl gap, one of which is linked to the widespread practice of vaccination. When vaccination levels were low (before the EPI), girls probably died more frequently from measles (and perhaps pertussis) than did boys. The elimination or reduction of the incidence of these two diseases thus proved more advantageous to girls than to boys. It appears that, in addition to antimeasles protection, the measles vaccine used produces a beneficial effect on child survival independent of the disease itself, perhaps through a nonspecific stimulation of the immune system, and that this effect was more pronounced in girls than in boys (Aaby et al., 1993).

Nutritional Status and Childhood Growth

The DHS-I and DHS-II took measurements of the weight and height of a sample of children aged 6-36 months. These data make it possible to

TABLE 5-7 Change in Age Pattern of Child Mortality in Selected Rural Areas

	Bandafassi		Niakhar-Ngayokhème		Mlomp			
Age (in months)	Cohort 1970-1985	Cohort 1986-1992	Cohort 1963-1967	Period 1984-1990	Cohort 1930-1964	Cohort 1965-1974	Cohort 1975-1984	Period 1985-1991
Probability of dying in 1-month period, by age group								
0	92	84	49	54	50	42	32	31
1-5	10.6	6.5	11.8	5.6	7.8	4.1	1.4	2.9
6-11	11.4	5.0	19.0	6.0	15.3	4.4	3.1	1.4
12-23	8.2	4.5	17.8	5.9	6.9	4.5	1.9	2.2
24-35	6.2	3.7	12.4		5.7	3.3	2.3	1.2
36-47	2.9	2.3	4.5		5.5	3.5	2.5	0.7
48-59	1.5	1.3	1.8		3.0	1.5	2.0	0.3
Probability of dying ($_1q_0$, $_4q_1$, and $_5q_0$)								
0-11 ($_1q_0$)	197	140	210	112	168	86	56	54
12-59 ($_4q_1$)	202	131	354	159	225	141	97	51
0-59 ($_5q_0$)	360	253	490	253	355	215	148	102

NOTE: See Appendix A for description of surveys.

SOURCES: Bandafassi: Lagarde et al. (forthcoming); Niakhar/Ngayokhème: Cantrelle et al. (1986) and Projet Niakar (1992); Mlomp: Lagarde et al. (forthcoming)

TABLE 5-8 Mortality Differences Between Male and Female Children, National Level and Selected Rural Areas

Population Covered and Period	$_5q_0$ (per 1,000)			$_4q_1$ (per 1,000)		
	Male	Female	Ratio m/f	Male	Female	Ratio m/f
National Level						
1970-1978	278	265	1.05	175	176	0.99
1981-1985	198	183	1.08	117	111	1.05
1988-1992	—	—	—	95	79	1.20
1987-1988 (urban)	—	—		47	40	1.17
1987-1988 (rural)	—	—		122	106	1.15
1987-1988 (national)	—	—		94	82	1.15
Niakhar/Ngayokhème						
1963-1981	431	421	1.02	305	291	1.05
1984-1988	298	263	1.13	192	171	1.12
1989-1991	186	184	1.01	108	111	0.97
Bandafassi						
1971-1985	415	412	1.01	248	255	0.97
1986-1992	267	228	1.17	139	122	1.14
Mlomp						
1985-1992	109	71	1.54	53	39	1.36

SOURCES: 1970-1978: 1978 WFS (Rutstein, 1983); 1981-1985: 1986 DHS-I (Ndiaye et al., 1988); 1987-1988: 1988 census (unpublished tables); 1988-1992: 1992-1993 DHS-II (Ndiaye et al., 1994); Niakhar/Ngayokhème, 1963-1981: Cantrelle et al. (1986); Niakhar/Ngayokhème, 1984-1991: Projet Niakhar (1992); Bandafassi: Pison et al. (1993); Mlomp: Lagarde et al. (forthcoming) assess the magnitude of malnutrition, and especially the frequency of wasting and stunting, in this age group. Wasting signifies low weight for height in relation to an international reference standard and may arise from recent or ongoing diseases, especially diarrhea and dehydration, as well as from acute food shortages. Low height for age, or stunting, indicates delayed growth, and may have multiple causes, in particular, a dietary deficiency over a long period, but also episodes of recurrent diseases. The generally adopted definitions of wasted and stunted are being more than two standard deviations below the median of a reference population (Waterlow et al., 1977), so by this definition, even within a well-nourished population some children may appear wasted or stunted.

The extent of wasting in the Senegalese population varies by season. Neither the DHS-I nor the DHS-II survey found particularly high levels of wasting among Senegalese children. The proportion of children aged 6-36 months in whom the weight/height ratio was more than two standard deviations below the reference median was only 6 percent in 1986 and 12 percent in 1992-1993 (Table 5-9). The prevalence of stunting was more frequent: nearly one in four of DHS-I and DHS-II children aged 6-36 months had a height for age more than two standard deviations below the reference median (Table 5-10).

The differences in the percentages of wasting among children aged 6-36 months in DHS-I and DHS-II may have several origins, and it is difficult to know the relative importance of any particular factor. Because the proportion of children who were stunted did not change appreciably, the increase in wasting is most likely due to short-term factors. Unfortunately, since both DHS-I and DHS-II were taken at different times of the year (DHS-I was in the field between April and July, 1986; DHS-II was in the field between November 1992 and March 1993), the short-term factors causing the differences in wasting are likely due to seasonal variation. Other possible causes for the differences may arise from (1) a difference in the measurement methods (of height or weight) and in the errors or biases between surveys; (2) annual variations in wastage due to epidemics (1992 was a measles epidemic year); or (3) the elimination of a supplementary feeding component to the national growth surveillance program in 1989. In the absence of more detailed information, it is not prudent to attribute the more frequent wasting of children in DHS-II to any single factor.

Stunting especially afflicts children aged 1 year or older. Before 1 year of age, children tend to rely on breastmilk and are infrequently affected. After age 1, when the child has been weaned, access to other sources of nutrition becomes important, and the incidence of stunting tends to be correlated with the household's socioeconomic status. Children in urban areas have a somewhat better dietary status than rural children, but the differences are not significant. More important differences relate to the literacy of the mother. Among children whose mothers know how to read, 1 percent were wasted and 14 percent stunted in 1986, as compared with 7 percent and 24 percent, respectively, of children of illiterate mothers.

Causes of Death

Reliable statistics for causes of death among children are unavailable at the national or regional level. DHS-I asked questions to determine cause of death for children; however, a detailed assessment of the quality of these data by DHS staff concluded that they should be used with caution (Boerma et al., 1994). Indeed, in 66 percent of cases of neonatal death and 42 percent of the cases of death under 5 years of age, the mother was unable to give a cause of death. Despite the problems in the data, they show that neonatal tetanus, which was attributed to 14 percent of all deaths, was the primary cause of death among neonatals. Diarrhea, malaria, acute respiratory infections, and measles were the leading causes of death for children between 1 and 4, accounting for 73 percent of childhood deaths (Boerma et al., 1994).

Data on causes of child mortality, based largely on verbal autopsy techniques, are also available from rural population studies such as those at Mlomp [10], Niakhar/Ngayokhème [11], and Bandafassi [8]. Table 5-11 (neonatal) and Table 5-12 (1 month to 5 years) give the breakdown of causes of death in these areas in the second half of the 1980s.

Neonatal tetanus and prematurity are the two principal causes of neonatal mortality in Bandafassi and Niakhar/Ngayokhème. Neonatal tetanus accounts for 19 and 37 percent, respectively, and prematurity accounts for 10 and 26 percent, respectively, of all neonatal mortality in these two study areas (see Table 5-11). These two causes represent nearly one-half of neonatal mortality, which is 51 and 78 per 1,000, for Niakhar/Ngayokhème and Bandafassi, respectively.

The situation in Mlomp is quite different although our knowledge of cause of death is based on far fewer cases than the two other areas. Deaths resulting from neonatal tetanus and prematurity are almost 10 times less frequent than in Niakhar/Ngayokhème or Bandafassi, an indication of the success of the pregnancy monitoring/maternity unit delivery policy in practice in the Mlomp area for several decades. Thus, Mlomp provides an indication of the gains to be expected from improved pregnancy and delivery conditions throughout Senegal. Today, however, the average situation in the rural areas is closer to that in Niakhar/Ngayokhème and Bandafassi than to that in Mlomp.

Three causes of death predominate for postneonatal mortality among children aged 1 month to 5 years (Table 5-12). The most important of these is the diarrhea-malnutrition complex, which causes approximately one out of three deaths in Mlomp and Niakhar/Ngayokhème, and almost one death out of five in Bandafassi. The two other principal causes of death are malaria and respiratory infections, each of which accounts for 6-20 percent of deaths in Niakhar/Ngayokhème and Bandafassi.

The insignificant role of measles and pertussis during the periods under consideration should be noted. These diseases were major causes of mortality in such rural areas in the past. Measles caused 28 percent of mortality among children aged 1 month to 5 years in Bandafassi during the period 1970-1985 (Pison and Desgrées du Loû, 1993). The pronounced decline of measles and pertussis as causes of death resulted from the EPI, particularly its acceleration campaign in 1987.

As in the case of neonatal mortality, postneonatal mortality in Mlomp is very different from that in the two other study areas. The mortality level resulting from all causes combined is four times lower in Mlomp, with lower risk of death from each of the causes except accident-related deaths, which are no less frequent in Mlomp than in the other two areas. The decline of malaria, malnutrition, and vaccine-preventable diseases (measles, pertussis) as causes of mortality is spectacular in Mlomp, and it again reflects the effectiveness of health programs, especially the antimalaria campaign and vaccinations.

Associations Between Socioeconomic Factors and Child Mortality

As with the fertility data reported in Chapter 4, the 1978 WFS, 1986 DHS-I, and 1992-1993 DHS-II allow the study of child mortality differentials by some important socioeconomic characteristics, such as place of residence, ethnicity, and level of instruction. The existence of the three comparable surveys allows us to analyze differences over time. In addition, the 1988 census allows us to analyze socioeconomic differences among departments of the country.

Tables 5-13 and 5-14 show variations in child mortality depending on the literacy of the mother and her ethnic group (Table 5-13), and according to urban or rural residence (Table 5-14).

Differences Resulting from Educational Level and Urban or Rural Setting

In the 1970s and early 1980s, children of illiterate mothers were between 2 and 2.5 times more likely to die before age 5 than those of literate mothers (Table 5-13). Children in rural areas died twice as often as those in urban areas (Table 5-14).

These differences in the probability of dying before age 5 are linked because the highest percentages of educated women live in urban areas.

TABLE 5-9 Nutritional Status of Children Aged 6-36 Months: Percentage Distribution in Percent of Weight for Height in Comparison with the International Distribution of Reference

	Standard Deviation from the Reference Median					
Sociodemographic Characteristic	At Least 2 Standard Deviations Below the Norm	Between 1 and 1.99 Standard Deviations Below the Mean	Between –0.99 and +0.99 Standard Deviations from the Mean	Between 1 and 1.99 Standard Deviations Above the Mean	More than 2 Standard Deviations Above the Mean	Sample Size
1986 DHS-I						
Age (in months)						
6-11	2.0	15.0	65.4	13.1	4.6	153
12-23	8.1	29.5	55.0	6.3	1.1	271
24-36	5.7	25.6	64.9	2.4	1.4	211
Residence						
Urban	3.5	21.2	65.8	6.5	3.0	231
Rural	7.2	26.7	57.9	6.7	1.5	404
Literacy of mother						
Does not know how to read	6.7	26.7	58.7	6.0	1.9	535
Knows how to read	1.0	14.0	72.0	10.0	3.0	100
Total	5.8	24.7	60.8	6.6	2.0	635

1992-1993 DHS-II						
Age (in months)						
6-11	12.3	—	—	—	—	470
12-23	15.8	—	—	—	—	816
24-36	7.5	—	—	—	—	743
Total	11.9					2029
			Normal Distribution[a]			
	2.3	13.6	68.0	13.6	2.3	

NOTE: See Appendix A for description of surveys.

[a]Reference distribution: National Center for Health Statistics/Centers for Disease Control/World Health Organization.

SOURCES: Ndiaye et al. (1988, 1994)

TABLE 5-10 Nutritional Status of Children Aged 6-36 Months: Percentage Distribution in Percent of Height for Age in Comparison with the International Distribution of Reference

	Standard Deviation from the Reference Median					
Sociodemographic Characteristic	At Least 2 Standard Deviations Below the Norm	Between −1 and −1.99 Standard Deviations Below the Mean	Between -0.99 and +0.99 Standard Deviations from the Mean	Between 1 and 1.99 Standard Deviations Above the Mean	More than 2 Standard Deviations Above the Mean	Sample Size
1986 DHS-I						
Age (in months)						
6-11	8.5	29.4	55.6	2.6	3.9	153
12-23	26.9	34.7	36.2	2.2	0.0	271
24-36	27.5	31.3	37.9	2.8	0.5	211
Residence						
Urban	17.7	26.4	52.8	2.6	0.4	231
Rural	25.5	35.6	34.9	2.5	1.5	404
Literacy of mother						
Does not know how to read	24.3	34.6	37.6	2.2	1.3	535
Knows how to read	14.0	20.0	62.0	4.0	0.0	100
Total	22.7	32.3	60.8	6.6	2.0	635

1992-1993 DHS-II						
Age (in months)						
6-11	10.9	—	—	—	—	470
12-23	23.4	—	—	—	—	816
24-36	28.8	—	—	—	—	743
Total	22.5					2029
		Normal Distribution[a]				
	2.3	13.6	68.0	13.6	2.3	

NOTE: See Appendix A for description of surveys.

[a]Reference distribution: National Center for Health Statistics/Centers for Disease Control/World Health Organization.

SOURCES: Ndiaye et al. (1988, 1994)

TABLE 5-11 Neonatal Mortality (probability of a child born alive dying before age 28 days), by Cause of Death: Comparison Among Three Rural Areas: Mlomp, Niakhar/Ngayokhème, and Bandafassi

	Mlomp 1985-1989		Niakhar/Ngayokhème 1984-1991		Bandafassi 1986-1990	
Cause of Death	Number of Deaths	Probability of Dying (per 1,000)	Number of Deaths	Probability of Dying (per 1,000)	Number of Deaths	Probability of Dying (per 1,000)
Congenital malformations	9	12.0	11	1.2	1	0.7
Complications of labor	3	4.2	3	0.3	5	3.6
Prematurity	2	2.8	128	13.8	14	10.1
Tetanus	1	1.4	180	19.4	26	18.8
Other cause	11	15.2	55	5.9	24	17.3
Undetermined	1	1.3	95	10.3	39	28.2
No information	6	—	20	—	30	—
Total	33	36	492	51	139	78

SOURCES: Mlomp: Pison et al. (1993); Niakhar/Ngayokhème: Projet Niakhar (1992); Bandafassi: Pison and Desgrées du Loû (1993)

TABLE 5-12 Probability of Dying Before Age 5 for a Child Alive at Age 1 Month, by Cause of Death: Comparison Among Three Rural Areas: Mlomp, Niakhar/Ngayokhème, and Bandafassi

	Mlomp 1985-1989		Niakhar/Ngayokhème 1984-1991		Bandafassi 1986-1990	
Cause of Death	Number of Deaths	Probability of Dying (per 1,000)	Number of Deaths	Probability of Dying (per 1,000)	Number of Deaths	Probability of Dying (per 1,000)
Gastroenteritis	14	15.7	470	56.5	24	19.8
Malaria, fever	2	2.2	199	23.9	37	30.4
Pneumonia	8	9.0	190	22.8	14	11.5
Malnutrition	0	0.0	176	21.2	20	16.5
Measles	0	0.0	74	8.9	1	0.8
Pertussis	1	1.1	74	8.9	2	1.6
Meningitis	1	1.1	40	4.8	13	10.7
Cholera	0	0.0	39	4.7	0	0.0
Accident	2	2.2	8	1.0	1	0.8
Other	7	7.9	59	7.1	11	9.1
Undetermined	6	6.7	380	45.7	95	78.2
No information	1	—	121	—	43	—
Total	42	46	1,830	205	261	179

SOURCES: Mlomp: Pison et al. (1993); Niakhar/Ngayokhème: Projet Niakhar (1992); Bandafassi: Pison and Desgrées du Loû (1993)

For example, in 1986, among women aged 15-49, 54 percent of urban dwellers had attended school for at least 1 year, compared with 6 percent of those living in rural areas (Ndiaye et al., 1988). In addition, the Dakar urban area probably contributes significantly to heightening the contrast between urban and rural areas because Dakar represents a large proportion of Senegal's total urban population, and mortality in Dakar is lower than anywhere else in Senegal.

Multivariate analysis allows the researcher to assess the independent effect of a set of explanatory variables on a dependent variable, which in this case is the probability of dying before age 5. A discrete-time hazard model has been applied to the WFS and DHS-I data because it permits us to model accurately both deaths and exposure to the risk of dying (see Tables 5-15 through 5-17. (Further detail on the methodology is provided in Appendix C). For example, area of residence and mother's educational level produce separate independent effects. Having a mother who attended school reduces by nearly one-third the probability of dying before age 5, independently of urban or rural residence. Similarly, the probability of dying before age 5 is from one-third to one-half lower in urban than in rural areas, controlling for level of education.

TABLE 5-13 Change in Child Mortality ($_5q_0$) According to Mother's Literacy and Ethnicity

	1968-1972		1976-1985	
Characteristic	$_5q_0$	Ratio[a]	$_5q_0$	Ratio[a]
Literacy				
Mother knows how to read	112		106	
Mother does not know how to read	277	2.5	225	2.1
Ethnicity				
Wolof	254		197	
Poular	231	0.9	212	1.1
Serer	289	1.1	226	1.1
Mandingo	392	1.5	261	1.3
Total	264		209	

NOTE: Results are from univariate analysis of data from national surveys 1978 WFS, 1986 DHS-I. See Appendix A for description of surveys.

[a]Ratio between $_5q_0$ of the category and $_5q_0$ of the first category.

SOURCES: 1968-1972: data from Guèye and Sarr (1985); 1976-1985: Ndiaye et al. (1988)

TABLE 5-14 Variations in Child Mortality (${}_5q_0$ or ${}_4q_1$) by Urban/Rural Residence

Residence	1968-1972 ${}_5q_0$	1968-1972 Ratio[a]	1976-1985 ${}_5q_0$ or ${}_4q_1$	1976-1985 Ratio[a]	1987-1988 ${}_4q_1$	1987-1988 Ratio[a]	1988-1992 ${}_5q_0$ or ${}_4q_1$	1988-1992 Ratio[a]
${}_5q_0$								
Urban	153		135		–		102	
Rural	314	2.1	250	1.9	–		184	1.8
${}_4q_1$								
Urban	–		71		41		50	
Rural	–		164	2.3	104	2.5	107	2.1

NOTE: Results are from univariate analysis of data from national surveys 1978 WFS, 1986 DHS-I, 1992-1993 DHS-II, and the 1988 census. See Appendix A for description of surveys.

[a]Ratio between ${}_5q_0$ of the category and ${}_5q_0$ of the first category.

SOURCES: 1968-1972: data from Guèye and Sarr (1985); 1976-1985: Ndiaye et al. (1988); 1987-1988: 1988 census (unpublished tables) 1988-1992: Ndiaye et al. (1994)

These findings differ somewhat from those of Cantrelle et al. (1986), who concluded, based on an analysis of data from the WFS, that the most important factor determining child mortality was urban or rural residence, and that the educational level of the parents, in particular of the mother, exerted only a modest influence.

The effects of mother's educational level became slightly more pronounced between the WFS (1973-1977) and the DHS-I (1981-1985), while the urban-rural differences declined. However, the disparities among regions persisted during the same period.

This finding appears to confirm in part the analysis of the 1986 DHS-I survey performed by Barbieri (1989), who concluded that educational level of the mother was the main factor explaining the variations in child mortality. For example, for mothers living in the same setting, urban or rural, attendance through the end of primary school halved the risk of mortality of their children before the age of 5. However, Barbieri found that, surprisingly, given the same educational level of the mother, children living in urban rather than rural areas faced a higher risk of death under age 5. No similar conclusion was drawn in our analysis. In both the WFS and DHS-I, the probability of dying by age 5 in urban areas is significantly lower than in rural areas after allowing for mother's education.

The survey conducted in 1986 in Pikine [15], a sprawling expansion of Dakar, further clarifies the respective influences of residence and mother's educational level on child mortality in the urban context (Antoine and Diouf, 1992). This survey gathered women's life histories while recording the changes in their socioeconomic status over their entire life span so as to learn of their situation at the time of each event, i.e., a birth or death of a child. This innovation allows the researcher to analyze the effects of different migration behaviors and changes in socioeconomic circumstances on mortality.

The Pikine population includes a major percentage of migrants, thereby making it possible to compare the migrant children's mortality with that of children born in Pikine. The rate for children born in rural areas was 2.5 times higher than the rate for children born in Pikine. However, Antoine and Diouf (1992) found that immigrant mothers rapidly adapt to urban living conditions. Their analysis suggests that it is not the place of origin (urban or rural) of the mothers that ultimately determines child mortality differences, but other factors, such as educational level.

Pikine provides further support for the effect previously estimated for the entire country of a one-third reduction in mortality when the mother has attended school. However, the education factor interacts with access to clean water. Children born in households that obtain their water from a standpipe have a 1.3 times higher probability of dying under age 5 than children born in households having an inside faucet. When the parents are illiterate, access to clean water does not affect the probability of child survival. Similarly, having educated parents does not lower mortality below that of the children of illiterate parents when water is obtained from a standpipe. An inside faucet produces lower child mortality only if at least one of the parents is literate, and the effect then becomes pronounced—mortality is halved.

The detailed multivariate analyses (Tables 5-15 for the period 1973-1977 and Table 5-16 for the period 1981-1985) reveal that regional differences, in particular the lower mortality in the western grand region in relation to the three other grand regions, stem from the larger urban population and higher level of maternal education in the former. However, urbanization and maternal education do not fully explain the child mortality differences. Even taking these two factors into account, gaps among the grand regions remain. Table 5-15 thus reveals, for 1973-1977, a north-south gradient, according to which mortality is lowest in the northeast. In the center, mortality is average and at the same level as in the west. In the south, it is the highest. This north-south gradient may be related to the fact that the northern regions are better served with water and electricity than those in the south (see the section Economic Background: Regional Disparities in Socioeconomic Indicators in Chapter 2).

Table 5-16, for the years 1981-1985, shows that small changes occurred in these patterns in 8 years. First, the differentials between the western region and the three others widened. This was the result of a decline in rural mortality in the west (in the rural areas of the region of Thiès, since the region of Dakar incorporates virtually no rural areas) that was more rapid than that in the other grand regions. Second, the center, and no longer the south, had the highest urban mortality in Senegal.

The 1988 census throws additional light on a more discriminating geographic scale, that of the departments.[4] Table 5-5 gives mortality rates for children aged 1-4 in 1987-1988 by administrative departments and rural/urban residence, according to the 1988 census. In the following analysis, we omit the three departments within the Dakar region, since either they have no rural population with which the urban population can be compared (Dakar and Pikine), or the rural population is extremely small (Rufisque). For the remaining departments, rural and urban mortality rates have a correlation coefficient of 0.50 (see Figure 5-8). Within a department, rural mortality is almost always greater than urban mortality, on average by 77 percent.

The contrast between urban and rural areas outside the Dakar region is often greatest in departments whose capital is a major city. Rural excess mortality is thus high in the departments of Louga (2.7); Thiès (2.6); Kaffrine (2.4); Tivaouane (2.4); Kolda (2.2); Kaolack (2.1); and Dagana, which includes Saint-Louis (2.0).[5] It is low or zero, and for some a slight urban

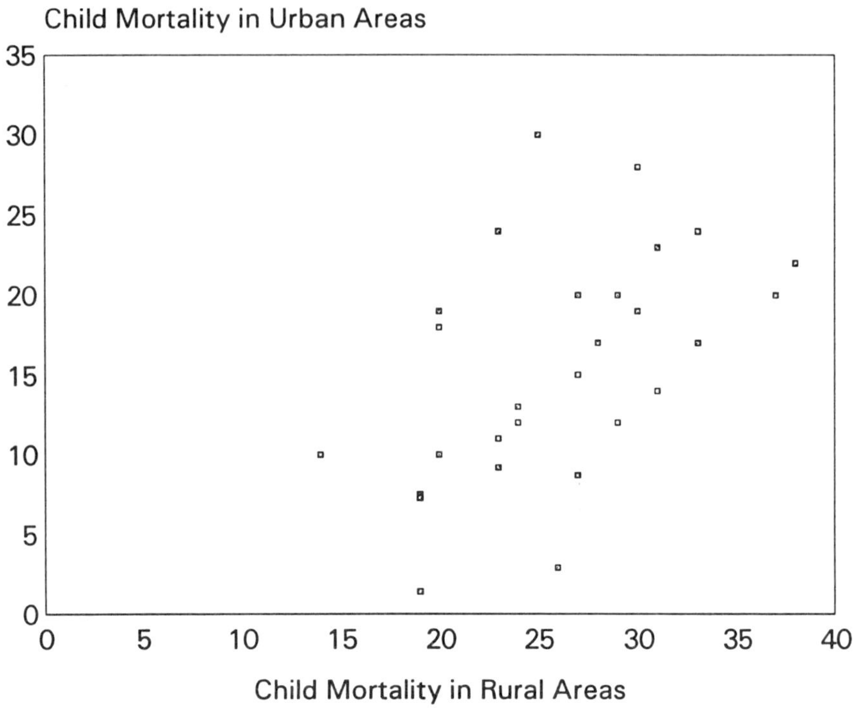

FIGURE 5-8 Relation between child mortality ($_4q_1$ per 1,000) in rural areas (x-axis) and in urban areas (y-axis) in the same department. NOTE: The three departments of the region of Dakar are not included because of the nonexistence, or small size, of the rural population. SOURCE: Unpublished tables, 1988 census.

excess mortality is even recorded, in the departments of Matam (0.8), Oussouye (1.0), Bakel (1.1), Nioro du Rip (1.1), and Linguère (1.1), whose capital towns are merely small cities.

Ethnic Differences

Compared with differences stemming from educational level or urban or rural residence, differences among ethnic groups are neither very pronounced nor very consistent at the national level. However, the excess mortality of Mandingo children in rural areas should be noted (Tables 5-15 and 5-16).

Measurements by ethnic group performed locally as part of small-scale population studies covering several ethnic groups reveal that the situation varies according to region and group. At Thiénaba and Fissel [16], there were, for example, no differences in mortality in 1981-1984 between the two ethnic groups represented, the Wolof and the Serer (Mbodji, 1988). In Bandafassi and Ndemene, on the other hand, mortality was lower among the Peul (belonging to the Poular group) than among the other major ethnic group in the region—the Malinké (belonging to the Mandingo group) in Bandafassi and the Wolof in Ndemene (Cantrelle et al., 1980; Pison et al., 1993). According to Cantrelle et al., the lower mortality rate among the Peul can be attributed to the fact that the Peul are predominantly cattle rearers and thus have more milk to give their children, which raises the children's nutritional status (Cantrelle et al., 1980). But these differences in mortality may also stem from differences in housing and household structure. The Peul tend to live in smaller households than other ethnic groups. In Bandafassi, for example, the average size of a Peul compound is 13 persons, as compared with 22 for the Malinké (Pison et al., 1993). In addition, the density in the Peul villages is lower than in the Malinké villages. Mortality due to certain infectious causes, such as measles, has been shown to increase with overcrowding and the frequency of intrafamily contagions (Aaby et al., 1993); these are more important in large households.

Quality of Housing and Household Facilities

Multivariate analysis of the data from the 1986 DHS-I shows a correlation between child mortality and the type of dwelling, toilet, and household water supply (see Table 5-17). Once these characteristics are considered, the type of place of residence, whether urban or rural, becomes insignificant, implying that the beneficial influence of living in urban as opposed to rural areas results largely from access to clean water and sanitation, as well as to better dwelling conditions.

The relative importance of these socioeconomic variables is not the same in rural as in urban areas. In rural areas, the type of dwelling is the only significant factor among the three. In urban areas, neither the type of dwelling nor the type of toilet is significant, but the type of household water supply is. Children living in households where water is drawn from an inside well or faucet or from a borehole or pump experience a nearly 40 percent lower probability of dying before age 5 as compared with those living in households obtaining their water from an outside well or faucet or a river.

TABLE 5-15 Variations in Mortality of Children Less Than 5 Years of Age (relative risk) According to Selected Demographic and Socioeconomic Characteristics, 1973-1977, Odds Ratios

		Models with Socioeconomic Variables and Regional Variables			Models with Socioeconomic Variables and Ethnic Variables		
Variable	Category	Senegal	Urban	Rural	Senegal	Urban	Rural
Sex	Male/female	1.09	1.05	1.10	1.08	1.05	1.09
Twins	Twin/singleton	1.38	2.28	1.21	1.22	2.50	0.98
Birth order	1	0.98	0.64	1.09	0.95	0.57	1.06
	2 to 6 (omitted)						
	7 or more	1.10	0.94	1.12	1.07	0.98	1.09
Age of mother	Less than 20 years	1.18	1.49	1.11	1.16	1.67	1.06
	20-34 years (omitted)						
	35 years	0.87	1.14	0.83	0.85	1.04	0.83
Survival of preceding child	Dead/surviving or no child	1.20[a]	0.85	1.26[a]	1.19[a]	0.76	1.24[a]
Mother's instruction	Instruction/no instruction	0.77[a]	0.83	0.65[a]	0.77[a]	0.86	0.62[a]
Residence	Urban/rural	0.46[a]	—	—	0.46[a]	—	—
Region	West (omitted)						
	Center	0.99	1.11	0.92	—	—	—
	Northeast	0.81	0.71	0.77	—	—	—
	South	1.26[a]	1.89[a]	1.15	—	—	—
Ethnicity	Wolof (omitted)						
	Poular	—	—	—	0.92	1.10	0.95
	Serer	—	—	—	1.09	1.48	1.10
	Mandingo	—	—	—	1.32[a]	1.02	1.47[a]
	Diola	—	—	—	0.93	1.61	0.92
	Other	—	—	—	0.78	0.33[a]	1.01

[a] $p < 0.05$, two-tailed test.

SOURCE: Multivariate analysis using WFS datafiles, period 1973-1977.

TABLE 5-16 Variations in Mortality of Children Less Than 5 Years of Age (relative risk) According to Selected Demographic, Geographic, and Ethnic Characteristics, 1981-1985, Odds Ratios

		Model with Socioeconomic Variables and Regional Variables			Model with Socioeconomic Variables and Ethnic Variables		
Variable	Category	Senegal	Urban	Rural	Senegal	Urban	Rural
Sex	Male/female	1.05	1.02	0.93	1.06	0.98	0.95
Twins	Twin/singleton	2.31[a]	2.62[a]	1.57	2.29[a]	2.58[a]	1.63
Birth order	1	1.05	0.72	1.17	1.05	0.79	1.15
	2 to 6 (omitted)						
	7 or more	0.94	0.75	0.84	0.91	0.68	0.81
Age of mother	Less than 20 years	1.01	1.32	1.04	1.01	1.39	1.06
	20-34 years (omitted)						
	35 years	0.94	1.04	1.08	0.93	0.87	1.09
Survival of preceding child	Dead/surviving or no child	0.99	0.62	0.96	1.04	0.69	0.97
Mother's instruction	Instruction/no instruction	0.65[a]	0.68	0.79	0.60[a]	0.66[a]	0.62
Residence	Urban/rural	0.78[a]	—	—	0.70[a]	—	—
Region	West (omitted)						
	Center	1.28[a]	1.62[a]	1.57[a]	—	—	—
	Northeast	1.00	0.67	1.31	—	—	—
	South	1.33[a]	1.11	1.48[a]	—	—	—
Ethnicity	Wolof (omitted)						
	Poular	—	—	—	0.88	0.48[a]	0.85
	Serer	—	—	—	0.87	0.49[a]	0.93
	Mandingo	—	—	—	1.08	0.53	1.30
	Diola	—	—	—	1.10	0.93	0.73
	Other	—	—	—	1.00	1.00	0.73

[a] $p < 0.05$, two-tailed test.

SOURCE: Multivariate analysis using DHS-I datafiles, period 1981-1985.

TABLE 5-17 Variations in Mortality of Children Less Than 5 Years of Age (relative risk) According to Selected Demographic and Socioeconomic Characteristics, 1981-1985, Odds Ratios

		Socioeconomic Variable and Variable on the Quality of Housing Considered Together		
Variable	Category	Senegal	Urban	Rural
Sex	Male/female	1.08	1.09	0.95
Twins	Twin/singleton	2.16[a]	2.64[a]	1.55
Birth order	1	1.05	0.74	1.15
	2 to 6 (omitted)			
	7 or more	0.92	0.75	0.82
Age of mother	Less than 20 years	0.96	1.19	1.02
	20-34 years (omitted)			
	35 years+	0.93	0.89	1.10
Survival of preceding child	Dead/surviving or no child	1.00	0.69	0.93
Mother's instruction	Instruction/no instruction	0.70[a]	0.78	0.89
Residence	Urban/rural	0.88	–	–
Quality of construction	Superior/inferior	0.71[a]	1.11	0.78[a]
Type of toilet	Superior/inferior	0.82[a]	1.06	0.84
Water supply	Superior/inferior	0.78[a]	0.63[a]	1.22

[a]$p < 0.05$, two-tailed test.

SOURCE: Multivariate analysis using DHS-I datafiles, period 1981-1985.

Associations Between Socioeconomic Level and Child Mortality from the 1988 Census

The 1988 census allows us to analyze associations between child mortality (measured by $_4q_1$) and selected socioeconomic variables at the department level.[6] But it is important to bear in mind that while associations may suggest, they do not prove, causal mechanisms. Not surprisingly, the correlation coefficients[7] between child mortality and all the socioeconomic indicators are negative; a higher socioeconomic status is related to lower child mortality (see Table 5-18).

In rural areas, the strongest indicator of child mortality seems to be whether households have electricity. In urban areas, however, having a latrine or toilet is the strongest indicator.

Figure 5-9, which shows the association between child mortality and the proportion of households having a latrine or toilet, is illustrative of the

TABLE 5-18 Correlation Coefficients Between Socioeconomic Indicators and Child Mortality ($_4q_1$)

Socioeconomic Indicator	Rural[a] (n = 28)	Urban[a] (n = 30)	National[a] (n = 30)	National[b] (n = 10)
Housing	–0.34	–0.44	–0.69	—
Electric	–0.45	–0.51	–0.77	—
Latrine	–0.10	–0.60	–0.71	—
Water	–0.30	–0.09	–0.68	—
Composite	–0.34	–0.44	–0.75	—
Ever school	—	—	—	–0.66
School enrollment rate (male)	—	—	—	–0.50
School enrollment rate (female)	—	—	—	–0.52

NOTE: See Chapter 2 for details on how the socioeconomic indicators were constructed.

[a]These coefficients are calculated using data at the departmental level. There are only 28 cases in the rural category because the departments of Dakar and Pikine do not have rural data.
[b]These coefficients are calculated using data at the regional level.

SOURCE: 1988 census (unpublished tabulations)

negative relationship between child mortality and socioeconomic status. Here, data for rural and urban residences for each department are shown.

Data on schooling are available only at the regional level, so there are only ten data points. However, a similar analysis reveals that child mortality is negatively related to various indicators of education. The strongest relationship is between child mortality and the proportion of the population aged 6 and older with some schooling.

Summary and Conclusions

Senegal has undergone a continuous decrease in child mortality since World War II, the only period for which data are available. In 45 years, from 1945-1990, the risk that a newborn would die before the age of 5 fell by a factor of three, declining from approximately 400 per 1,000 to 130 per 1,000. This decrease accelerated toward the end of the 1970s and the beginning of the 1980s. A new health policy, which emphasized primary health care and was implemented during this period, may have played a role. The proliferation of health infrastructures (which had previously been highly concentrated in Dakar) in the various regions and the implementation of the Expanded Programme on Immunization (EPI) probably contributed significantly to the accelerated decline.

Acceleration of the mortality decline accompanied implementation of

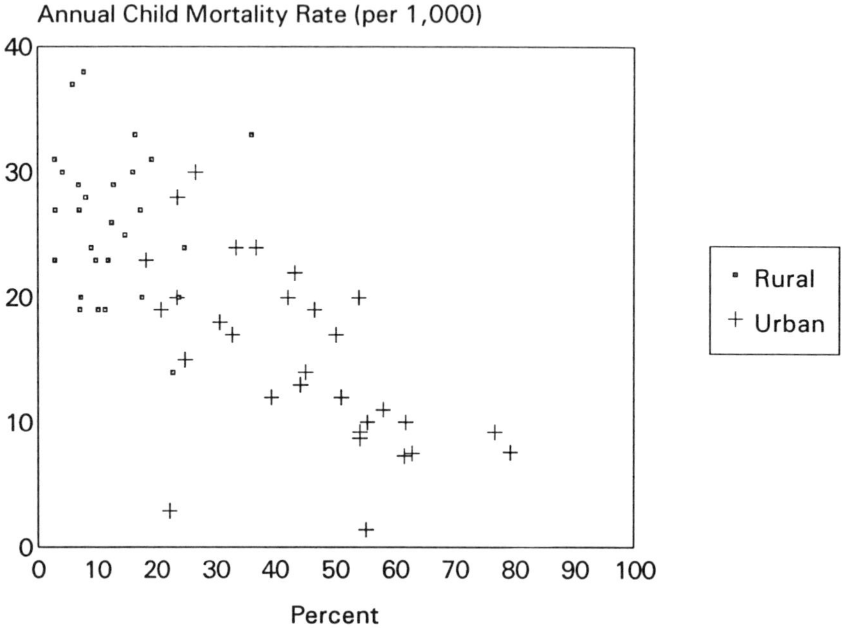

FIGURE 5-9 Relationship between child mortality ($_4q_1$) and level of sanitation, 1988. SOURCE: Unpublished tables, 1988 census.

the structural adjustment policies carried out in the early 1980s, an indication that the policies as implemented did not produce the adverse effect that might have been imagined.[8] Public and private assistance programs set up by nongovernmental organizations undoubtedly made an important contribution in this regard.

Urban and rural areas experienced different rhythms of mortality change. Urban areas, with Dakar in the lead, had already experienced a significant decline in mortality in the first half of the century. Conversely, mortality remained high in rural areas until much later. The decline began in earnest in these areas only in the 1970s or 1980s. This trend, which started in the rural areas surrounding Dakar, gradually expanded to include the most remote regions. Once the decline had begun in rural areas, it spread rapidly, thereby narrowing the gap between rural and urban areas. Acceleration of the EPI in 1987 contributed heavily to this narrowing of the gap.

In the 1970s and 1980s, the principal differences in child mortality occurred according to the educational level of the parents and urban or rural residence. In the late 1980s, mortality in the rural areas was appreciably higher in the southern half of Senegal than in the northern half, perhaps because of the stronger impact of malaria in the former region. Socioeconomic differences, while perceptible, were not very great on the local level, a sign of relative equality of opportunity and of the important role of infrastructure and health programs in the observed levels and trends.

Continued mortality decreases in the coming years will depend substantially on the continuation of health programs, in particular of the sustained vaccination initiative, improved pregnancy monitoring, and enhanced conditions of delivery. Much remains to be done in all three of these areas.

ADULT MORTALITY

Three broad types of data are used here to estimate adult mortality in Senegal: changes in cohort size from one census to another, information on deaths by age and sex in the 12 months before the 1988 census, and information on survival of parents from the 1988 census (see Table 5-19). Further details on each method are given below.

Data Sources

A number of data sources provide information about adult mortality in Senegal. First, intercensal survival methods can be used with the population estimates from the 1960-1961 DS [1] and the 1970-1971 NDS [2] and counts from the 1976 [17] and 1988 [18] censuses. Second, the 1988 census collected information on household deaths in the year before the census, by age and sex. In combination with the census populations, the information on deaths can be used to calculate age-specific mortality rates (ASMRs), and from them all other life table parameters. Third, the 1988 census also collected data on the survival of mothers and fathers, the basic information needed to apply the orphanhood method of adult mortality estimation (Timæus, 1991). Finally, the small-scale population studies [8-16] conducted in various parts of the country collected detailed prospective information on deaths by age and sex.[9] Results obtained using these four sources are discussed below.

Results

Intercensal Survival Methods

A number of methods have been developed for deriving adult mortality estimates from successive census counts (United Nations, 1983a; Preston

TABLE 5-19 Methods for Calculating Adult Mortality

Method	Data Required	Source
1. Intercensal survival methods		
(a) intercensal survival probabilities	Age distribution by sex from two consecutive censuses.	United Nations (1983a)
(b) intercensal growth rates	Intercensal growth rates for 5-year age groups.	Preston and Bennett (1983)
2. Distribution of deaths by age		
(a) direct calculation	Deaths in a year, classified by 5-year age group and sex.	Shryock and Siegel (1976)
(b) growth balance methods	Midyear population classified by 5-year age groups and sex; see 2(a).	Brass (1975); United Nations (1983a); Hill (1987)
3. Survival of Parents		
(a) maternal orphanhood data: Brass method	Survival probabilities of mother alive (or dead), classified by 5-year age groups of women. Mean age of childbearing.	United Nations (1983a)
(b) paternal orphanhood data: Timæus method	Survival probabilities of father alive (or dead), classified by 5-year age groups of men. Mean age of childbearing.	Timæus (1991)

and Bennett, 1983). The Preston and Bennett method, which uses age-specific growth rates in its computation, is particularly appropriate for the 12-year intercensal period in Senegal. However, single-year survivorship ratios were calculated first to explore data quality and revealed systematic age-reporting bias.

Figure 5-10 shows the observed single-year survivorship ratios, for females and males. The ratios are extremely erratic. The points appear to divide into three sets: one set of very high ratios (corresponding to ages ending in 7 in 1976, and thus ending in 9 in 1988, such as 47-59); one set of very low ratios (corresponding to ages ending in zero in 1976, and thus ending in 2 in 1988, such as 50-62); and one set of values in between. This pattern is most unusual. In most African (and other developing country) census age distributions, there is a strong tendency for ages ending in zero (and, to a lesser extent, 5) to be inflated at the expense of ages ending in 9 and 1. In the 1988 census, this overreporting of age affects ages ending in 9, accounting for the high survivorship ratios for ages ending in 9 in 1988, whereas in 1976 the typical pattern is observed, accounting for the low survivorship ratios for ages ending in zero in 1976.

Neither pattern is correct, of course. It is not the case that there were really more people with ages ending in 9 than ages ending in other digits in 1988, or that there were more people with ages ending in zero in 1976. The error is one of ascribing to some convenient age a number of people of surrounding ages who do not know their ages exactly. The change in reporting pattern is inconvenient for analytical purposes, however. For data tabulations by standard 5-year age groups, heaping on zero tends to exaggerate the true age of the population of a 5-year age group (because those of ages close to, but below, the figure ending in zero are categorized in the higher 5-year age group), whereas heaping on 9 categorizes people at ages below their true ones. Thus the change in age-reporting practice makes comparisons between 1976 and 1988 particularly problematic.

To make the 1988 data correspond to standard patterns, these data have been "repreferenced," with the excess numbers reported on ages ending in 9 being shifted to the next higher age ending in zero. The repreferencing was performed by subtracting from ages ending in 9 (and those ending in 4) the difference between the observed number and the average of the four single ages on either side and adding this difference to the adjacent age ending in zero (or 5).

The corrective measures taken into account for the 12-year intercensal period, as well as for age misreporting, allow comparison of the survival ratios with the Coale-Demeny West family of model life tables. Along with the 1976-1988 survivorship ratios from the censuses, Figure 5-10 shows the survivorship ratios from levels 5, 10, 15, and 20 of the Coale-Demeny West family of model life tables. It is immediately clear that the data suffer from

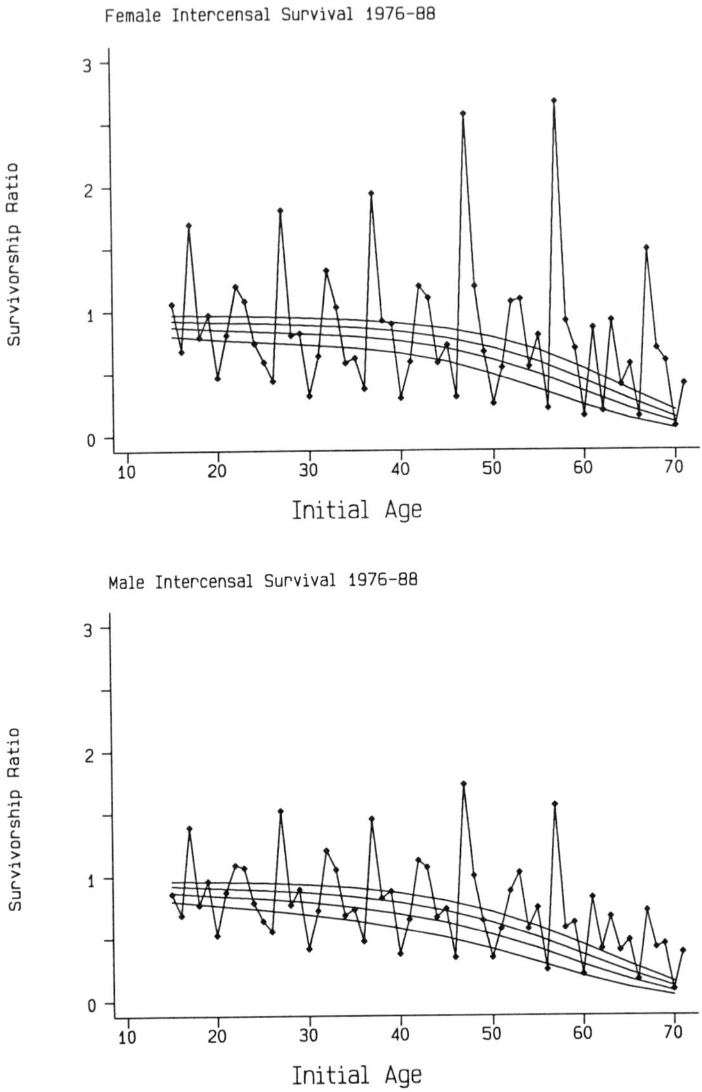

FIGURE 5-10 Observed single-year survivorship ratios and ratios from various levels of Coale-Demeny "West" life tables.

distortions more serious than just erratic noise. The survivorship ratios decline much less sharply with age than any of the model patterns, such that for young adults, the ratios suggest levels of adult mortality in the range of levels 10-15 in the Coale-Demeny tables (e[15]—life expectancy at age 15—in the range 40-50 years), but the ratios for older adults indicate adult mortality well below any of the models shown. Since we know from the various small-scale studies that age patterns of adult mortality resemble the models quite closely, the census data are probably distorted by substantial age exaggeration, particularly from middle age onwards.

The Preston-Bennett technique has been applied to the three intersurvey periods, 1960-1970, 1970-1976, and 1976-1988. Essentially, this method uses intercensal growth rates for each age group to convert an average of the age distributions into a stationary (or life-table) age distribution, from which expectations of life at each age can be obtained. This method, as well as being convenient for census intervals that are not multiples of five, is also relatively robust to local age misreporting patterns, such as digital preference, that are repeated from one census to the next (since age-specific growth rates are little affected by such repeated misreporting), though it is sensitive to substantial biases in age reporting and to changes in coverage completeness.

The expectations of life at each age from 15-55 estimated by the Preston-Bennett method are shown by sex and time period in Table 5-20; also shown are the corresponding Coale-Demeny West model life-table levels. The model life-table levels provide a convenient index for comparing estimates across ages and sexes.

The intercensal survival results are disappointing. The 1960-1970 survival data are not entirely implausible, but the male/female difference (median Coale-Demeny levels of 12.2 for females, 5.8 for males) and the extreme variability in estimated levels across age groups (suggesting massive age misreporting) do not inspire confidence. The 1970-1976 period is far worse: the mortality estimates are uniformly ridiculously low. The growth rates of both the male and female population over age 70 exceed 10 percent per year, and for males the rates of growth of the population over 45 all exceed 6 percent per year. The 1970 population estimate and the 1976 census count are clearly not consistent. Such an outcome is not uncommon with population totals coming from sample surveys analyzed together with those from censuses; censuses have often been found to do a substantially better job of coverage than surveys.

The mortality estimates obtained from an intercensal survival analysis of the 1976 and 1988 censuses are surprisingly high. For both males and females, the levels for ages 40 and below are modestly consistent (in the range of 7.9 to 9.1 for males, 6.1 to 10.5 for females), both between ages

TABLE 5-20 Intercensal Survival Estimates of Adult Mortality

	1960-1970				1970-1976				1976-1988			
	Male		Female		Male		Female		Male		Female	
Age	e(x)	Level	e(x)	Level	e(x)	Level	e(x)	Level	e(x)	Level	e(x)	Level
15	62.6	>24	53.0	17.1	83.5	>>24	73.4	>>24	39.1	7.9	44.7	10.5
20	48.4	19.3	38.8	8.8	75.5	>>24	64.9	>>24	36.2	8.5	38.4	8.4
25	35.2	10.7	30.9	4.9	73.4	>>24	56.2	>>24	33.3	8.9	33.4	6.9
30	27.6	6.6	28.8	5.5	75.8	>>24	49.4	>24	30.3	9.1	29.5	6.1
35	23.1	5.0	29.6	9.4	81.1	>>24	44.2	>24	26.9	9.1	27.4	7.0
40	19.4	3.8	28.4	12.2	83.9	>>24	37.6	23.2	23.6	9.0	24.9	7.6
45	16.7	3.5	26.2	14.6	84.0	>>24	32.5	22.9	22.0	11.3	24.0	10.9
50	14.7	4.3	22.8	14.4	74.5	>>24	28.8	23.6	20.0	13.8	22.5	14.5
55	13.1	5.8	20.2	17.8	60.3	>>24	26.5	>24	17.5	15.8	19.9	16.9
60	n.a.	n.a.	n.a.	n.a.	n.a.	n.a.	n.a.	n.a.	14.5	16.5	16.9	18.7
65	n.a.	n.a.	n.a.	n.a.	n.a.	n.a.	n.a.	n.a.	12.0	18.2	14.0	20.2
70	n.a.	n.a.	n.a.	n.a.	n.a.	n.a.	n.a.	n.a.	10.4	22.3	12.6	23.9

NOTE: See Appendix A for description of surveys and censuses; n.a., not available.

and between sexes. The estimated mortality is very high, implying a probability of surviving from age 15-60 of less than 50 percent. Above age 40, the model levels rise (mortality level falls) steeply with age, exceeding level 20 by age 70. Clearly, the estimates based on the population above age 40 are affected by systematic age exaggeration, whereby people report themselves to be older than they really are (over and above any local age misreporting).

The very high estimates of adult mortality (based on the population below age 40), higher than those from any of the small-scale area studies, suggest yet another problem with the data from the two censuses. It is likely that the 1976 census had relatively higher coverage than the 1988 census, giving rise to the impression of high intercensal mortality. The coverage change could have come about as a result of either overenumeration in 1976 or underenumeration in 1988; the comparisons available do not address the question of which census is relatively better, but merely demonstrate that they are different.

In summary, the available age distribution data suffer from three patterns of error that affect adult mortality estimation: the inconvenient but not disastrous preference for ages ending in certain digits, with the unusual wrinkle of a preference for ages ending in 9 in 1988; a disastrous (from the point of view of adult mortality estimation) tendency to exaggerate age; and a disastrous (from the same point of view) change in census coverage. However one interprets the relative coverage of the various sources, it remains the case that essentially no conclusions about levels or trends of adult mortality can be obtained from the available sequence of population estimates or counts.

Age-Specific Mortality Rates Based on Deaths Reported in the Year Before the 1988 Census

The 1988 census included a series of questions on deaths in the household in the previous 12 months. (The French version of the census questionnaire asks for deaths in the previous 12 months, but in practice interviewers are believed to have asked for events since "la Korité," an important Muslim holiday, the date of which fell almost to the day 1 year before the reference day of the census; see Chapter 4, footnote 6 for more details.) Information collected included the name, sex, and age at death of each deceased.

The data resulting from these questions permit the direct calculation of ASMRs, and thus of all standard life-table functions (see, for example, Shryock and Siegel, 1976). Although it is clear that the operative age preference affecting age at death is for ages ending in zero,[10] the reported 1988 population age distribution, despite its anomalous digital preference for ages ending with 9, has been used in the denominators. Table 5-21 shows the ASMRs, the life-table survivorship column, the expectation of life at each age from 15-70, and the corresponding Coale-Demeny model life-table level corresponding to each expectation of life.

The consistency of the model life-table levels implied by the expectations of life at adult ages is remarkable, especially if one omits from consideration the 70+ age group, which is affected by assumptions about the age distribution of the elderly. Reasonable consistency is not very surprising, of course, since computing a survivorship function from a set of age-specific death rates, and then computing expectations of life at successive ages, imposes a substantial degree of smoothing on the raw data.

An attempt to assess the completeness of death reporting through growth balance methods was overwhelmed by biases in age reporting (see Appendix D). However, the evidence discussed above that reporting of deaths of children aged 1-5 was close to complete, combined with the consistency of the age-specific estimates between the ages of 15-70, suggest that the 1988 death data are of usable quality for ages after infancy. Thus the 1987-1988 life table is accepted as a reasonable estimate of adult mortality for the period for Senegal. Almost 30 percent of males and about 27 percent of females die between the ages of 15 and 60. Although male risks are higher, males do slightly better than females in terms of Coale-Demeny model levels, implying that the male disadvantage is slightly smaller in Senegal than in the historical experience embodied in the models.

Estimates Based on Survival of Parents

The 1988 census included questions for all respondents on survival of mother and father. The proportion of respondents of a given age with mother still alive reflects the female adult survivorship from roughly the average age of childbearing to that age plus the age of the respondents. Proportions with father still alive provide similar measures for adult males. Standard methods exist for converting proportions with surviving mother or father into conventional life-table measures. The methods used here are those described by United Nations (1983a) for mothers and by Timæus (1991) for fathers.

Table 5-22 shows proportions with mother surviving, implied survivorship from age 25, implied Coale-Demeny West mortality level, and time reference period for respondents aged 15-19 to 45-49. The estimates cover the period 1971-1980. Early in the period, mortality was high (West level around 12.5, probability of dying from age 15-60 around 37 percent), but appears to have improved dramatically by 1980 (West level around 16, probability of dying between ages 15 and 60 around 28 percent).

Table 5-23 shows proportions with father surviving, implied survivorship from age 35, implied Coale-Demeny West mortality level, and time reference period for respondents aged 5-9 to 35-39. The estimates cover the period 1974-1983. Early in the period, adult male mortality was quite high (West level around 15, probability of dying between ages 15 and 60 around 37 percent), but appears to have fallen sharply over the period for which estimates are available, to quite low levels in the early 1980s (West level about 19, probability of dying between ages 15 and 60 around 26 percent).

These rates of change in adult mortality in quite a short period are very high, and though they are theoretically possible, the potential role of typical data errors must be taken into account. Mortality estimates based on reports of parental survival by young respondents are often distorted downward; this is often due to an adoption effect, whereby young children, one of whose parents has died, are adopted by a relative who is treated, at least for all data collection purposes, as the true parent. The effect of this error for older respondents is limited, however, because the parent, whether true or adoptive, dies within the respondent's own memory span. Thus the most accurate adult mortality estimates from data on survival of parents are those based on older respondents. On this basis, the orphanhood data indicate that in the early 1970s, the probability of dying between the ages of 15 and 60 was about 37 percent, for both males and females.

The orphanhood estimates combined with the 1988 life table indicate substantial declines in adult mortality. For males, the probability of dying between 15 and 60 fell from 37 to 30 percent from the early 1970s to the late 1980s. For females, the decline was even more pronounced, from 37 to 27 percent over the same period. The corresponding increases in expectation of life at age 15 are from about 48.3 to 50.0 for males and from about 47.0 to 51.5 for females.

Evidence from Small-Scale Studies

Senegal is unusual by African standards of demographic data availability with respect to the number of small-scale, intensive population studies that have been conducted [8-16]. Data from three of these studies are discussed here. The earliest such population study was established in the arrondissement of Niakhar [11] in 1962[11]; Bandafassi [8], in eastern Senegal, has been observed since 1970, and Mlomp [10], in the south, has been under observation since 1984. All three areas provide mortality information collected longitudinally, typically by annual rounds of data collection and are thus less prone than retrospective data to omission, misplacement of events in time, and event-related age misreporting. On the other hand, the populations under observation are quite small, so it is not possible to follow trends closely, at least in adult mortality. Nor can these local-area mortality measures be regarded as representative of Senegal as a whole. However,

TABLE 5-21 Adult Mortality Indicators, 1988 Census: Deaths in Last 12 Months

Age	Deaths 1987-1988	Population 1988	Population 1976	Mid-Year Population 1987-1988[a]	ASMR	l(x)[b]	$_5L_x$[c]	e(x)[d]	"West" Level
Males									
15-19	1,214	333,468	246,856	329,344	.00369	.8335	4.1309	50.01	16.9
20-24	1,130	260,066	202,963	257,416	.00439	.8183	4.0486	45.89	17.1
25-29	1,092	239,588	170,075	236,212	.00462	.8005	3.9585	41.85	17.2
30-34	1,169	181,011	128,383	178,454	.00655	.7822	3.8505	37.77	17.3
35-39	900	158,738	121,084	156,971	.00573	.7570	3.7335	33.94	17.7
40-44	963	105,298	107,486	105,398	.00914	.7356	3.5990	29.85	17.8
45-49	837	106,186	94,850	105,697	.00792	.7027	3.4479	26.13	18.4
50-54	1,160	83,553	77,424	83,296	.01393	.6754	3.2677	22.08	18.1
55-59	1,042	79,531	65,454	78,895	.01321	.6299	3.0525	18.48	18.3
60-64	1,683	58,463	55,569	58,345	.02885	.5895	2.7568	14.57	16.7
65-69	1,233	51,690	35,135	50,870	.02424	.5100	2.4098	11.44	16.0
70+	9,277	70,302	70,882	70,331	.13190	.4516	3.4237[e]	7.58	9.3
unknown		—	5,209						

Females										
15-19	1,269	376,720	264,355	371,215	.00342	.8619	4.2744	51.60	16.0
20-24	1,194	299,951	224,342	296,354	.00403	.8473	4.1958	47.44	16.1
25-29	1,197	292,445	202,120	287,989	.00416	.8304	4.1108	43.36	16.1
30-34	1,226	198,166	154,403	196,123	.00625	.8133	4.0063	39.21	16.0
35-39	995	180,976	136,742	178,882	.00556	.7882	3.8893	35.38	16.3
40-44	932	113,623	117,486	113,786	.00819	.7666	3.7592	31.30	16.3
45-49	787	113,075	89,241	111,969	.00703	.7358	3.6181	27.50	16.6
50-54	1,086	80,670	74,150	80,390	.01351	.7104	3.4404	23.39	16.3
55-59	846	80,400	52,797	79,006	.01071	.6639	3.2363	19.85	16.9
60-64	1,348	49,944	49,591	49,931	.02700	.6292	2.9548	15.80	15.7
65-69	838	46,281	27,586	45,296	.01850	.5495	2.6305	12.72	16.2
70+	8,035	70,069	66,794	69,906	.11494	.5008	4.3571	8.70	11.1
unknown		—	2,302						

NOTE: Probability of dying, 15-60, ${}_{45}q_{15}$ (= 1 - l(60)/l(15)) = .293 for males and .270 for females.

[a]Computed by calculating age-specific growth rate, reducing 1988 population by half year's growth.
[b]Separation factor of 2.6 used throughout; ${}_5q_x = 5 * {}_5ASMR_x / (1 + (5 - 2.6) * {}_5ASMR_x)$.
[c]${}_5L_x = 2.6 * l(x) + 2.4 * l(x + 5)$.
[d]$e(x) = \Sigma^w_x \, {}_5L_x / l_x$.
[e]$L(70+) = l(70+) / {}_wASMR_{70+}$.

SOURCE: 1988 census (unpublished tables); Coale and Demeny (1983)

TABLE 5-22 Adult Female Mortality Estimated from Survival of Mother, 1971-1980

Age	N	Proportion with Mother Alive	l(25+N)/ l(25)	Mortality Level	Reference Date
15-19	20	0.9034	0.8940	16.1	1980.6
20-24	25	0.8577	0.8491	15.6	1978.7
25-29	30	0.7825	0.7751	14.4	1977.0
30-34	35	0.7076	0.7011	14.1	1975.6
35-39	40	0.5793	0.5688	12.6	1974.0
40-44	45	0.4665	0.4474	12.3	1972.8
45-49	50	0.3466	0.3131	12.3	1971.7

SOURCE: Coale and Demeny (1983); 1988 census (unpublished tabulations)

age patterns of mortality and broad patterns of change over time may well reflect a wider reality than the areas themselves.

Table 5-24 shows the Coale-Demeny West model life-table levels implied by the expectation of life at each age from 15-75 for the life tables from Ngayokhème (1963-1981), Niakhar-II (1984-1991), Bandafassi (1971-1991), and Mlomp (1985-1990). Figure 5-11 plots age- and sex-specific mortality rates against the rates from the four regional families of the Coale-Demeny (1983) model life-table systems, the model life-table levels being selected on the basis of the expectation of life at birth of the observed tables. Although the observed mortality rates fluctuate somewhat, no doubt because of the small numbers of observations, in most cases they track the West family mortality pattern fairly closely. The exception is the 1963-1981 Niakhar/Ngayokhème life table, which has clearly lower mortality in old age, given the level in early and middle age, than any of the model families. The life table also has lower rates in old age than the later 1984-1991 life table for Niakhar/Ngayokhème, despite substantially higher rates at earlier ages. Rather than assume that mortality at advanced ages increased while mortality at younger ages fell, and that the initial mortality pattern was very different from model patterns, it is concluded that the Ngayokhème pattern is affected by considerable exaggeration of age at initial data collection. Such exaggeration means mortality rates that appear to be for, say, those aged 60 are actually for, say, those aged 50, thus giving the appearance of low older-age mortality.

Although the mortality levels implied by the expectations of life rise at old ages in most of the tables, consistent with continued effects of age exaggeration, the levels at younger ages are reasonably consistent, with only two exceptions. Thus between ages 15 and 50, the male e(x) values fall in the range of Coale-Demeny West levels 16.7 to 18.1 for Niakhar-II

TABLE 5-23 Adult Male Mortality Estimated from Survival of Father, 1974-1983

Age	N	Proportion with Father Alive	l(35+N)/ l(35)	Mortality Level	Reference Date
5- 9	10	0.956	0.9678	21.3	1983.7
10-14	15	0.915	0.9471	21.9	1981.7
15-19	20	0.821	0.8425	18.1	1979.9
20-24	25	0.718	0.7269	16.2	1978.2
25-29	30	0.582	0.6021	15.6	1976.7
30-34	35	0.456	0.4505	14.8	1975.1
35-39	40	0.314	0.2918	13.9	n.a.
40-44	n.a.	0.205	n.a.	n.a.	n.a.

NOTE: Calculations assume mean age of childbearing = 37.3

SOURCE: Coale and Demeny (1983); 1988 census (unpublished tabulations)

1984-1991, and 16.9 to 18.0 for Mlomp 1985-1990; at the national level, the 1987-1988 census life table implies a West level of about 17.5. For females between the same ages, the range is 14.7 to 19.8 for Ngayokhème 1963-1981, 16.5 to 17.1 for Niakhar-II 1984-1991; 10.3 to 11.9 for Bandafassi 1971-1991, and 17.2 to 19.0 for Mlomp 1985-1990. At the national level, orphanhood estimates indicate a level of about 12.6 in the early 1970s, and the 1987-1988 census life table implies a West level of about 16.4. The exceptions to consistency are the values for Ngayokhème 1963-1981 males and Bandafassi males, both of which show a strong upward trend in model levels, from 14.2 at age 15 to 15.7 at age 50 in Ngayokhème, and from 13.4 at age 15, to 16.1 at age 50, to 18.6 at age 65 in Bandafassi.

Although the numbers of observations are not large, two of the small-scale studies provide some evidence of trends in adult mortality. For Ngayokhème, expectation of life at age 15 increases by about 3 years from its average for the period 1963-1981 to its average for the period 1984-1991, an increase of about one-fifth of a year per year if the decline was reasonably steady over time (see Table 5-25). For Bandafassi, Malinké villages have been under observation for 20 years, with expectation of life at age 20 increasing from 36 years in the period 1971-1976 to 43 years in the period 1986-1991 (Pison and Desgrées du Loû, 1993), an increase of almost half a year per year in a heavier mortality environment. Thus the regional-level studies do suggest substantial declines in adult mortality.

The small-scale studies also provide the only information available on the cause-of-death structure in Senegal. Verbal autopsies have been used to try to identify the probable cause of death in Niakhar-II from 1984-1990. Unfortunately, 50 percent of all deaths of persons over age 5 were from

TABLE 5-24 Coale-Demeny West Levels Implied by Expectations of Life at Each Age, Four Regional Studies:

Age	Male				Female			
	Niakhar/Ngayokhème 1963-1981	Niakhar/Ngayokhème 1984-1991	Bandafassi 1971-1991	Mlomp 1985-1990	Niakhar/Ngayokhème 1963-1981	Niakhar/Ngayokhème 1984-1991	Bandafassi 1971-1991	Mlomp 1985-1990
15	14.2	16.9	13.4	18.0	14.7	16.7	11.6	18.9
20	14.4	17.0	13.5	17.8	14.8	16.5	11.4	19.0
25	14.0	16.7	14.3	17.5	15.8	16.7	11.9	18.6
30	14.2	17.0	14.2	16.9	16.5	16.9	11.5	18.5
35	15.0	17.6	14.0	17.5	16.8	16.7	11.0	18.7
40	15.8	17.5	13.7	17.7	18.3	16.7	10.3	18.7
45	15.6	18.0	14.8	17.7	19.1	16.6	11.0	18.8
50	15.7	18.1	16.1	17.3	19.8	17.1	11.9	17.2
55	16.3	18.6	17.4	18.9	20.7	17.3	10.7	17.8
60	16.2	19.3	18.3	17.9	22.0	17.9	11.2	17.6
65	18.2	18.6	18.6	16.0	22.9	17.6	10.7	17.2
70	22.2	18.4	17.3	12.8	23.1	18.0	13.1	20.8
75	>24	20.8	23.0	14.3	>24	18.2	20.3	21.1

SOURCES: Niakhar/Ngayokhème, 1963-1981: Cantrelle et al. (1986); Niakhar/Ngayokhème, 1984-1991: Projet Niakhar (1992); Bandafassi: Pison and Desgrées du Loû (1993); Mlomp: Lagarde et al. (forthcoming)

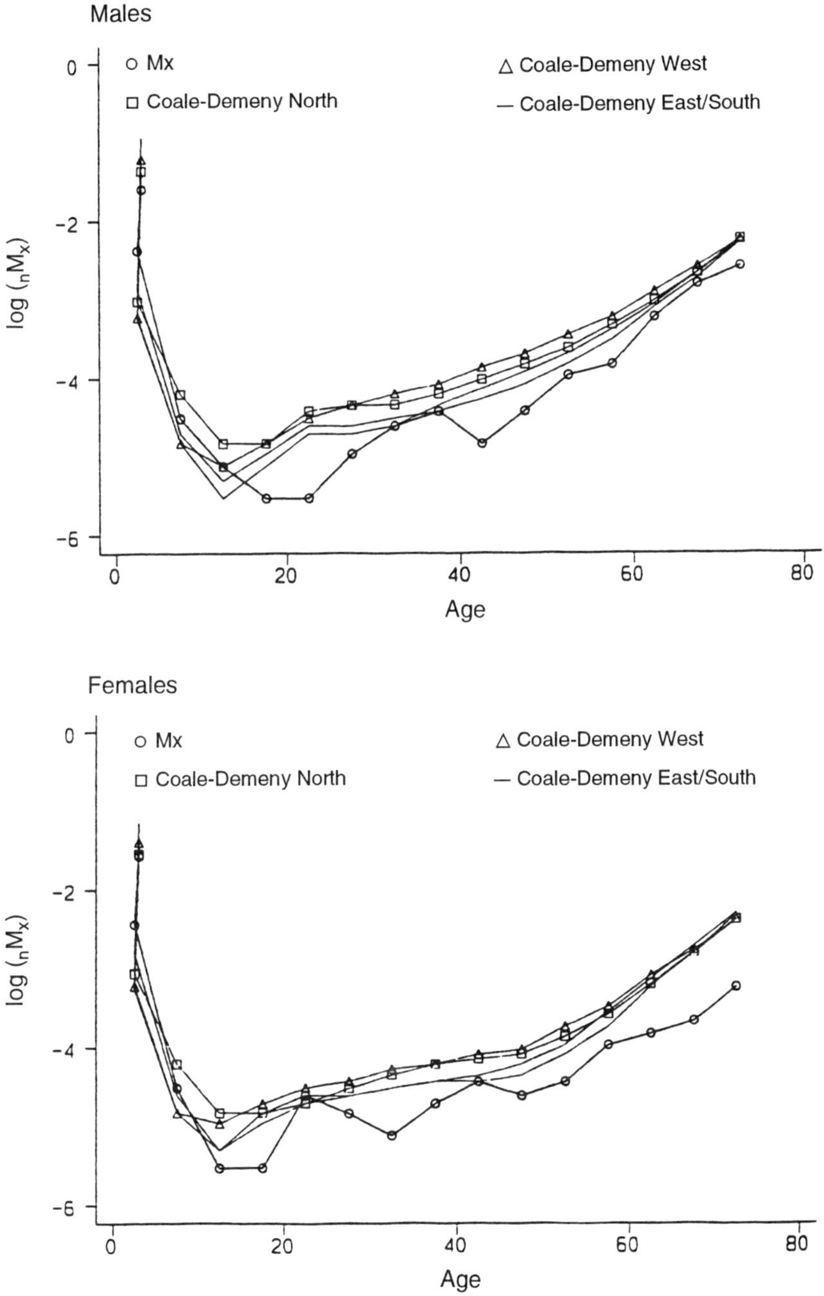

FIGURE 5-11a Ngayokhème life table 1963-1981 versus Coale-Demeny level 8 models.

Males

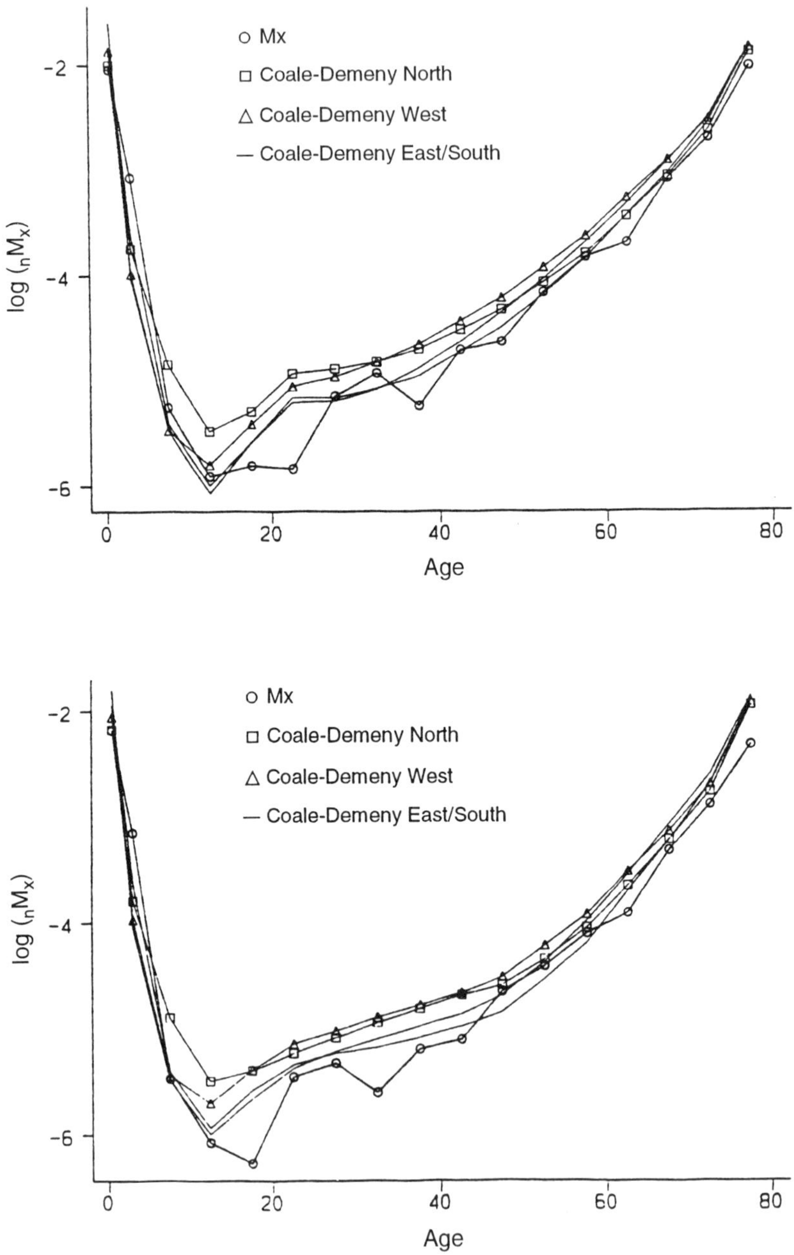

FIGURE 5-11b Niakhar life table 1984-1991 versus Coale-Demeny level 13 models.

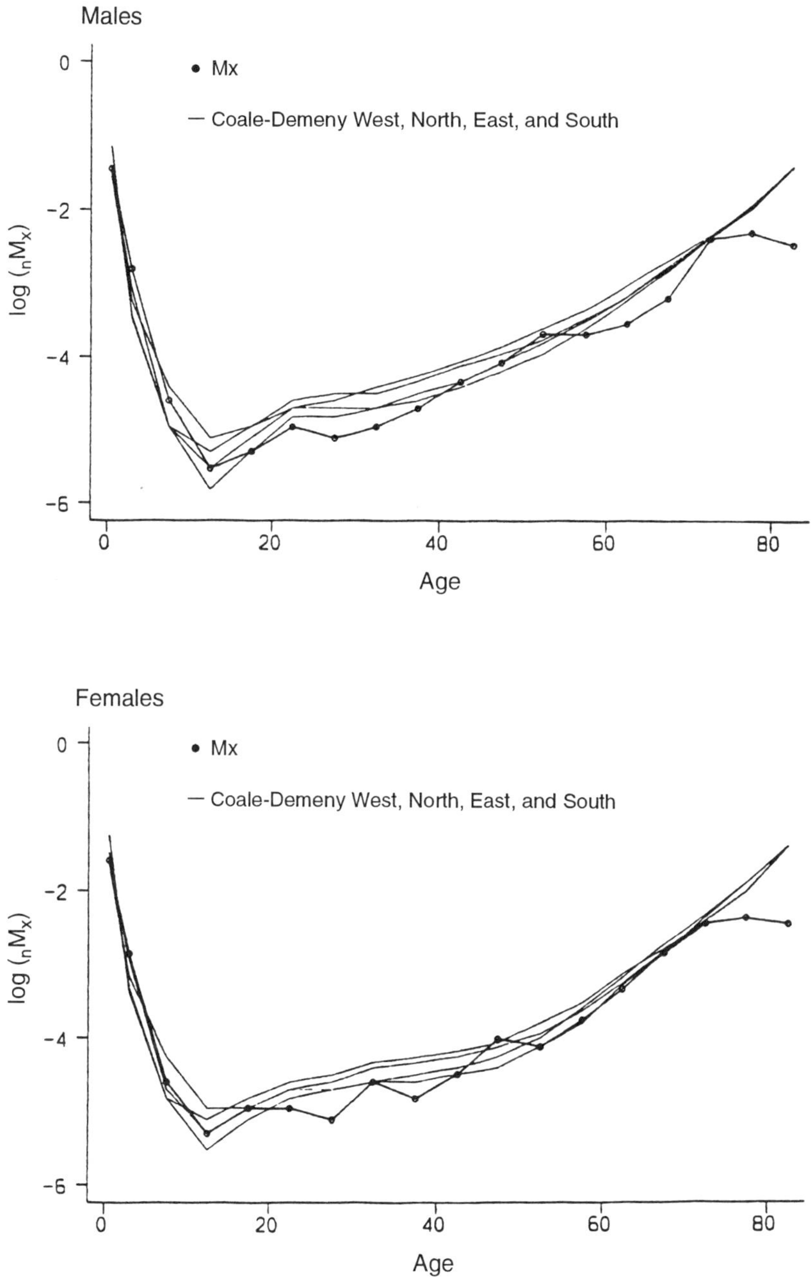

FIGURE 5-11c Bandafassi life table 1970-1990 versus Coale-Demeny level 9 (males) and level 8 (females) models.

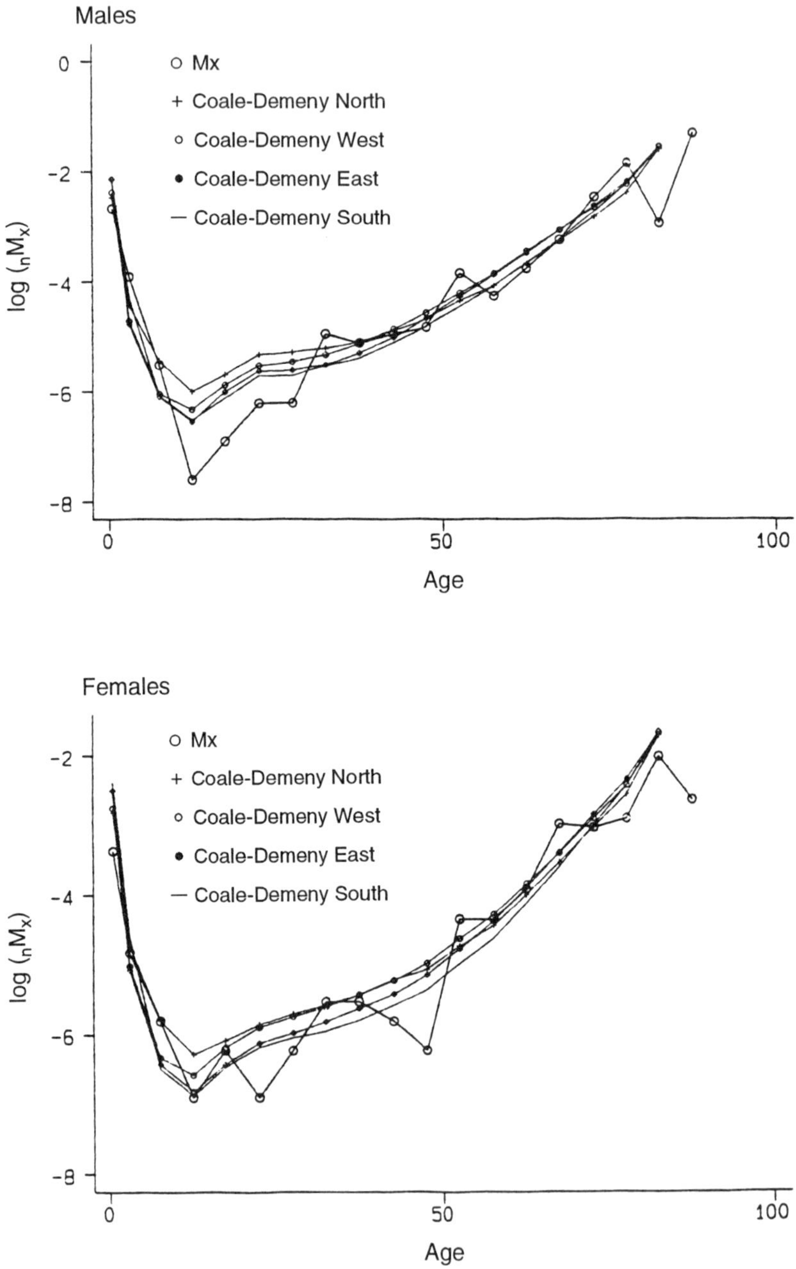

FIGURE 5-11d Mlomp life table 1985-1990 versus Coale-Demeny level 17 (males) and level 18 (females) models.

TABLE 5-25 Estimates of Adult Mortality, National- and Regional-Level Sources

Study	Reference Date	Male $_{45}q_{15}$	Male e(15)[a]	Female $_{45}q_{15}$	Female e(15)
National					
	1970	n.a.	47.5	n.a.	48.5
	1978	n.a.	48.9	n.a.	51.5
Orphanhood, 1988 census	1976	0.354	48.3	n.a.	n.a.
Orphanhood, 1988 census	1972	n.a.	n.a.	0.375	47.1
Deaths in year before 1988 census	1987-1988	0.295	49.9	0.271	51.5
Regional					
Ngayokhème	1963-1981	0.386	46.9	0.361	49.8
Niakhar	1984-1990	0.331	50.0	0.279	52.4
Bandafassi	1971-1991	0.434	46.0	0.411	46.0
Mlomp	1985-1990	0.291	51.3	0.200	55.3

[a]The table in Cantrelle et al. (1986) refers to this figure as e(10), whereas the text refers to it as e(15); the magnitudes of the differences between these values and the e(0)s cited indicate that they are probably e(15)s.

SOURCES: Local data for Ngayokhème, Niakhar, Bandafassi and Mlomp same as Table 5-24); 1988 census (unpublished tables); Cantrelle et al. (1986).

unidentified causes, and for another 10 percent no information was provided. The largest single probable cause of death recorded was cholera, which was a major killer in 1985 and 1987. Maternal mortality was the probable cause of 3 percent of deaths, diarrhea and malaria of 2 percent each, diseases of the lung nearly 5 percent, other infectious diseases nearly 4 percent, and accidents 2 percent.

Civil registration in the city of Saint-Louis has a long tradition of high quality, and deaths by cause have been tabulated for the period 1970-1988. The three largest groups, each contributing over 15 percent of deaths over age 20, are infectious and parasitic diseases, diseases of the circulatory system, and diseases of the digestive system. Accidents account for some 5 percent of deaths among males aged 20 and over, but only about 2.5 percent of female deaths.

Three tentative conclusions can be drawn from the small-scale studies. First, the age pattern of adult mortality in Senegal is fairly well approximated by the Coale-Demeny West family of model life tables. Second, female adult mortality seems to be somewhat higher (relative to the historical differences embodied in the Coale-Demeny model life tables) than male adult mortality, except in Mlomp, where females seem to do slightly better than males. Third, for the areas under study for a sufficient period, adult mortality has fallen substantially through the 1960s, 1970s, and 1980s.

Variations in Adult Mortality by Region

Two types of information allowing the calculation of regional variations in adult mortality are available from the 1988 census: orphanhood data and deaths within the last 12 months. One problem with using orphanhood data for subnational populations is migration: the residence of the respondent (child) is not necessarily the same as the residence of the person exposed to risk (parent). To minimize this problem, special tabulations of survival of parents by region were produced from the census data, including only those respondents born in the same region as that in which they were resident at the time of the enumeration. These data were then analyzed using the procedures described above.

It has been noted that the time trends in adult mortality indicated by data on survival of parents are unreasonably fast, particularly for males. The same problem affects most of the regions also, being especially marked in areas with initially high mortality. Table 5-26 summarizes the regional estimates of adult mortality derived from information on survival of parents. For adult male mortality, indicators of reference date, Coale-Demeny level, and implied ${}_{45}q_{15}$ have been obtained by averaging the results for two broad age groups—a "recent" estimate based on respondents aged 10-14 to 25-29, and an "earlier" estimate based on age groups 25-29 to 40-44. The presentation is similar for female adult mortality, except that the two age ranges used are 20-24 to 30-34 for the "recent" estimate, and 35-39 to 45-49 for the "earlier" estimate. Note that although the age ranges differ substantially, the reference dates of the "recent" and "earlier" periods differ by only about 5 years.

Discussion here focuses on the "earlier" estimates because of concerns that the "recent" estimates have been substantially distorted, but not equally for all regions. The female estimates are for mortality in the early 1970s, whereas the male estimates are for the mid-1970s. There are sharp differences in adult mortality among regions: in the two high-mortality regions (Tambacounda and Kolda), the probability of dying between the ages of 15 and 60 is around 50 percent; in the five middle-mortality regions (Diourbel, Fatick, Kaolack, Louga, and Ziguinchor), it is around 35 percent; and in the three low-mortality regions (Dakar, Saint-Louis, and Thiès), it is around 20 percent.

There is a strong correlation between the mortality conditions for males

TABLE 5-26 Estimates of Adult Mortality by Region Based on Survival of Parents

Parent and Region	Recent Period			Earlier Period[a]		
	Date	Level	${}_{45}q_{15}$	Date	Level	${}_{45}q_{15}$
Fathers (male mortality)						
Dakar	80.2	21.8	0.181	76.8	21.3	0.197
Ziguinchor	80.2	20.3	0.225	76.0	17.5	0.301
Diourbel	80.1	19.7	0.241	75.5	15.7	0.349
Saint-Louis	80.4	21.4	0.193	77.0	19.9	0.235
Tambacounda	79.6	15.8	0.346	73.1	9.4	0.525
Kaolack	80.0	19.2	0.254	75.3	15.0	0.367
Thiès	80.3	22.1	0.171	76.7	19.4	0.249
Louga	80.2	21.5	0.190	76.1	18.0	0.287
Fatick	80.0	19.0	0.260	75.3	15.1	0.364
Kolda	79.7	16.9	0.317	73.8	11.0	0.477
Mothers (female mortality)						
Dakar	77.9	21.3	0.145	76.0	21.3	0.145
Ziguinchor	77.3	16.3	0.275	73.0	12.7	0.367
Diourbel	77.2	15.7	0.291	72.8	12.6	0.370
Saint-Louis	77.5	18.0	0.231	74.1	16.3	0.275
Tambacounda	76.2	9.6	0.454	70.2	6.6	0.544
Kaolack	77.1	15.3	0.301	72.6	12.3	0.378
Thiès	77.8	20.1	0.176	74.4	19.8	0.184
Louga	77.3	16.7	0.265	73.7	15.0	0.309
Fatick	77.3	16.5	0.270	73.3	14.1	0.332
Kolda	76.3	9.7	0.452	70.1	6.5	0.547

[a]For male mortality, "recent period" is based on age groups 10-29, "earlier period" on age groups 25-44; for female mortality, "recent period" is based on age groups 20-34, "earlier period" on age groups 35-49.

and females. Using the probability of dying between the ages of 15 and 60 as the indicator, the relationship is shown in the top panel of Figure 5-12. The strong correspondence by sex is powerful evidence that the measures are not hopelessly biased. It may be noted, however, from Table 5-26, that the relationship between male and female mortality levels appears to depend on the overall level of mortality. In the two regions with very heavy mortality, females do relatively much worse than males, with Coale-Demeny levels around 6 for females as against around 10 for males. For the five middle-level mortality regions, females do a bit worse than males (female levels around 13, male levels around 16). For the three low-mortality regions the male and female levels are quite similar.

Deaths by age reported in the year before the 1988 census provide another, and much more recent, source of information about adult mortality differences among regions. Table 5-27 shows the regional indicators of adult mortality calculated from the deaths reported in the census. The lower panel of Figure 5-12 plots the resulting female probabilities of dying between the ages of 15 and 60 against those for males by region. There is reasonable agreement between the sex-specific regional estimates, though the ranges of the estimates, for both males and females, are smaller than is the case for the orphanhood-based estimates.

Figure 5-13 compares the orphanhood-based mortality estimates with those based on deaths in 1987-1988. For males, there is no clear relationship, but for females a higher mortality estimate from survival of mother is associated with a higher mortality estimate from deaths in 1987-1988, though the relationship is not very strong. Orphanhood estimates have a broader range from best to worst and may be better measures of regional differentials than deaths in 1987-1988, for which omission might be lowest in low-mortality regions and highest in high-mortality regions, thus narrowing the differentials.

Figure 5-14 compares regional estimates of adult mortality with regional estimates of child mortality, in both cases using deaths in 1987-1988. Both for male and female adult mortality, there is a fairly clear positive relationship between child and adult mortality, though child mortality varies more in relative terms among regions than does adult mortality. These comparisons suggest that the regional adult mortality measures are of reasonably good quality.

Impact of Acquired Immunodeficiency Syndrome in Senegal

The HIV seroprevalence rate is unknown for Senegal as a whole. For four cities—Dakar, Saint-Louis, Kaolack, and Ziguinchor—a surveillance program was started in late 1989. It provides an estimate of the seroprevalence rate among pregnant women, which is a proxy for the rate in the general

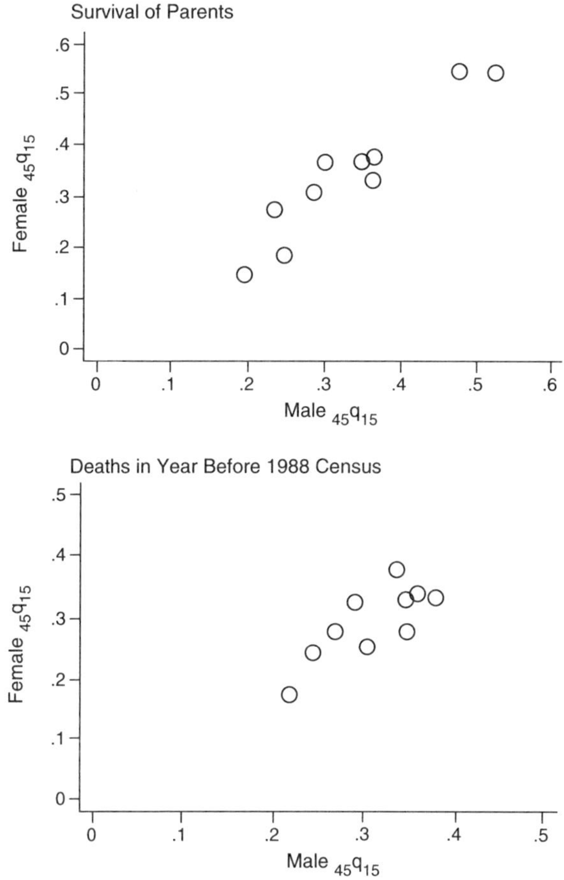

FIGURE 5-12 Comparison of regional estimates of male and female adult mortality ($_{45}q_{15}$) using data on survival of parents and data on deaths the year before 1988 census. SOURCE: Unpublished tables, 1988 census.

population for these cities. For the period 1989-1992, the city of Saint-Louis, in the north, had the lowest prevalence rate (0.1 percent). The three other cities had similar rates, all between 1 and 2 percent: Dakar (1.0 percent), Kaolack (1.6 percent), and Ziguinchor (1.7 percent) (Comité National de Prévention du SIDA, 1991, 1993). Both strains of HIV (HIV-1 and HIV-2) are present in Senegal, but HIV-2 infection is more frequent, accounting for 70 percent of infections among pregnant women in Dakar, 81 percent in Kaolack, and 91 percent in Ziguinchor. The prevalence rate among pregnant women seems to have been stable over the period 1989-1992. In rural areas, local studies during the period 1986-1990 show very

TABLE 5-27 Regional Estimates of Adult Mortality Calculated from Deaths in the 12 Months Before the 1988 Census

	Male		Female	
Region	e(15)	$_{45}q_{15}$	e(15)	$_{45}q_{15}$
Dakar	50.7	0.220	52.8	0.173
Diourbel	45.7	0.346	46.5	0.325
Fatick	44.6	0.380	46.4	0.328
Kaolack	48.3	0.268	48.7	0.273
Kolda	46.2	0.336	44.7	0.374
Louga	49.6	0.244	50.3	0.240
Saint-Louis	46.1	0.348	48.2	0.275
Tambacounda	47.5	0.290	46.6	0.322
Thiès	47.9	0.304	49.5	0.250
Ziguinchor	45.8	0.359	46.2	0.336

low levels of HIV infection among the adult population, between 0 and 1 percent, with a gradient from north to south—the rates being higher in the south (Le Guenno et al., 1992).

Senegal is in the low range of African countries in terms of the AIDS epidemic in the general population in 1989-1992. Data on causes of death are not available, but it is unlikely that the impact of the epidemic on mortality was very high over this period. Even if HIV becomes much more prevalent, the impact on the age structure of the population and the population growth rate are not likely to be very large. (See Stoto [1993] for a discussion of the likely effects of HIV on the population of Africa.)

Socioeconomic Factors Linked to Adult Mortality

Adult mortality estimates have been developed only at the regional level. Consequently, there are only 10—not 30—observations of associations between adult mortality and all the socioeconomic indicators. This shortage of observations makes it more difficult to identify associations between adult mortality outcomes and socioeconomic indicators.

Table 5-28 shows the correlation coefficients between adult mortality and the same socioeconomic indicators discussed above by region. As is the case for child mortality, all of the relationships between adult mortality and socioeconomic indicators are negative. Interestingly, the negative relationships are stronger for female than for male mortality for all of the socioeconomic indicators used. In addition, the education indicators, particularly the current school enrollment rates, show a weaker relationship with adult mortality than do the housing indicators, of which water supply and electricity show the strongest relationships.

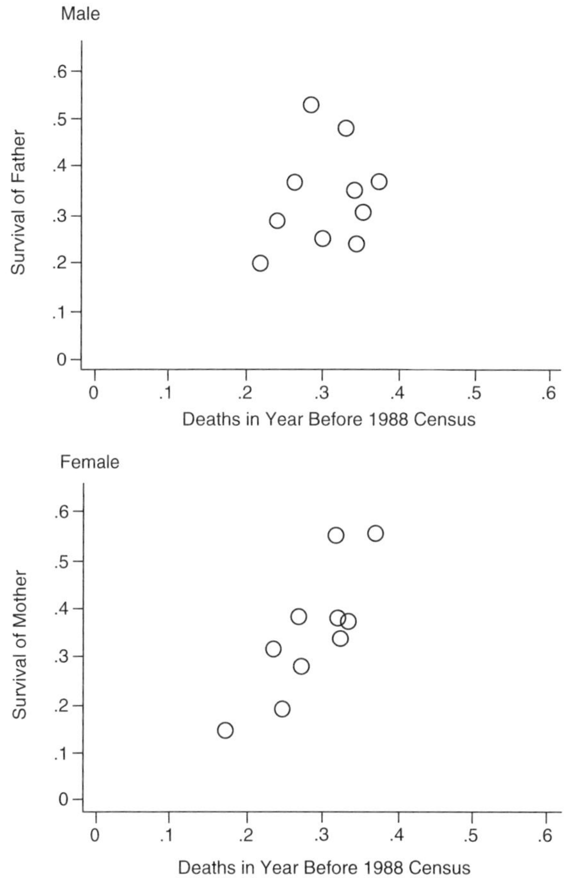

FIGURE 5-13 Comparison of orphanhood estimates of adult mortality ($_{45}q_{15}$) and estimates of adult mortality based on deaths in year before 1988 census, males and females, regional data. SOURCE: Unpublished tables, 1988 census.

Table 5-28 also shows the correlation coefficients between the same socioeconomic indicators and adult mortality for all the regions except Dakar. It is clear that the relatively high socioeconomic status of Dakar, coupled with the relatively low adult mortality, accounts for the relatively strong correlations seen in Table 5-28. When Dakar is excluded, all of the correlation coefficients that remain negative weaken. Moreover, several of the associations become positive.

Both mortality and the socioeconomic indicators reviewed above refer to the late 1980s, and can thus be regarded as coincident. Figure 5-15, however, relates the regional change in adult mortality—simply the differ-

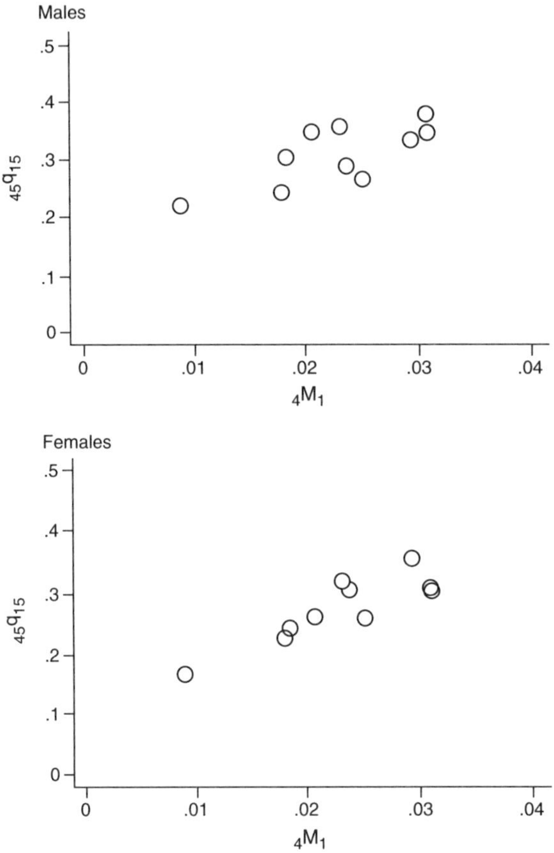

FIGURE 5-14 Comparison of regional estimates of male and female adult mortality with regional estimates of child mortality using data on deaths in year before 1988 census. SOURCE: Unpublished tables, 1988 census.

ence between the probability of dying between the ages of 15 and 60 in the early 1970s and that in the late 1980s—to the change in the proportion of females aged 15-49 with some education. To the extent that there is a relationship, it appears to be in a counterintuitive direction: regions with large changes in educational stock had small or negative declines in adult mortality, while regions with large changes in adult mortality had small increases in educational stock. Regions with very high mortality in the early 1970s apparently enjoyed large survivorship gains, while regions with low adult mortality experienced only small gains.

TABLE 5-28 Correlation Coefficients Between Socioeconomic Indicators and Adult Mortality ($_{45}q_{15}$)[a]; All Regions and All Regions Excluding Dakar

	All Regions		All Regions Excluding Dakar	
Indicator	Female	Male	Female	Male
Housing	–0.77	–0.41	–0.49	0.17
Electric	–0.80	–0.61	–0.69	–0.20
Latrine	–0.70	–0.61	–0.15	–0.17
Water	–0.84	–0.57	–0.66	–0.21
Composite	–0.82	–0.57	–0.63	–0.09
Urban	–0.73	–0.52	–0.00	0.32
Ever school	–0.53	–0.28	0.10	0.38
School enrollment rate (male)	–0.35	–0.10	0.08	0.40
School enrollment rate (female)	–0.37	–0.10	–0.31	0.10

NOTE: See Chapter 2 for details on how the socioeconomic indicators were constructed.

[a]These coefficients are calculated using data from the regional level, $n = 10$.

SOURCE: 1988 census (unpublished tabulations)

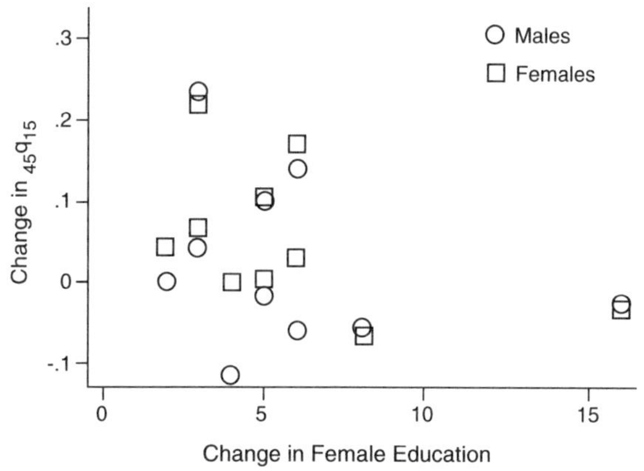

FIGURE 5-15 Relationship between change in male and female survivorship and change in the proportion of females with some education, ca. 1970-1988. SOURCE: Unpublished tables, 1988 census.

Summary and Conclusions

Table 5-25 summarizes the national adult mortality estimates regarded as being of acceptable quality, together with estimates from local studies. A varicty of methods applied to a variety of data give rise to a puzzling variety of estimates of adult mortality in Senegal. Intercensal survival methods applied to the 1960, 1970, 1976, and 1988 surveys and censuses lead to very variable estimates of mortality. The estimates appear to have been affected by changes in population coverage from 1970-1976, and again from 1976-1988, the latter change being estimated on the order of 20 percent. Deaths in the year before the 1988 census give rise to mortality patterns that are highly consistent with model patterns, indicating an expectation of life at age 15 of about 50 years for males and 51.5 years for females, corresponding to probabilities of dying between ages 15 and 60 of about 30 percent and about 27 percent, respectively. Estimates of adult mortality based on survival of parents show sharply, indeed implausibly sharply, falling mortality over time, particularly for males. However, the parental survival estimates of mortality for the early 1970s seem quite reasonable. Female expectation of life at age 15 was probably about 47 years (probability of dying between ages 15 and 60 about 37 percent), whereas male expectation of life at age 15 around 1976 was probably about 48.3 years (probability of dying between ages 15 and 60 about 36 percent).

National data sources indicate a decline in adult mortality from the early 1970s to the late 1980s, with expectation of life at age 15 increasing by about 2 years for males between the mid-1970s and the late 1980s, and by about 4 years for females over the slightly longer period from the early 1970s to the late 1980s. The Niakhar/Ngayokhème study suggests a rather similar rate of increase in e(15) of around 2.5 years from the early 1970s to the late 1980s. Bandafassi data indicate a more rapid reduction of mortality, with e(20)—not very different from e(15)—rising by 7 years from the early 1970s to the late 1980s, though from substantially higher initial mortality levels.

Mortality declines have not, however, resulted in homogenous levels of adult mortality throughout Senegal. In fact, orphanhood measures, which may give the best indication of regional differences, show that these differences are sharp. Adult mortality is highest in the southeastern part of the country, where the probability of dying between ages 15 and 60 is around 50 percent, and lowest in the western part of the country, where it is about 20 percent.

APPENDIX
HEALTH INFRASTRUCTURE AND PROGRAMS

Health Infrastructures

Health statistics make it possible to monitor the progress of the health infrastructure in Senegal during the last 30 years (see Table 5-29). The number of hospitals increased threefold between 1960 and 1988, reflecting the policy to equip each region with a hospital and to divide some hospitals into two in the large cities. The number of hospital beds has not grown proportionally; it has not even kept pace with population growth. Thus, despite the proliferation of hospitals, the supply of beds per inhabitant has declined.

The number of health centers has not changed much, continuing to reflect the policy of having one center for every departmental capital. Such centers are normally run by a physician and are equipped with hospital beds. The number of dispensaries, on the other hand, has increased sharply, having more than tripled between 1960 and 1988. These dispensaries, which are run by nurses, are found throughout the country. They are normally located in the district ("arrondissement") capitals or rural communities.

Maternity clinics, of which there are not very many, were concentrated in the towns until 1977. Beginning in 1978, the primary health care policy led to the construction of a large number of such clinics in rural areas. In 1988, there were nearly as many rural maternity clinics as dispensaries, according to health statistics. In addition, the number of family planning clinics increased substantially in the late 1980s (Osmanski et al., 1991). (See the section Contraception in Chapter 4 for more discussion of family planning.)

Though Senegal's health infrastructure has not always kept pace with population growth (as in the case of hospital beds), it was decentralized during the period 1960-1988 by virtue of hospital, dispensary, and maternity clinic construction virtually everywhere in the country. In 1960, the Dakar region, which had 14 percent of the population, had 3 out of 5 hospitals (60 percent) and the vast majority of hospital beds. In 1988, Dakar had 22 percent of the population, but only 6 out of 16 hospitals (38 percent) and one-half of the hospital beds (Table 5-30). The distribution of facilities between Dakar and the rest of the country, while remaining unequal, appears to have improved appreciably. Nevertheless, health personnel remain very concentrated in Dakar, where two-thirds of the country's physicians, pharmacists, and dentists, and approximately one-half of its nurses and midwives, are found (Table 5-30). Thus while the distribution of health resources in Senegal has improved over time, the Dakar region has remained relatively overserved, with more than 50 percent of resources serving less than one-quarter of the population as of 1988.

TABLE 5-29 Change in Health Infrastructure, 1960, 1980, 1988

Infrastructure	1960	1980	1988
Hospitals	5	12	16
Hospital beds	2,400	3,523	5,179
Inhabitants per hospital bed	1,300	1,580	1,650
Health center[a]	34	35	47
Dispensary[b]	201	376	659
Rural maternity clinic	—	189	502
Population (in millions)	3.1	5.6	6.9

[a]Headed by a physician.
[b]Headed by a nurse.

SOURCES: République du Sénégal (1988); Osmanski et al. (1991)

Health Programs

Before 1978

As noted above, Senegal introduced primary health care in 1978. Before that time, public health programs to improve hygienic conditions and control disease had been developed primarily in the towns, building on existing health infrastructures. Rural areas, poorly served by these infrastructures, benefited only from periodic visits of mobile teams from the Major Endemic Diseases Department.[12] However, the activities of these mobile teams began to deteriorate following independence in 1960.

Numerous programs were implemented before 1978. However, each carried out a specific activity: for example, smallpox eradication and control of leprosy were carried out by mobile teams; maternal and child health (MCH) services were provided by MCH centers in the towns beginning in the 1950s, and growth monitoring and distribution of supplementary foodstuffs were done by the Nutrition and Health Protection Program[13] beginning in the 1960s. Two of these specific programs, the antimalaria campaign and vaccinations, are discussed in greater detail below.

Antimalaria Campaign Malaria, which is endemic in Senegal and one of the major causes of child mortality, was the focus of specific eradication programs beginning in 1953 (Cantrelle et al., 1986). Between 1953 and 1961, an eradication trial was conducted in the region of Thiès and the western part of the region of Fatick, in which homes were sprayed with

TABLE 5-30 Public and Private Health Resources Located in the Region of Dakar, 1988

Resource	Total for Senegal	Total for the Region of Dakar	Percentage in the Region of Dakar
Health Infrastructure			
Hospitals	16	6	38
Hospital beds	5,179	2,565	50
Health centers	47	7	15
Dispensaries	659	78	12
Medical Personnel			
Doctors	407	280	69
Pharmacists	200	133	67
Dentists	58	42	72
Nurses	934	375	40
Midwives	474	239	50
Population (in millions)	6.9	1.5	22

SOURCES: République du Sénégal (1988)

DDT combined, after 1957, with chemoprophylaxis. This program was a failure. In 1963, another antimalaria program, using chloroquine-based chemoprophylaxis (and named "chloroquinization"), was launched throughout Senegal. It appears to have been marked by both failures and successes and to have affected the various regions unevenly, though there was little follow-up or evaluation. On the whole, its effects on morbidity and mortality due to malaria appear to have been limited (Garenne et al., 1985). This program, as well as the eradication trial, nevertheless helped popularize chemoprophylaxis in the affected regions. In 1979, this program ended. Thereafter, malaria prevention was incorporated into primary health care.

Vaccinations Until the Expanded Programme on Immunization (EPI) was instituted in 1981, vaccinations had been administered in two ways. The first was through mass campaigns conducted in successive operations by mobile teams combing the rural and urban areas. For example, smallpox vaccination campaigns were implemented as part of the worldwide eradication effort against this disease. Vaccinations against yellow fever and meningitis were also organized during epidemic upsurges of these diseases. In addition, measles vaccinations were administered between 1967 and 1969 throughout the country.

The second method of administering vaccinations was through MCH centers. These centers dispensed standard vaccines against tuberculosis (BCG), diphtheria, pertussis, and tetanus (DPT), and polio, as well as measles, beginning in 1968. Unlike the vaccinations given through the mass campaign system, these vaccinations were administered on a regular basis: mothers brought their children to the MCH centers on the days scheduled for vaccination sessions. Since the MCH centers existed only in the towns, this system benefited primarily the urban population. The only exception was the rural area of Khombole in the region of Thiès, which had the only rural MCH center in the country, built in 1958 by the Dakar Medical School.

After 1978

In 1978, following the recommendations of the Alma-Ata Conference on primary health care, Senegal reformulated its health care policy with an emphasis on primary health care. Paralleling the effort towards decentralization of the major health facilities (hospitals and dispensaries), this policy led to the training of community health workers and the establishment of village pharmacies and maternity clinics.

The EPI, a component of primary health care, was organized as a separate program. It was given special attention in Senegal, since this country was a testing ground for assessing the ability to achieve EPI objectives in an African country. Data gathered to assess the program's effectiveness are examined in detail in the following section.

Expanded Programme on Immunization (EPI)

Organization

The EPI was initiated in Senegal in 1981. The program was designed to extend vaccination coverage to rural areas, which were at that time not well served, and to improve coverage in urban areas. Its objective was to protect children against seven diseases: tuberculosis, diphtheria, tetanus, pertussis, polio, measles, and yellow fever. It relied on fixed vaccination centers and mobile teams to achieve this objective.

In urban areas, the MCH centers operated as fixed centers, as they had done previously. Their activities were supplemented in the rural areas by dispensaries, which began to administer vaccinations systematically at fixed sites. In addition, the rural dispensaries provided coverage for people within a 15-km radius by means of traveling vaccination teams. Mobile teams were established in rural areas to administer vaccinations beyond the 15-km radius served by the fixed dispensary centers. Vaccinations were administered to young children and pregnant women, the latter being given tetanus vaccinations to protect their newborns against neonatal tetanus.

Since its beginning, the EPI has undergone two major acceleration efforts, one in early 1987 and the other in early 1990. These initiatives led to training and mobilization of administrative and health personnel, media information campaigns (especially radio), and the outfitting of dispensaries with new equipment, especially in 1987.

Changes in Vaccination Coverage

No reliable measurements of vaccination coverage before 1984 are available for Senegal at the national level.[14] In 1984, 1987, and 1990, however, three national vaccination coverage surveys [5] were conducted (Claquin et al., 1987; OCCGE-Muraz, 1990). These surveys, along with the 1986 DHS-I [4] and the 1992-1993 DHS-II [7], supply measurements of vaccination coverage (Ndiaye et al., 1988; Ndiaye et al., 1994).

The vaccination coverage surveys show that the percentage of children aged 12-23 months who were completely vaccinated[15] increased from 18 percent in July 1984 to 35 percent in July 1987, and to 55 percent in June 1990 (see Table 5-31). The 1987 and 1990 percentages probably represent maxima for the period 1987-1990. Indeed, in both years the surveys were carried out just after an acceleration phase, and the average for the period is likely somewhat lower. Detailed analysis of vaccination dates confirms that the increased coverage rate coincided with the two acceleration campaigns that took place in the first trimester of 1987 and the first trimester of 1990.

Data from the DHS-I and DHS-II are not strictly comparable, either with each other or with the vaccination coverage surveys, because of their differing treatment of children who lacked health or immunization cards. However, both surveys confirm the substantial increase in vaccination coverage between 1986—just before the first EPI acceleration campaign—and 1992-1993.

Table 5-31 shows that, in 1987 and 1990, the vast majority of children in Senegal were vaccinated against at least one disease; 92 percent had received the BCG vaccine. The much lower proportion of completely vaccinated children is attributable mainly to the fact that many of these children did not receive the required second or third dose of DPT and polio vaccines, and that some of them were not vaccinated against measles (or received it at an improper age). The same situation was noted in 1986. These discrepancies, of major importance in 1986 and 1987, were partly overcome in 1990, and this contributed to the appreciable rise in the proportion of completely vaccinated children—from 35 percent in 1987 to 55 percent in 1990. Coverage for each particular vaccine (with the exception of DPT3 and polio 3) increased less than the percentage receiving all vacci-

TABLE 5-31 Vaccination Coverage of Children Aged 12-23 Months (in percent) According to the Date and the Vaccine[a]

Vaccine	Demographic and Health Survey[b]		Vaccination Coverage Survey (standard World Health Organization method)[b]		
	May-July 1986	December 1992 -March 1993[c]	July 1984	July 1987	June 1990
BCG	27	84	—	92	94
DPT1 + Polio 1[d]	27	77	—	81	91
DPT2 + Polio 2[d]	18	69	—	69	83
DPT3 + Polio 3[d]	10	59	—	47	63
Measles	20	57	—	63	76
Yellow fever	19	55	—	72	75
Completely vaccinated children[e]	7	49	18	35	55

[a]Measure based only on the information contained on health cards or vaccination cards. When these documents were lost, the child was not counted as being vaccinated. These estimations are, therefore, the minimum. The only exception is the 1992-1993 DHS-II, where when the child did not have the documentation, the mother's statement was taken into consideration. Also, for this survey, the percentages are calculated for all of the children, whether they had documentation or not.

[b]Because of differences in survey methodologies, the absolute rates are not comparable; their relative variations from one vaccination to another are, however.

[c]Among all children, whether they have a health card or not, the proportion of them who have received each vaccination according to the health card or mother's statement.

[d]In 1986 and 1992-1993, only DPT.

[e]In 1987 and 1990, children vaccinated against seven diseases; in 1986 and 1992-1993, children vaccinated against six diseases (excluding the yellow fever vaccination). The definition of completely vaccinated children is not known for 1984.

SOURCES: May - July 1986: Ndiaye et al. (1988); December 1992-March 1993: Ndiaye et al. (1994); July 1984: Claquin et al. (1987); July 1987: Claquin et al. (1987); June 1990: OCCGE-Muraz (1990)

nations. The coverage rate for the BCG vaccine, already remarkably high, did not change much, rising from 92 to 94 percent. The coverage rate for measles vaccine increased only slightly—from 63 to 76 percent.

Vaccination coverage appears to have declined between June 1990 and December 1992-March 1993. The actual decline may be greater than that indicated in Table 5-31. The 1990 measurement is a minimum estimate. In that year, a child who did not have a vaccination card was considered not to be vaccinated. On the contrary, in 1992-1993, if a child did not have a vaccination card, the statements of the mother concerning vaccination were taken on faith. This and other methodological differences between DHS-I and DHS-II make it difficult to draw firm conclusions.

By region in the order of children completely vaccinated in 1990, Table 5-32 gives the proportions of children aged 12-23 months who were vaccinated against measles in 1987 and 1990, along with the proportion of children completely vaccinated in the same years. The regions receiving the poorest overall coverage in 1990 were Tambacounda, which also had the lowest coverage in 1987, Saint-Louis, Diourbel, Kaolack, and Louga. Ziguinchor was the region with the highest level of vaccination coverage in 1990, ahead, notably, of the region of Dakar.

The regional differentials in vaccination coverage were more pronounced in 1990 than in 1987. In 1990, they ranged from 26 percent completely vaccinated in the region of Tambacounda to 70 percent in Ziguinchor, and from 54 percent vaccinated against measles in Tambacounda to 87 percent in Kolda. In 1987, they ranged from 25 percent completely vaccinated in Tambacounda to 57 percent in Ziguinchor, and from 54 percent vaccinated against measles in Kolda to 74 percent in Ziguinchor.

Table 5-33 traces the progress of vaccination coverage in urban and rural areas between July 1984 and July 1987. In the region of Dakar, vaccination coverage increased only from 32 to 39 percent. In other urban areas, it rose from 25 to 37 percent. The strong vaccination campaign that took place in early 1987 thus had only a moderate impact in urban areas. Conversely, in rural areas, where coverage was relatively low in 1984, the accelerated campaign had a very strong impact, increasing coverage almost threefold from 12 to 34 percent. Speeding up the program in 1987 ultimately had as a consequence, in addition to a doubling of overall vaccination coverage, virtual elimination of the inequalities between urban and rural areas. This was, in fact, one of the objectives of the accelerated campaign—to reach all of the children in Senegal.

We do not have separate measurements for urban and rural areas for the 1990 survey, so we do not know whether the additional 50 percent increase in vaccination coverage at the national level between 1987 and 1990 occurred equally in urban and rural areas; however, some speculation can be offered. The acceleration campaign of 1990 was inspired primarily by the realization that the progress made in areas of high population density, in urban areas in general and in Dakar in particular, had been so weak. Consequently, the initiative centered on these areas. It is therefore a virtual certainty that the 50 percent increase at the national level seen in Table 5-32 resulted from the combination of a strong increase in urban areas and a lesser increase (or even decrease) in rural areas. Thus the gaps between the urban and rural areas that were virtually eliminated by the 1987 acceleration have probably reemerged.

The vaccination coverage survey conducted in 1992 in the Bandafassi

TABLE 5-32 Variations in Vaccination Coverage of Children Aged 12-23 Months (in percent), by Region and Year, 1987 and 1990

	Vaccinated Against Measles		Completely Vaccinated	
Region[a]	July 1987	June 1990	July 1987	June 1990
Ziguinchor	74	83	57	70
Kolda	54	87	27	63
Dakar	58	73	39	62
Thiès	64	85	31	62
Fatick	66	76	35	61
Louga	59	76	31	57
Kaolack	67	74	29	56
Diourbel	65	74	34	47
Saint-Louis	68	74	39	35
Tambacounda	63	54	25	26
Senegal	63	76	35	55

NOTE: A child is considered to be completely vaccinated if he/she has received vaccinations for the seven following diseases: tuberculosis, diptheria, tetanus, pertussis, polio, measles, and yellow fever.

[a]In decreasing order according to the proportion of children completely vaccinated in June 1990.

SOURCES: July 1987: Claquin et al. (1987: adapted from Table 2, p. 24); June 1990: OCCGE-Muraz (1990)

TABLE 5-33 Change in Vaccination Coverage of Children Aged 12-23 Months (in percent) Between 1984 and 1987, According to Residence

	Percentage of Children Completely Vaccinated	
Region	July 1984	July 1987
Region of Dakar	32	39
Urban (outside of Dakar)	25	37
Rural	12	34
Senegal	18	35

NOTE: The 1990 vaccination coverage survey report does not give the results by the characteristics used in this table.

SOURCES: Claquin et al. (1987:6 and Table 2, p. 24).

study area within the region of Tambacounda [8] furnishes an example of progress in a rural district during this period (Desgrées du Loû and Pison, 1994). Complete vaccination coverage, which was close to zero before 1987, rose to 45 percent for children aged 12-23 months (and 85 percent for children receiving at least one vaccination) after the first acceleration campaign in early 1987. Coverage declined thereafter, falling to 22 percent of children completely vaccinated (and 44 percent of children receiving at least one vaccination) in 1992, though there was a temporary increase in 1990. In this study area, the main factor determining the variation in the probability that a given child would be vaccinated was the distance from a dispensary. The progress in vaccination coverage was, therefore, quite different from village to village, depending on the distance from a dispensary. Villages located less than 10 km from a dispensary saw improved vaccination coverage between 1987 and 1992. In villages located a moderate distance away, 10-15 km, coverage remained constant into 1991, then deteriorated in 1992. In villages more than 15 km from a dispensary, the coverage rate declined rapidly over the 5-year period, with virtually no children receiving all vaccinations in 1992. This deterioration resulted mainly from the fact that the mobile teams, who were theoretically responsible for vaccinations in the villages and whose rounds in 1987 allowed almost the entire population to be served, did not make new rounds after 1987.

In Senegal, as in many countries, improvements due to the EPI thus depend on the strengthening of activities in rural areas and in areas with the most difficult access through revitalizing and increasing the effectiveness of mobile teams. This high-priority task has been neglected since 1987.

As noted above, the EPI includes the vaccination of pregnant women to protect newborns against the risk of neonatal tetanus. This work was evaluated by the 1990 vaccination survey, as well as the DHS-I and DHS-II. The 1990 survey revealed that, in all of Senegal, 37 percent of women who delivered during the preceding year had received two injections of the antitetanus vaccine (OCCGE-Muraz, 1990). Since it is believed that two injections give 80 percent protection, and since some unvaccinated women had some protection as a result of vaccinations during previous pregnancies, at least 32 percent of newborns ultimately received protection. The differentials among regions were highly pronounced: only 11 percent of newborns in the regions of Tambacounda and Kaolack were protected, as compared with 62 percent of those in the region of Dakar.

The data supplied by the DHS are not easily compared with the data from the vaccination-specific surveys. The DHS-I indicates, however, that among children born during the 5-year period preceding the survey, between 1981 and 1986, mothers received at least one tetanus shot in 31 percent of cases. The DHS-II reveals that, for births during the period

1987-1992, the proportion was 71 percent, thus indicating a strong increase in tetanus vaccinations among pregnant women over a 7-year period.

NOTES

1. The term "grand region" is used throughout this report in reference to the four WFS and DHS regions, as opposed to the ten administrative regions.

2. This atypical mortality pattern has been observed in other sub-Saharan African countries as well, but it was discovered first in the Niakhar-Ngayokhème region in Senegal in the 1960s by Cantrelle.

3. Male/female mortality differentials vary by age. Analysis using traditional age groups indicate that during the neonatal period, males usually experience a higher mortality than females, but that this differential often is reversed later in childhood. The reader is referred to Baye (1994), Desgrées du Loû (forthcoming), and Desgrées du Loû et al. (forthcoming) for a discussion of mortality differentials using nonclassical age groups.

4. Recall that when using the census data, we restrict the study of mortality to the 1-4 age group, excluding those less than age 1, for whom the mortality data gathered from the census are unreliable.

5. The departments of Kébémer and Podor have surprisingly low urban mortality rates, for unknown reasons. They have been omitted from these calculations.

6. See Chapter 2 for a detailed description of the socioeconomic variables discussed in this section.

7. A correlation coefficient is a measure of the association between two nonrandom variables.

8. The structural adjustment policies implemented by Senegal are discussed in Chapter 2. See Rouis (1994) for an excellent description of these policies. See Working Group on Demographic Effects of Economic and Social Reversals (1993) for a discussion of the demographic responses.

9. The quality of the data on adult mortality is uneven and needs to be evaluated before conclusions can be drawn. Much of the evaluation was conducted in terms of the age pattern of adult mortality, since such age patterns are sensitive to typical data errors. The small-scale studies in Bandafassi, Mlomp, and Niakhar/Ngayokhème, though not nationally representative, provide a reasonable basis for determining the true age pattern of adult mortality. These studies suggest that the age pattern of adult mortality in Senegal is well approximated by the Coale-Demeny "West" family. Available national data will thus be compared with the West family for checks of data quality.

10. Deaths in age groups starting with zero, such as 50-54, are typically as numerous as those in the previous age group starting with 5, 45-49 in the example.

11. The boundaries of the study area changed somewhat over the years. However, during 1963-1981 data was collected consistently in Ngayokhème, a part of the total study area. After 1984, the Niakhar study area changed again, extending farther north, but not as far south, as the old region. We refer to the latter study area as Niakhar-II to emphasize the minor change in the baseline population.

12. Service des Grandes Endémies.

13. Programme de Protection Nutritionnelle et Sanitaire.

14. Routine health service statistics are available, but they are not reliable and show a strong tendency to overestimate actual vaccination coverage (OCCGE-Muraz, 1990).

15. A child was considered completely vaccinated if he/she had been vaccinated against seven diseases: tuberculosis, diphtheria, tetanus, pertussis, polio, measles, and yellow fever.

6

Conclusions

Over the last two decades, child mortality has declined rapidly in Senegal, while changes in fertility have been small. According to the 1992-1993 DHS-II, the total fertility rate in the 4 years before the survey was 6.1, while the probability of dying by age 5 in the 5 years before the survey was 131 per 1,000 live births. These two figures imply a rate of natural increase of close to 3 percent per year, and since we find no evidence of major net migration, the actual rate of population growth is also likely to be close to 3 percent. This rapid growth can be attributed to both sustained high fertility—on average each woman bears approximately six children—and declining mortality. What are the prospects for future change?

FERTILITY

Two recent reviews of fertility transition in Asia and Latin America underscore the point that no unique characteristic or combination of characteristics represents necessary and sufficient conditions for substantial fertility decline in a population over the course of economic development (Casterline, 1994; Guzman, 1994). However, several elements appear particularly important: low child mortality, high female education, well-organized national family planning programs, and the existence of a desire to have fewer children.

In Senegal, child mortality is falling rapidly, but it is not yet low;

female education remains low; family-size desires are falling quite rapidly, but they are still close to actual fertility; and the family planning program is quite weak. In 1982, family planning efforts in Botswana, Kenya, Senegal, and Zimbabwe were all quite weak, and the Ross-Mauldin Index[1] for all countries was very similar: between 23 and 28 percent of the maximum score. By 1989, however, the family planning programs in Kenya and Zimbabwe had increased in strength to between 56 and 58 percent of the maximum score, and the program in Botswana had increased in strength to 75 percent of the maximum score, making it among the strongest programs in the developing world. In Senegal, the score had increased somewhat—to 44 percent of the maximum—but not enough to avoid classification as a weak program.

Not surprisingly, the decline in fertility in Senegal has been quite modest: national demographic surveys indicate that fertility declined about one child per woman between 1975-1978 and 1989-1992, and most of that decline took place among urban women. The driving force behind these changes appears to have been a trend towards later marriage and later first birth, and the decline in fertility occurred almost entirely among women under age 30. Little of the fertility decline in Senegal appears to be attributable to either a decrease in ideal family size or an increase in the use of modern contraception, although the proportion of women using modern contraception has increased over the very recent past. Current preferences for number of children still lie very close to the physiological maximum level, given a continued regime of delayed marriage and long birth intervals.

Assuming Senegal achieves further increases in primary and secondary school enrollment for women, as well as greater urbanization, further fertility declines can be expected to occur in the near future. In rural areas, further declines in actual fertility can still be achieved through the mechanism of later marriage. However, in urban areas, particularly Dakar, most of the decline in actual fertility that is achievable solely by an increase in age at marriage has already occurred, so that future fertility reductions must await greater coverage of modern contraception.

MORTALITY

The *World Development Report 1993: Investing in Health* (World Bank, 1993b) identifies three key factors in the dramatic mortality declines of the twentieth century: income growth; improvements in medical technology; and the implementation of public health measures, including both infrastructure and the spread of knowledge. Income growth allows the purchase of more food, better housing, and more health care. Advances in medical technology have increased the amount of health improvement achievable through a given expenditure on health, although they can have a beneficial effect only among a population with access to services. Public health infrastructure improvements, including primary health care services, as well as water supply and sanitation, have reduced exposure to pathogens and contributed to disease prevention. The spread of knowledge about disease prevention and treatment has also contributed greatly to mortality decline worldwide, and has been accelerated by rising levels of education, particularly among mothers.

Senegal has experienced particularly rapid declines in child mortality over the last two decades. The probability of dying by age 5 (per 1,000 live births) declined from about 265 in 1975 to about 135 in 1990. Child mortality decline started in urban areas in the 1950s, but did not spread to all rural areas until the late 1970s. Income gains in Senegal over the last two or three decades have been negligible, as documented in Chapter 2, and can have contributed little to the mortality decline. Nor can improvements in medical technology explain the sudden decline in child mortality in the mid-1970s. There are large differentials in child mortality by education of mother in Senegal, though overall educational levels remain low, and improvement has been quite slow: 73 percent of women of reproductive age had no education in the 1992-1993 DHS-II, as compared with 77 percent in the 1986 DHS-I. The decline in child mortality in Senegal, at least in rural areas, appears to be most closely linked to the improved health infrastructure, particularly the primary health care policy introduced in 1978 and the implementation of the World Health Organization Expanded Programme on Immunization starting in 1981. The experience of one rural area, Mlomp in southern Senegal, provides support for this conclusion. Mortality decline in Mlomp, well documented by a population observatory, was both early and very rapid, and appears to have resulted from the establishment of a private dispensary and maternity clinic in the area. Thus of the three key factors in mortality decline identified by the *World Development Report*, improvement in the health infrastructure, particularly the provision of primary health care, appears to have been the most important in Senegal's mortality decline.

THE DEMOGRAPHIC TRANSITION IN SENEGAL IN AN AFRICAN CONTEXT

The above picture of demographic change suggests that Senegal's small fertility decline is unlike the recent declines in other sub-Saharan African countries. In Botswana, Kenya, and Zimbabwe—usually considered the three countries in the vanguard of African fertility transition—fertility declines have been associated with increased use of modern contraception. Botswana, Kenya, and, to a lesser extent, Zimbabwe have also experienced a decline in teenage marriages, but fertility rates under age 20 have not changed much. Consequently, these countries have experienced an increase in nonmarital fertility. This separation of marriage and fertility has had the effect of reducing the influence of marriage on fertility rates (Working Group on the Social Dynamics of Adolescent Fertility, 1993). In Senegal, fertility has fallen because marriage has been delayed, and marriage and fertility have remained linked.

The Senegalese pattern matches more closely, though not exactly, the pattern found in certain northern African countries during the first phase of their fertility declines. For example, most of the initial decline in fertility observed in countries such as Algeria, Egypt, and Tunisia can be attributed to later age at first marriage (Fargues, 1989; National Research Council, 1982). In these countries, the initial phase of fertility decline was immediately followed by a second phase linked to a substantial decline in the demand for children and a corresponding increase in use of modern contraception among married women.

Though we cannot know for certain what the demographic future of Senegal will be, it may be revealing to compare Senegal with another country that is further along in its demographic transition to see what may lie ahead. Because the emerging pattern of fertility change in Senegal appears to be more similar to the changes that have occurred in the countries of northern Africa than to those that have occurred in sub-Saharan Africa, it may be useful to compare Senegal with a northern African country. For the sake of discussion, we have selected Tunisia, the country of northern Africa that has progressed furthest towards reduced fertility and child mortality.

A comparison of the decline in child mortality in the two countries indicates that the rate of decline in Senegal after 1975 is very similar to that in Tunisia from 1960 on. In Tunisia, mortality before age 5 declined steadily from about 250 per 1,000 live births in 1960 to around 100 in 1980, to around 45 in 1990 (Hill and Yazbeck, 1994). Using the same trend-fitting methodology, mortality before age 5 in Senegal declined from about 300 in 1960 to about 265 in 1975, to about 135 in 1990. Thus, Senegal is currently following a child mortality pattern similar to that followed about 15 years earlier by Tunisia.

The parallels between the subsequent fertility declines in the two countries are also clear, though the time lag is greater—close to 20 years.[2] In Tunisia, total fertility (between the ages of 15 and 35) was about 5.3 in the early 1960s. It fell to 4.2 by the mid-1970s and to about 3.4 by the mid-1980s. In Senegal, total fertility (ages 15-35), which had not changed appreciably since the 1960s, was 5.3 in the mid-1980s, a figure closely resembling that in Tunisia 20 years earlier. In 1991, total fertility in Senegal had fallen to 4.5[3]—a level comparable to that in Tunisia 16 years earlier.

The initial decline in fertility in northern Africa, as in Senegal, can be attributed to a later age at first marriage and first birth: in northern Africa, this initial decline was immediately followed by a second stage, characterized by falling ideal family size and rising contraceptive use. An analysis, using Senegalese data, of the variables associated with Tunisia's continued fertility decline may allow speculation about fertility change in Senegal in the future.

Fertility differentials may be harbingers of fertility trends, and differentials in median age at first birth in Senegal suggest the potential for rapid change. For women aged 25-29 in 1992-1993, the median age at first birth for urban women was 20.8, compared with 18.5 in rural areas. The contrast was even more pronounced by education: 24.5 years for women with secondary or higher education versus 18.7 years for women with no education. In Tunisia in 1988, the urban-rural medians were 25.1 and 23.5, respectively, and the secondary+ education versus no education medians were 25.7 and 23.4, respectively. Thus for well-educated women, patterns of entry into childbearing are not very different in Senegal than in Tunisia, though the differences among less-educated women are very large.

Differences between actual fertility and fertility preferences should also provide insights into future change. At the time of the Tunisia WFS in 1978, total fertility (ages 15-49) was 5.9, but desired family size was only 4.2, and rate of use of modern contraceptives among married women was 25 percent. By 1988, total fertility had dropped to 4.4, desired family size had fallen to 3.5, and rate of use of modern contraception had increased to 40 percent. In Senegal, total fertility in 1978 was 7.1, while desired family size was 8.3, and rate of use of modern contraception was less than 1 percent. By 1986, total fertility reportedly had fallen to 6.6, desired family size had fallen to 6.8, and rate of use of modern contraception had increased to 2 percent. By 1992-1993, total fertility had reportedly fallen to 6.0, desired family size had fallen to 5.9, and modern contraceptive prevalence had increased to nearly 5 percent. Thus it is only in the most recent period that desired family size in Senegal has fallen below actual fertility, and that use of modern contraception has increased above trivial levels.

Changes in desired family size in Senegal have been particularly rapid for women with primary education (falling from about 7.5 children in 1978 to about 4.9 children in 1992-1993), though women with no education show sharp declines as well (from 8.5 to 6.4). Desired family size for women with secondary or higher education was already relatively low in 1978, at 5.0, and declined only to 4.1 by 1992-1993. In Tunisia in 1978, desired family size for women with no education was as low as 4.4, declining slightly to 3.8 by 1988; the change for women with secondary or higher education was even smaller, from 3.1 to 2.8. Fertility measures and family-size preferences in 1992-1993 in Senegal are clearly higher than in Tunisia 15 years earlier, so fertility decline is further behind than child mortality decline. However, all educational categories of women in Senegal, except those with no education at all, now have a desired family size below the current fertility rate. Given that over a quarter of women of reproductive age in Senegal in 1992-1993 had some education, there is a potential for a substantial decline in fertility within marriage over the next 5 years.

Such fertility decline as has occurred in Senegal appears to have resulted from rising age at first marriage, rather than from control of fertility within marriage. This pattern bears some resemblance to the fertility decline in northern Africa in the 1960s and 1970s. Comparisons of Senegal and Tunisia indicate that the pace of child mortality decline has been very similar in the two countries, with Senegal about 15 years behind. In terms of fertility variables—age at first birth, contraceptive use, and family-size desires—Senegal seems to be somewhat more than 15 years behind Tunisia. However, sharply declining family-size preferences among women with primary education or less over the period 1978 to 1992-1993 suggest that fertility change through contraceptive use may occur in the near future in Senegal.

NOTES

1. The Ross-Mauldin Index is a commonly used metric to grade national family planning programs for level of effort. Programs are graded on a series of program components, and a final score is given as a percentage of the maximum possible score. Scores of over 65 generally indicate a strong family planning program, scores of 50 and above indicate moderate family planning program effort, and scores under 50 indicate weak programs.

2. The 1978 Tunisia Fertility Survey and 1988 Tunisia DHS provide estimates of fertility trends in the period from the early 1960s to the late 1980s that are methodologically comparable to the information available from the 1978 WFS and the 1986 and 1992-1993 DHSs.

3. There is some question about the accuracy of this most recent figure.

Appendix A

Data Sources

The surveys and censuses referenced in this report are described in this appendix. The numbers appearing in brackets beside the name of each source have been used to cite the sources in the text. Figure A-1 indicates the site where each of the subnational surveys was conducted. The figure also delineates the World Fertility Survey (WFS) and Demographic and Health Survey (DHS) regions used in this report (referred to in the report as the "grand" regions).

NATIONAL-LEVEL SURVEYS

1960-1961 Demographic Survey (DS) [1]

This was the first national-level sample survey conducted in Senegal. It surveyed 5 percent of the population in urban areas and had variable sampling rates (from 1/20 to 1/160) in rural areas. (See République du Sénégal, 1964, for more information.)

1970-1971 National Demographic Survey (NDS) [2]

This was a multiround survey that had three rounds at 6-month intervals and a sample size of approximately 150,000 persons. (See République du Sénégal, 1974, for more information.)

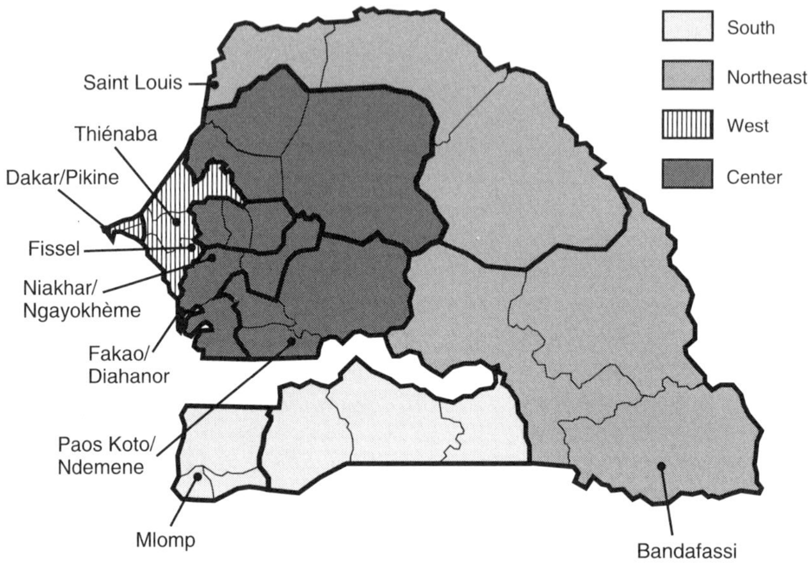

FIGURE A-1 Geographic location of subnational surveys and WFS and DHS grand regions (south, northeast, west, and center). NOTE: The other divisions shown on this map correspond to regional and departmental administrative divisions at the time of the 1988 census. See Figure 2-2 for names of administrative divisions.

1978 World Fertility Survey (WFS) [3]

This was a multistage sample survey that collected retrospective birth histories from 3,985 woman aged 15-49 years. It was conducted by the Direction de la Statistique du Ministère de l'Economie et des Finances in collaboration with the International Statistical Institute. (See République du Sénégal, 1981, for more information.)

1986 Demographic and Health Survey in Senegal (DHS-I) [4]

This was a multistage sample survey that collected complete birth histories from 4,415 women aged 15-49. It was conducted by the Direction de la Statistique du Ministère de l'Economie et des Finances in collaboration with the Institute for Resource Development/Westinghouse. (See Ndiaye et al., 1988, for more information.)

1984, 1987, and 1990 National Vaccination Coverage Surveys [5]

These were national-level surveys undertaken in 1984, 1987, and 1990 using standard World Health Organization methodologies. The target population was children aged 12-23 months and women who had given birth in the preceding year. (See Claquin et al., 1987, and OCCGE-Muraz, 1990, for more information.)

1991-1992 Enquête Sur les Priorités [6]

This survey included approximately 10,000 households and was undertaken between November 1991 and January 1992. The collection of information on the effects of structural adjustment programs on households was one of the major goals of this survey.

1992-1993 Demographic and Health Survey in Senegal (DHS-II) [7]

This was a multistage sample survey that collected complete birth histories from 6,310 women aged 15-49. It was conducted by the Direction de la Statistique du Ministère de l'Economie et des Finances in collaboration with Macro International, Inc. (See Ndiaye et al., 1994, for more information.)

REGIONAL-LEVEL SURVEYS

These surveys consist of a number of subnational studies through which accurate birth and death registers have been maintained over several years. Although the small study areas are not representative of the entire country, they yield estimates of fertility that are thought to be more accurate than those from large-scale surveys and censuses. Hence, these small-scale studies can provide a useful independent check on the accuracy of the other estimates.

Bandafassi Study Area (1970-present) [8]

This rural area has been monitored by annual rounds in Malinké villages since 1970, Peul villages since 1975, and Bedik villages since 1980. It included a population of 8,155 inhabitants as of March 1, 1991. (See Pison and Desgrées du Loû, 1993, for more information.)

Cap-Vert (Dakar) Fertility Survey (1972) [9]

This survey was a round added to the third round of the NDS. It involved systematic sampling stratified according to age, and included complete birth histories of 1,460 women 13-54 years old. (See Ferry, 1977, for more information.)

Mlomp Demographic Monitoring (1984-present) [10]

This rural area is monitored through annual rounds. It included a population of 6,435 persons as of October 1990. (See Lagarde et al., forthcoming and Pison et al., 1993, for more information.)

Niakhar/Ngayokhème (1962-present) [11]

Niakhar-I, 1962-1967: included a population of 35,187 persons as of January 1, 1966. (See Cantrelle, 1969; Cantrelle and Léridon, 1971; and Projet Niakhar, 1992, for more information.)

Niakhar-II, 1983-present: included 26,496 persons as of March 1, 1992. (See Projet Niakhar, 1992, for more information.)

Ngayokhème Area (included in the Niakhar-I and Niakhar-II areas), 1963-present: included 5,947 persons as of March 1, 1991. (See Waltisperger, 1974; and Pison, 1978, for more information.)

Paos Koto/Ndemene (1963-1978) [12]

Included a population of 18,988 persons as of January 1, 1966. The Paos Koto survey was monitored from 1963-1965, and Ndemene from 1963-1978. (See Cantrelle, 1969; and Cantrelle et al., 1980, for more information.)

Fakao and Diahanor (ca 1940 - ca 1966) [13]

These studies reconstituted families by retranscribing parish certificates and surveys among resident women in 1965-1966. Diahanor included 284 persons as of June 1, 1966; Fakao included approximately 3,000 persons as of January 1, 1966. (See Lacombe, 1973, for more information.)

Sine-Saloum Demographic Survey (1982) [14]

This survey involved multistage cluster sampling of the rural population of Sine-Saloum (the current regions of Fatick and Kaolack), a retrospective survey among 1,894 women aged 15-44 having been married or had one live birth, with the birth history being cut off at 6 years. (See Goldberg et al., 1984, for more information.)

Dakar-Pikine Survey (1986) [15]

This survey collected retrospective data from 1,856 households (including 2,812 women) on infant and child mortality in Pikine during March and April 1986. (See Antoine and Diouf, 1989, 1992; and Bocquier, 1991, for more information.)

Survey on Child Mortality in the Sahel (EMIS) (1981-1984) [16]

This was a longitudinal study of women who had had children. It consisted of eight interviews between the time the children were born to age 2 years and 4 months. It was conducted in the areas of Fissel and Thiénaba in the region of Thiès between 1981 and 1984. (See Mbodji, 1988, for more information.)

NATIONAL CENSUSES

1976 Senegal Census [17]

This was the first national census, taken in April 1976. (See République du Sénégal, no date, for more information.)

1988 Senegal Census [18]

This was the second national census. It included questions on births and deaths during the preceding 12 months. The census date (May 27, 1988) was chosen to take advantage of the end of Ramadan, the Korité, as a temporal indicator for marking the beginning of the 12-month reference period. (See République du Sénégal, 1989, for more information.)

Appendix B

Correcting the Fertility Estimates in the 1988 Census

The 1988 census [18] questionnaire contained a single question to women about their births in the last 12 months. Unfortunately, because of mistakes in coding and processing, these data were not published in official census publications, and to this day, fertility estimates from the 1988 census remain unpublished. In an attempt to resolve this problem, members of the working group traveled to Senegal to work for a week on a team with officials from the Government of Senegal's Directorate of Statistics. The team analyzed the programs used to construct the fertility rates and reviewed the program used to clean the data before the final data analysis began. The Directorate of Statistics also made available to the team the raw data for a 10-percent sample in one department (Fatick) so that it could be carefully scrutinized.

The team identified the major problem to be that blank entries in the coded data were subject to two interpretations: blanks could signify either that there were no data for the women or that the women had not had a birth in the last 12 months. On closer examination, the team found that:

- Boys and girls had been coded separately on the 1988 census data file. If either the number of boys or the number of girls was recorded as a blank on the data file, the program calculating the fertility rates excluded the birth(s) of the other sex.
- If both entries were blank, the responses were treated as 0,0 (i.e., no boys, no girls).

The team used the 10-percent sample of Fatick to examine the importance of these findings for the fertility rates. They discovered that although the interviewers were supposed to have recorded the number of boys and girls born to all women in the 12 months before the census, the responses were missing for many women. Missing data were coded as two blank entries. There were also a considerable number of cases where one column contained data and the other was blank. Furthermore, the distribution of blank entries varied by the age of the women (with older and younger women having higher-than-average levels), but there seemed to be an underlying level of blank entries across all ages.

Based on this analysis, the age-specific fertility rates (ASFRs) were then reestimated using two methods: (1) assuming none of the blanks were missing births, and (2) assuming all of the blanks were missing births. At the national level, the interpretation of the blank entries altered the estimate of the total fertility rate (TFR) by approximately 0.3 of a birth. Although the difference in ASFRs between the two methods was not large, it confirmed the team's earlier finding that there was a distinct pattern to the blanks in the coded data. Subsequently, the ASFRs for each department were adjusted by the smallest ratio of [ASFR(ALL)/ASFR(NONE)], which was taken as the best estimate of the underlying level of nonresponse (π) in that department. Hence, the best estimate of the ASFRs in each region became:

$$\text{Adjusted ASFR} = \pi * \text{ASFR(NONE)}.$$

These adjusted ASFRs are provided in Tables B-1 through B-11.

TABLE B-1 Age-Specific Fertility Rates, National, 1988 Census

	Place of Residence		
Age Group	Urban	Rural	Total
10-14	0.005	0.016	0.012
15-19	0.075	0.193	0.142
20-24	0.203	0.295	0.254
25-29	0.253	0.288	0.274
30-34	0.242	0.244	0.243
35-39	0.182	0.153	0.164
40-44	0.083	0.074	0.078
45-49	0.024	0.028	0.026
50-54	0.009	0.013	0.012

TABLE B-2 Age-Specific Fertility Rates, Dakar, 1988 Census

	Department			
Age Group	Dakar	Pikine	Rufisque	Region
Total				
10-14	0.003	0.006	0.005	0.004
15-19	0.048	0.086	0.068	0.063
20-24	0.147	0.233	0.206	0.182
25-29	0.202	0.284	0.278	0.238
30-34	0.206	0.264	0.259	0.236
35-39	0.161	0.200	0.205	0.179
40-44	0.078	0.094	0.117	0.088
45-49	0.021	0.025	0.024	0.023
50-54	0.006	0.013	0.005	0.009
Urban				
10-14	0.003	0.006	0.004	0.004
15-19	0.048	0.086	0.049	0.063
20-24	0.147	0.233	0.178	0.184
25-29	0.202	0.284	0.252	0.241
30-34	0.206	0.264	0.248	0.235
35-39	0.161	0.200	0.207	0.182
40-44	0.078	0.094	0.107	0.088
45-49	0.021	0.025	0.024	0.023
50-54	0.006	0.013	0.004	0.009
Rural				
10-14	—	—	0.007	0.007
15-19	—	—	0.125	0.125
20-24	—	—	0.285	0.284
25-29	—	—	0.344	0.343
30-34	—	—	0.286	0.286
35-39	—	—	0.199	0.198
40-44	—	—	0.142	0.142
45-49	—	—	0.026	0.026
50-54	—	—	0.008	0.008

NOTE: —, not applicable

TABLE B-3 Age-Specific Fertility Rates, Diourbel, 1988 Census

	Department			
Age Group	Bambey	Diourbel	Mbacké	Region
Total				
10-14	0.015	0.015	0.013	0.014
15-19	0.159	0.150	0.147	0.152
20-24	0.263	0.268	0.259	0.263
25-29	0.270	0.281	0.265	0.271
30-34	0.218	0.231	0.231	0.227
35-39	0.127	0.141	0.136	0.135
40-44	0.054	0.060	0.057	0.057
45-49	0.025	0.025	0.025	0.025
50-54	0.020	0.006	0.012	0.013
Urban				
10-14	0.010	0.009	0.006	0.008
15-19	0.084	0.098	0.102	0.098
20-24	0.216	0.218	0.222	0.220
25-29	0.288	0.249	0.257	0.257
30-34	0.249	0.236	0.240	0.240
35-39	0.198	0.162	0.131	0.156
40-44	0.087	0.073	0.065	0.072
45-49	0.011	0.019	0.028	0.021
50-54	0.013	0.008	0.008	0.009
Rural				
10-14	0.016	0.020	0.014	0.016
15-19	0.166	0.191	0.156	0.167
20-24	0.266	0.306	0.266	0.274
25-29	0.268	0.301	0.266	0.274
30-34	0.214	0.228	0.228	0.223
35-39	0.120	0.126	0.138	0.129
40-44	0.050	0.051	0.056	0.053
45-49	0.026	0.029	0.024	0.026
50-54	0.021	0.005	0.013	0.014

TABLE B-4 Age-Specific Fertility Rates, Fatick, 1988 Census

	Department			
Age Group	Fatick	Foundiougne	Gossas	Region
Total				
10-14	0.006	0.013	0.010	0.009
15-19	0.181	0.192	0.164	0.179
20-24	0.336	0.321	0.301	0.320
25-29	0.330	0.323	0.302	0.319
30-34	0.283	0.274	0.257	0.272
35-39	0.212	0.172	0.181	0.191
40-44	0.081	0.074	0.067	0.075
45-49	0.034	0.022	0.029	0.030
50-54	0.012	0.010	0.012	0.011
Urban				
10-14	0.001	0.004	0.007	0.004
15-19	0.063	0.086	0.122	0.091
20-24	0.277	0.281	0.258	0.271
25-29	0.304	0.302	0.290	0.299
30-34	0.262	0.287	0.271	0.272
35-39	0.211	0.208	0.209	0.210
40-44	0.062	0.078	0.047	0.059
45-49	0.030	0.006	0.023	0.023
50-54	0.017	0.007	0.007	0.011
Rural				
10-14	0.006	0.014	0.010	0.010
15-19	0.201	0.203	0.172	0.192
20-24	0.344	0.324	0.308	0.327
25-29	0.333	0.325	0.304	0.321
30-34	0.285	0.273	0.254	0.272
35-39	0.212	0.168	0.176	0.189
40-44	0.083	0.073	0.070	0.077
45-49	0.035	0.024	0.031	0.031
50-54	0.012	0.010	0.012	0.012

TABLE B-5 Age-Specific Fertility Rates, Kaolack, 1988 Census

	Department			
Age Group	Kaffrine	Kaolack	Nioro du Rip	Region
Total				
10-14	0.022	0.013	0.028	0.020
15-19	0.212	0.141	0.246	0.194
20-24	0.294	0.246	0.331	0.285
25-29	0.280	0.264	0.314	0.283
30-34	0.223	0.221	0.245	0.227
35-39	0.131	0.154	0.142	0.142
40-44	0.062	0.059	0.065	0.062
45-49	0.024	0.023	0.021	0.023
50-54	0.013	0.012	0.014	0.013
Urban				
10-14	0.018	0.007	0.001	0.008
15-19	0.139	0.083	0.095	0.089
20-24	0.281	0.202	0.271	0.212
25-29	0.236	0.249	0.253	0.248
30-34	0.230	0.212	0.222	0.215
35-39	0.113	0.169	0.172	0.163
40-44	0.040	0.062	0.084	0.062
45-49	0.020	0.025	0.030	0.025
50-54	0.005	0.013	0.006	0.011
Rural				
10-14	0.023	0.020	0.030	0.024
15-19	0.216	0.212	0.255	0.227
20-24	0.295	0.305	0.335	0.308
25-29	0.282	0.280	0.317	0.292
30-34	0.223	0.231	0.246	0.231
35-39	0.133	0.136	0.140	0.136
40-44	0.063	0.056	0.063	0.061
45-49	0.024	0.021	0.021	0.023
50-54	0.013	0.011	0.015	0.013

TABLE B-6 Age-Specific Fertility Rates, Kolda, 1988 Census

	Department			
Age Group	Kolda	Sédhiou	Vélingara	Region
Total				
10-14	0.021	0.019	0.024	0.020
15-19	0.237	0.226	0.245	0.234
20-24	0.318	0.302	0.306	0.309
25-29	0.283	0.270	0.283	0.278
30-34	0.221	0.218	0.225	0.221
35-39	0.135	0.132	0.131	0.133
40-44	0.066	0.066	0.061	0.065
45-49	0.024	0.029	0.024	0.027
50-54	0.016	0.011	0.008	0.012
Urban				
10-14	0.015	0.008	0.006	0.012
15-19	0.151	0.096	0.204	0.151
20-24	0.287	0.320	0.302	0.298
25-29	0.300	0.293	0.322	0.305
30-34	0.251	0.231	0.260	0.250
35-39	0.168	0.186	0.158	0.171
40-44	0.060	0.103	0.078	0.073
45-49	0.022	0.060	0.021	0.030
50-54	0.018	0.007	0.006	0.013
Rural				
10-14	0.023	0.019	0.026	0.022
15-19	0.256	0.232	0.250	0.243
20-24	0.325	0.301	0.306	0.310
25-29	0.280	0.269	0.279	0.275
30-34	0.213	0.217	0.220	0.217
35-39	0.127	0.129	0.128	0.128
40-44	0.068	0.064	0.059	0.064
45-49	0.024	0.028	0.024	0.026
50-54	0.016	0.011	0.009	0.012

TABLE B-7 Age-Specific Fertility Rates, Louga, 1988 Census

	Department			
Age Group	Kébémer	Linguère	Louga	Region
Total				
10-14	0.013	0.018	0.012	0.014
15-19	0.155	0.196	0.133	0.157
20-24	0.259	0.275	0.254	0.261
25-29	0.251	0.278	0.278	0.269
30-34	0.203	0.241	0.259	0.235
35-39	0.107	0.141	0.157	0.136
40-44	0.053	0.071	0.071	0.065
45-49	0.018	0.023	0.023	0.022
50-54	0.009	0.015	0.016	0.013
Urban				
10-14	0.002	0.004	0.006	0.005
15-19	0.065	0.107	0.078	0.080
20-24	0.204	0.238	0.218	0.220
25-29	0.259	0.285	0.289	0.285
30-34	0.213	0.265	0.282	0.271
35-39	0.138	0.178	0.201	0.190
40-44	0.053	0.074	0.086	0.080
45-49	0.007	0.021	0.025	0.022
50-54	0.000	0.007	0.012	0.010
Rural				
10-14	0.015	0.019	0.015	0.016
15-19	0.162	0.204	0.155	0.172
20-24	0.263	0.278	0.270	0.270
25-29	0.251	0.277	0.274	0.266
30-34	0.202	0.238	0.247	0.228
35-39	0.106	0.138	0.141	0.127
40-44	0.053	0.070	0.065	0.062
45-49	0.019	0.023	0.023	0.021
50-54	0.010	0.016	0.017	0.014

TABLE B-8 Age-Specific Fertility Rates, Saint-Louis, 1988 Census

Age Group	Department: Dagana	Matam	Podor	Region
Total				
10-14	0.007	0.012	0.014	0.011
15-19	0.112	0.144	0.163	0.136
20-24	0.245	0.257	0.277	0.256
25-29	0.284	0.273	0.293	0.282
30-34	0.270	0.237	0.263	0.258
35-39	0.209	0.149	0.197	0.184
40-44	0.107	0.079	0.091	0.093
45-49	0.029	0.030	0.032	0.030
50-54	0.009	0.014	0.013	0.011
Urban				
10-14	0.003	0.003	0.002	0.003
15-19	0.071	0.084	0.074	0.072
20-24	0.230	0.237	0.208	0.230
25-29	0.277	0.226	0.208	0.272
30-34	0.269	0.209	0.220	0.264
35-39	0.217	0.131	0.216	0.212
40-44	0.106	0.042	0.099	0.101
45-49	0.023	0.023	0.032	0.024
50-54	0.008	0.000	0.017	0.008
Rural				
10-14	0.013	0.013	0.015	0.014
15-19	0.167	0.146	0.168	0.158
20-24	0.268	0.258	0.281	0.268
25-29	0.292	0.275	0.297	0.286
30-34	0.272	0.238	0.264	0.255
35-39	0.199	0.150	0.196	0.176
40-44	0.109	0.080	0.090	0.090
45-49	0.034	0.030	0.032	0.032
50-54	0.009	0.014	0.012	0.012

TABLE B-9 Age-Specific Fertility Rates, Tambacounda, 1988 Census

Age Group	Department			Region
	Bakel	Kédougou	Tambacounda	
Total				
10-14	0.023	0.014	0.025	0.022
15-19	0.202	0.197	0.229	0.215
20-24	0.278	0.252	0.296	0.282
25-29	0.260	0.226	0.275	0.261
30-34	0.230	0.149	0.234	0.215
35-39	0.151	0.108	0.125	0.129
40-44	0.071	0.044	0.055	0.058
45-49	0.031	0.015	0.027	0.026
50-54	0.015	0.012	0.014	0.014
Urban				
10-14	0.002	0.003	0.010	0.008
15-19	0.144	0.139	0.154	0.151
20-24	0.264	0.241	0.283	0.273
25-29	0.240	0.254	0.302	0.287
30-34	0.300	0.174	0.285	0.267
35-39	0.141	0.131	0.150	0.145
40-44	0.084	0.076	0.071	0.075
45-49	0.020	0.015	0.016	0.017
50-54	0.000	0.009	0.020	0.014
Rural				
10-14	0.024	0.017	0.029	0.025
15-19	0.206	0.207	0.248	0.226
20-24	0.279	0.254	0.300	0.284
25-29	0.261	0.222	0.269	0.257
30-34	0.224	0.145	0.219	0.205
35-39	0.152	0.104	0.119	0.127
40-44	0.069	0.036	0.050	0.054
45-49	0.032	0.015	0.030	0.027
50-54	0.016	0.013	0.012	0.014

TABLE B-10 Age-Specific Fertility Rates, Thiès, 1988 Census

	Department			
Age Group	Mbour	Thiès	Tivaouane	Region
Total				
10-14	0.008	0.007	0.009	0.008
15-19	0.123	0.097	0.141	0.118
20-24	0.287	0.235	0.274	0.261
25-29	0.308	0.279	0.288	0.290
30-34	0.285	0.264	0.261	0.269
35-39	0.199	0.195	0.163	0.186
40-44	0.099	0.095	0.078	0.091
45-49	0.031	0.024	0.027	0.027
50-54	0.009	0.009	0.011	0.010
Urban				
10-14	0.006	0.003	0.004	0.004
15-19	0.086	0.062	0.061	0.069
20-24	0.247	0.195	0.214	0.212
25-29	0.289	0.245	0.253	0.260
30-34	0.271	0.249	0.271	0.259
35-39	0.199	0.187	0.188	0.191
40-44	0.092	0.093	0.076	0.091
45-49	0.030	0.023	0.025	0.026
50-54	0.008	0.007	0.012	0.008
Rural				
10-14	0.009	0.011	0.011	0.010
15-19	0.148	0.148	0.156	0.152
20-24	0.311	0.288	0.284	0.293
25-29	0.319	0.314	0.293	0.306
30-34	0.292	0.281	0.259	0.275
35-39	0.198	0.202	0.159	0.183
40-44	0.102	0.098	0.078	0.091
45-49	0.031	0.025	0.028	0.028
50-54	0.009	0.012	0.011	0.011

TABLE B-11 Age-Specific Fertility Rates, Ziguinchor, 1988 Census

	Department			
Age Group	Bignona	Oussouye	Ziguinchor	Region
Total				
10-14	0.010	0.008	0.008	0.009
15-19	0.183	0.157	0.128	0.152
20-24	0.328	0.355	0.270	0.300
25-29	0.307	0.354	0.309	0.312
30-34	0.286	0.288	0.269	0.278
35-39	0.185	0.221	0.185	0.188
40-44	0.104	0.101	0.080	0.093
45-49	0.042	0.040	0.032	0.038
50-54	0.022	0.011	0.014	0.018
Urban				
10-14	0.005	0.004	0.007	0.007
15-19	0.108	0.058	0.117	0.109
20-24	0.245	0.403	0.261	0.249
25-29	0.247	0.307	0.302	0.281
30-34	0.211	0.237	0.269	0.248
35-39	0.148	0.184	0.187	0.172
40-44	0.083	0.039	0.067	0.066
45-49	0.026	0.000	0.031	0.028
50-54	0.007	0.000	0.012	0.010
Rural				
10-14	0.011	0.009	0.012	0.011
15-19	0.200	0.180	0.197	0.198
20-24	0.343	0.347	0.351	0.346
25-29	0.316	0.361	0.372	0.335
30-34	0.299	0.295	0.308	0.301
35-39	0.190	0.225	0.204	0.198
40-44	0.107	0.107	0.121	0.110
45-49	0.044	0.044	0.038	0.042
50-54	0.023	0.012	0.018	0.021

Appendix C

Methodology for Analysis of Child Mortality

The procedure used for analyzing child mortality, Poisson regression, has been described in detail in the volume entitled *Demographic Effects of Economic Reversals in Sub-Saharan Africa* (Working Group on Demographic Effects of Economic and Social Reversals, 1993:42-43) and is reiterated in large part here.

Poisson regression is essentially a methodology for the multivariate analysis of counts of occurrences, in this case, of child deaths. The method assumes some underlying risk or hazard of the event occurring in some category of duration of exposure, in this case an age group of children. In our model, the natural logarithm of the hazard, h_{ia}, for observation *i* of age group *a* is assumed to be given by an additive expression including the base hazard for the age group, h_a, and the effects of a series of other variables, *X*, that are assumed to influence the hazard:

$$\ln(h_{ia}) = h_a + \tau' X_i \ .$$

Note that in our model, the effects of the variables *X* are assumed not to vary with age.

The expected number of events or deaths, D'_{ia}, observed for individuals with a particular set of characteristics in duration-of-exposure category *a*, will be the hazard multiplied by the exposure time of such individuals in the exposure category, E_{ia}. Thus for individuals with characteristics *i* and age *a*,

$$\ln(D'_{ia}) - \ln(E_{ia}) = h_a + \tau' X_i \ .$$

The logarithm of the exposure term E_{ia} is commonly referred to as the "offset," which standardizes cell counts for varying exposure times. We set up the data for Poisson analysis by counting events (deaths) and exposure time in each cell of a matrix defined by age a, time t, and a vector of control variables X.

Appendix D

Growth Balance Methods for Estimating Coverage of Adult Deaths

Brass (1975) proposed a method for assessing the coverage of death recording by comparing the age pattern of deaths with the age pattern of the population. In a stable population with no migration, the growth rate at each age is constant, so the difference between the entry rates and exit rates of successive age groups must be identical. A straight line fitted through the points has a slope determined by the reciprocal of death-reporting coverage and an intercept equal to the constant annual growth rate. This method has been applied to the 1988 adjusted population and 1988 deaths in the year before the census [18]. The results are not very encouraging: the points (see Figure D-1) do not lie on a straight line, the estimated growth rates are 3.5 percent per year for females and 3.8 percent for males, and the estimated coverage of deaths is in excess of 200 percent for both males and females.

The intercensal survival estimates of adult mortality have been seen to suggest very high levels of adult mortality, and one possible reason put forward to explain this is a change in census coverage between 1976 and 1988. The General Growth Balance method (Hill, 1987), developed for nonstable population applications from the Brass Growth Balance Method (Brass, 1975), provides a convenient way of assessing change in census coverage when the age pattern of adult mortality is reasonably well established.

In essence, the method compares two estimates of the death rate above a range of ages x—one estimate obtained from an age pattern of deaths, and

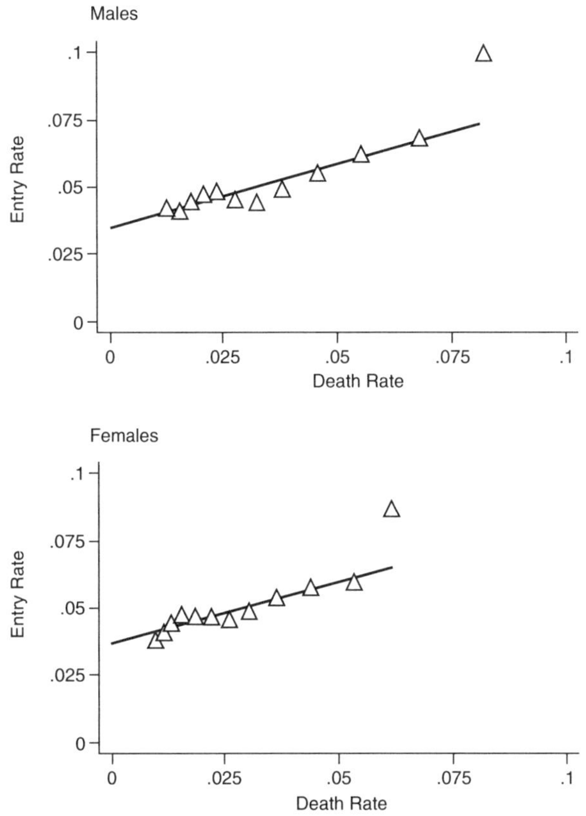

FIGURE D-1 Brass growth balance method for estimating coverage of adult deaths, robust regression. SOURCE: Unpublished data, 1988 census. NOTE: Each point represents a particular age group (i.e., 0+, 5+, 10+).

the other as the residual of the entry rate and population growth rate above age x. For the present application, the deaths in the 12 months before the 1988 census have been used with the 1976 and adjusted 1988 age distributions. Figure C-2 shows the plots of the application of the method. In terms of census coverage, the ratio of coverage in the 1976 census [17] to that in 1988 is 1.18 for males and 1.23 for females. As suggested earlier, either the 1976 census was a substantial overcount or the 1988 census was a substantial undercount. The estimates of coverage of deaths are less satisfactory: for males, relative to the coverage of the 1976 census, deaths were overreported by nearly 60 percent, whereas for females the corresponding figure is in excess of 170 percent. These estimates are most implausible. It is probably the case that the exaggeration of age in the census age distribu-

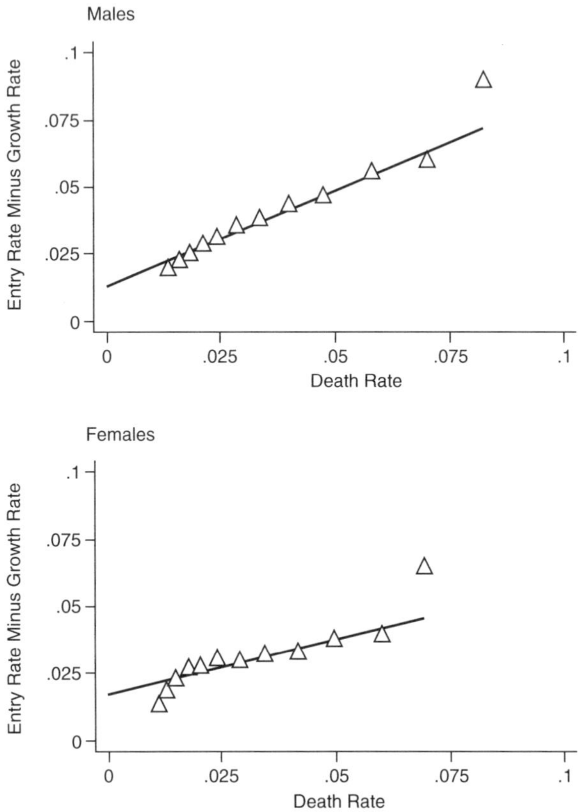

FIGURE D-2 General growth balance method for estimating coverage of adult deaths, robust regression. SOURCES: Unpublished data, 1976 and 1988 censuses. NOTE: Each point represents a particular age group (i.e., 0+, 5+, 10+).

tions and deaths has greatly distorted the estimate of death coverage. As seen above, the age patterns of the adult mortality estimates based on deaths in 1987-1988 are very consistent with model patterns, and in the absence of any strong indication of systematic error, the data are accepted as being reasonably accurate.

References

Aaby, P., B. Samb, F. Simondon, K. Knudsen, A.M. Seck, J. Bennett, and H. Whittle

1993 Divergent mortality for male and female recipients of low-titer and high-titer measles vaccines in rural Senegal. *American Journal of Epidemiology* 138:(9)746-755.

Aloui, T., A. Mouhamed, and H. Fourati

1989 *Enquête Démographique et de Santé en Tunisie 1988.* Ministère de la Santé Publique, Office National de la Famille et de la Population, Direction de la Population Tunis, Tunisie. Columbia, Md.: Institute for Resource Development/Macro Systems, Inc.

Anker, R., and J. Knowles

1982 *Fertility Determinants in Developing Countries: A Case Study of Kenya.* Liège, Belgium: Ordina.

Antoine, P., and P.D. Diouf

1989 Indicateurs de mortalité des enfants et conditions socio-économiques en milieu urbain: Premiers résultats d'une enquête menée à Pikine. Pp. 505-514 in G. Salem and E. Jeannee, eds., *Urbanisation et Santé dans le Tiers-Monde: Transition Epidémiologique, Changement Social et Soins de Santé Primaires.* Paris: ORSTOM.

1992 Un exemple de mesure des différences de mortalité en milieu urbain: Pikine (Sénégal). *Démographies et Différences* Congrès de l'Association Internationale des Démographes de Langue Française. Vol. 4, no. 4, pp. 311-321. Paris: Presses Universitaires de France.

Antoine, P., and F.G. Mbodji

1991 La mortalité des enfants au Sénégal: Une synthèse des données. *Etude de la Population Africaine* 5 (January):18-35.

Antoine, P., and J. Nanitelamio

1991 More single women in African cities: Pikine, Abidjan and Brazzaville. *Population: An English Selection* 3:149-169.

Arnold, F.
1990 Assessment of the quality of birth history data in the Demographic and Health Surveys. Pp. 83-111 in *An Assessment of DHS-I Data Quality*. Demographic and Health Surveys Methodological Reports No. 1. Columbia, Md: Institute for Resource Development/Westinghouse.

Arnold, F., and A.K. Blanc
1990 Fertility trends and levels. *Demographic and Health Surveys Comparative Studies 2: Fertility*. Columbia, Md.: Institute for Resource Development/Westinghouse.

Barbieri, M.
1989 The Determinants of Infant and Child Mortality in Senegal: An Analysis of DHS Data. Unpublished Ph.D. dissertation, Graduate Group in Demography, Program in Population Research, University of California, Berkeley.

Barro, I.
1991 Impact de la Nouvelle Politique Industrielle sur le Secteur Informel. Banque Internationale de Reconstruction et Développement. Paper presented at the Symposium National sur l'Emploi, Dakar, July, 15-18.

Baye, M.
1994 Inégalités Sexuelles en Matière de Santé, de Morbidité et de Mortalité dans l'Enfance dans Trois Pays de l'Afrique de l'Ouest. Hypothèses, Mesures d'Explication des Mécanismes. Unpublished Ph.D. dissertation, Louvain Catholic University, France.

Becker, C., and M. Mbodji
1994 Perspectives historiques. Pp. 31-58 in Y. Charbit and S. Ndiaye, eds., *La Population du Sénégal*. Paris: Centre d'Etudes et de Recherches sur les Populations Africaines et Asiatiques.

Becker, G.S.
1981 *A Treatise on the Family*. Cambridge, Mass.: Harvard University Press.

Berg, E.
1990 *Ajustement Ajourné: Réformes de la Politique Economique du Sénégal dans les Années 80*. Washington, D.C.: U.S. Agency for International Development.

Bocquier, P.
1991 Les relations entre mortalité des enfants et espacement des naissances dans la banlieue de Dakar (Sénégal). *Population* (July-August) 46(4):813-831.

Boerma, J.T., A.E. Sommerfelt, and J.K. van Ginneken
1994 Causes of death in childhood: An evaluation of the results of verbal autopsy questions used in seven DHS surveys. Pp. 145-157 in *An Assessment of the Quality of Health Data in DHS-I Surveys*. DHS Methodological Reports, No. 2. Calverton, Md.: Macro International, Inc.

Bongaarts, J.
1978 A framework for analyzing the proximate determinants of fertility. *Population and Development Review* 4(1):105-132.

Bongaarts, J., and R.G. Potter
1983 *Fertility, Biology, and Behavior: An Analysis of the Proximate Determinants*. New York: Academic Press.

Bongaarts, J., O. Frank, and R. Lesthaeghe
1984 The proximate determinants of fertility in sub-Saharan Africa. *Population and Development Review* 10(3):511-537.

Boone, C.
1993 Rise and Decline of Senegal's Light Industry. Pp. 269-282 in *Année Africaine 1992-1993*. Paris: Centre d'Etudes d'Afrique Noire and Editions de Pédone.

Brass, W.
1975 *Methods of Estimating Fertility and Mortality from Limited and Defective Data*.

Occasional Publication. Chapel Hill, N.C.: International Program of Laboratories for Population Statistics.

Brass, W., and F. Juarez
1983 Censored cohort parity progression ratios from birth histories. *Asian and Pacific Census Forum* 10(1):5-13.

Caicedo, E.
1990 *Tableau de Bord de la Situation Sociale au Sénégal.* Dakar: U.N. Development Programme.

Cantrelle, P.
1969 Etude démographique dans la région du Sine-Saloum (Sénégal): Etat civil et observations démographiques, 1963-65. *Travaux et Documents de l'ORSTOM*, No. 1. Paris: ORSTOM.

Cantrelle, P., and B. Ferry
1979 Approches de la fécondité naturelle dans les populations contemporaines. Pp. 315-370 in H. Léridon and J. Menken, eds., *Natural Fertility: Patterns and Determinants of Natural Fertility.* Liège, Belgium: Ordina.

Cantrelle, P., and H. Léridon
1971 Breastfeeding, mortality in childhood and fertility in a rural zone of Senegal. *Population Studies* 25(3):505-533.

Cantrelle, P., H. Léridon, and P. Livenais
1980 Fécondité, allaitement et mortalité infantile: Différences ethniques dans une même région (Saloum, Sénégal). *Population* 3:623-648.

Cantrelle, P., I.L. Diop, M. Garenne, M. Guèye, and A. Sadio
1986 The profile of mortality and its determinants in Senegal, 1960-80. Pp. 86-116 in *Determinants of Mortality Change and Differentials in Developing Countries: The Five-Country Case Study Report.* New York: United Nations.

Casterline, J.
1994 Fertility transition in Asia. Pp. 69-86 in T. Locoh and V. Hertrich, eds., *The Onset of Fertility Transition in Sub-Saharan Africa.* Liège, Belgium: Ordina.

Charbit, Y., L. Guèye, and S. Ndiaye
1985 *Nuptialité et Fécondité au Sénégal.* Paris, France; Institut National d'Etudes Démographiques

Claquin, P., F. Diouf, B. Floury, and M. Garenne
1987 *Rapport d'Evaluation de la Couverture Vaccinale des Enfants de 12 à 23 Mois en République du Sénégal au 1er Juillet 1987.* Dakar: ORSTOM and Ministère de la Santé Publique.

Coale, A.J., and P. Demeny
1983 *Regional Model Life Tables and Stable Populations*, 2nd ed. New York: Academic Press.

Coeytaux, F.M.
1988 Induced abortion in sub-Saharan Africa: What we do and do not know. *Studies in Family Planning* 19(3):186-190.

Cohen, B.
1993 Fertility levels, differentials, and trends. Pp. 8-67 in K. Foote, K. Hill, and L. Martin, eds., *Demographic Change in Sub-Saharan Africa.* Panel on the Population Dynamics of Sub-Saharan Africa, Committee on Population, National Research Council. Washington, D.C.: National Academy Press.

Comité National de Prévention du SIDA
1991 *Bulletin Epidémiologique HIV.* No. 3, Dakar.
1993 *Bulletin Epidémiologique HIV.* No. 4, Dakar.

Condé, J., and P. Diagne
1986 *Les Migrations Internationales Sud-Nord. Une Etude de Cas: Les Migrants Maliens, Mauritaniens, et Sénégalais de la Vallée du Fleuve Sénégal en France.* Paris: Development Centre, Organisation for Economic Co-operation and Development.

Davis, K., and J. Blake
1956 Social structure and fertility: An analytic framework. *Economic Development and Cultural Change* 4:211-235.

Delaunay, V.
1994 *L'Entrée dans la Vie Féconde. Expression Démographique des Mutations Socio-Economiques d'un Milieu Rural Sénégalais* . Les Etudes du Centre Français sur la Population et le Developpement, no. 7. Paris: Centre Français sur la Population et le Developpement.

Desgrées du Loû, A.
Forth - coming *Le rôle des vaccinations dans la baisse de la mortalité des enfants en Afrique: Résultats d'une enquête longitudinale menée dans la zone rurale de Bandafassi, au Sénégal, entre 1970 et 1993.* Les Etudes du Centre Français sur la Population et le Developpement. Paris: Centre Français sur la Population et le Developpement.

Desgrées du Loû, A., G. Pison, and P. Aaby
Forth- coming The role of immunisations in the recent decline in childhood mortality and the changes in the female/male mortality ratio in rural Senegal. *American Journal of Epidemiology.*

Desgrées du Loû, A., and G. Pison
1994 Barriers to universal child immunization in rural Senegal, five years after the accelerated expanded program on immunization. *Bulletin of the World Health Organization* 72(5):751-759.

Diop, F.P., and O. Dieng
1985 *Les Migrations Rurales au Sénégal. Effets sur les Structures Agraires.* Rome: Food and Agriculture Organization.

Diop, I.L.
1990 Etude de la Mortalité à Saint-Louis du Sénégal à Partir des Données de l'Etat Civil. Thèse de doctorat de 3ème cycle, Université Paris I.

Diop, N.
1993 La Fécondité des Adolescentes au Sénégal. Unpublished working paper. Department of Demography, University of Montreal.

Diouf, P.D.
1994 L'Avortement à Pikine. Pp. 409-418 in Y. Charbit and S. Ndiaye, eds., *La Population du Sénégal.* Dakar: Direction de la Prévision et de la Statistique; Paris: Centre d'Etudes et de Recherches sur les Populations Africaines et Asiatiques.

Duruflé, G.
1994 *Le Sénégal peut-il Sortir de la Crise? Douze ans d'Ajustement Structurel au Sénégal.* Paris: Karthala.

Enel, C., and G. Pison
1992 Sexual relations in the rural area of Mlomp (Casamance, Senegal). Pp. 249-267 in T. Dyson, ed., *Sexual Behaviour and Networking: Anthropological and Socio-cultural Studies on the Transmission of HIV.* Liège, Belgium: Ordina.

Enel, C., G. Pison, and M. Lefebvre
1989 Migrations et évolution de la nuptialité. L'exemple d'un village Joola du sud du Sénégal, Mlomp. *Dossiers et Recherches.* No. 28. Paris: Institut National d'Etudes Démographiques, Muséum National d'Histoire Naturelle.
1994 Migration and marriage change: A case study of Mlomp, a Joola village in south-

ern Senegal. Pp. 92-113 in C. Bledsoe and G. Pison, eds., *Nuptiality in Sub-Saharan Africa: Contemporary Anthropological and Demographic Perspectives.* Oxford: Clarendon Press.

Fargues, P.
1989 The decline of Arab fertility. *Population: English Selection* 44 (September):147-175.

Fargues, P., and M. Khlat
1989 Child mortality in Beirut: Six indirect estimates based on data collected at the time of a birth. *Population Studies* 43(3):497-513.

Ferry, B.
1976 Données récentes sur la fécondité à Dakar (Sénégal). *Population* 31(3):717-722.
1977 *Etude de la Fécondité à Dakar: Objectifs, Méthodes, et Résultats.* Dakar: ORSTOM.
1981 The Senegalese surveys. Pp. 265-273 in H.J. Page and R. Lesthaeghe, eds., *Child-Spacing in Tropical Africa: Traditions and Change.* New York: Academic Press.

Frank, O.
1983 Infertility in sub-Saharan Africa: Estimates and implications. *Population and Development Review* 9(1):137-144.

Garenne, M.
1994 Mortality in sub-Saharan Africa: Trends and prospects. Pp. 167-186 in W. Lutz, ed., *The Future Population of the World: What Can We Assume Today?* London: International Institute for Applied Systems Analysis.

Garenne, M., and E. van de Walle
1989 Polygyny and fertility among the Sereer of Senegal. *Population Studies* 43:267-283.

Garenne, M., and J. van Ginneken
1994 Enquêtes rétrospectives et suivi longitudinal: Comparaisons sur les Serer. Pp. 385-407 in Y. Charbit and S. Ndiaye, eds., *La Population du Sénégal.* Paris: Centre d'Etudes et de Recherches sur les Populations Africaines et Asiatiques.

Garenne, M., P. Cantrelle, and I.L. Diop
1985 Le cas du Sénégal. Pp. 307-330 in J. Vallin and A. Lopez, eds., *La Lutte Contre la Mort.* Paris: Institut National d'Etudes Démographiques, Presses Universitaires de France.

Garenne, M., P. Cantrelle, and I. Sarr
1992 Estimation of Mortality Trends in Urban and Rural Senegal. Center for Population and Development Studies, Harvard University. Unpublished.

Goldberg, H., J.S. Friedman, F. M'Bodji, and A. Sow
1984 Final Report: Sine-Saloum Family Health Survey, 1982. Atlanta, Georgia: Centers for Disease Control.

Gordon, E., ed.
1988 *Senegal in Pictures*, rev. ed. Minneapolis, Minn.: Lerner Publications Company.

Guèye, L.
1984 *Evaluation de l'Enquête Sénégalaise sur la Fécondité 1978.* World Fertility Study Scientific Report No. 50. London: World Fertility Study.

Guèye, L., and B. Ferry
1985 Les déterminants proches de la fécondité. Pp. 105-127 in Y. Charbit, L. Guèye, and S. Ndiaye, eds., *Nuptialité et Fécondité au Sénégal.* Paris: Institut National d'Etudes Démographiques.

Guèye, C.
1989 Migrations inter-régionales au Sénégal: 1960-1980. *Historiens et Géographes du Sénégal* 4-5 (2nd semester):24-33.

Guèye, M., and A. Sarr

1985 La mortalité infanto-juvénile. Pp. 141-145 in Y. Charbit, L. Guèye, and S. Ndiaye, eds., *Nuptialité et Fécondité au Sénégal*, Cahier No. 112. Paris: Institut National d'Etudes Démographiques, Presses Universitaires de France.

Guillaumont, S.

1992 Les Difficultés de la Mesure du Taux de Change Réel: L'exemple du Sénégal. Paper presented at Colloque Association Française de Science Economique, Clermont-Ferrand, France.

Guzman, J.H.

1994 The onset of fertility decline in Latin America. Pp. 46-67 in T. Locoh and V. Hertrich, eds., *The Onset of Fertility Transition in Sub-Saharan Africa*. Liège, Belgium: Ordina.

Hill, A.L.L.

1992 Trends in childhood mortality in Sub-Saharan Africa. Pp. 10-31 in E. van de Walle, G. Pison, and M. Sala-Diakanda, eds., *Mortality and Society in Sub-Saharan Africa*. Oxford, England: Clarendon Press.

1993 Trends in childhood mortality. Pp. 153-217 in K.A. Foote, K.H. Hill, and L.G. Martin, eds., *Demographic Change in Sub-Saharan Africa*. Panel on the Population Dynamics of Sub-Saharan Africa, Committee on Population, National Research Council. Washington, D.C.: National Academy Press.

Hill, K.

1987 Estimating census and death registration completeness. *Asian and Pacific Population Forum* 1(3):8-13.

Hill, K., and A. Yazbeck

1994 Trends in child mortality, 1960-90: Estimates for 84 developing countries. *World Development Report 1993: Investing in Health*. Background Paper No. 6. Washington, D.C.: The World Bank.

Hugon, P.

1993 *L'Economie de l'Afrique*. Paris: La Découverte.

International Labour Organization

1989 *African Employment Report 1988*. Addis Ababa: Jobs and Skills Programme for Africa.

1991 *Towards Social Adjustment: Labour Market Issues in Structural Adjustment*. Geneva: International Labour Office.

International Monetary Fund

1993a *Balance of Payments Statistics Yearbook*. Washington, D.C.: International Monetary Fund.

1993b *International Financial Statistic Yearbook*. Washington, D.C.: International Monetary Fund.

Jolly, C., and J. Gribble

1993 The proximate determinants of fertility. Pp. 68-116 in K. Foote, K. Hill, and L. Martin, eds., *Demographic Change in Sub-Saharan Africa*. Panel on the Population Dynamics of Sub-Saharen Africa, Committee on Population, National Research Council. Washington, D.C.: National Academy Press.

Lacombe, B.

1972 Fertility and development in Senegal. Pp. 123-124 in S.H. Ominde and C.N. Ejiogu, eds., *Population Growth and Economic Development in Africa*. London: Heinemann.

1973 La fécondité des villages de Diahanor (Sénégal). *Cahiers ORSTOM: Série Sciences Humaines* 10(4):333-341.

Lagarde, E., G. Pison, C. Enel, and M. Lefebvre

Forthcoming Mlomp (Sénégal): Niveaux et tendances démographiques, 1985-1992. *Dossiers et Recherches* No. X. Paris: Institut National d'Etudes Démographiques.

Le Guenno, B., G. Pison, C. Enel, E. Lagarde, and C. Seck
1992 HIV2 seroprevalence in three rural regions of Senegal: Low levels and heterogeneous distribution. *Transactions of the Royal Society of Tropical Medicine and Hygiene* 86:301-302.

Lesthaeghe, R., G. Kaufmann, and D. Meekers
1989 The nuptiality regimes in sub-Saharan Africa. Pp. 238-337 in R. Lesthaeghe, ed., *Reproduction and Social Organization in Sub-Saharan Africa.* Berkeley: University of California Press.

Logeay, D.
1990 L'Industrie Sénégalaise: Perspectives après la nouvelle politique industrielle. Working Paper published in *Notes et Etudes.* Paris: Caisse Centrale de Cooperation Economique.

Mbodji, F.G.
1988 *Enquête sur la Mortalité Infantile dans le Sahel (EMIS).* Rapport d'analyse, Vol. 3. Dakar: Direction de la Statistique du Sénégal; Bamako, Mali: Centre D'Etudes et de Recherches sur la Population pour le Développement.

Mboup, G.
1993 Etude des Déterminants Socio-Economiques et Culturels de la Fécondité au Sénégal à Partir de l'Enquête Sénégalaise sur la Fécondité (ESF, 1978) et l'Enquête Démographique et de Santé (EDS, 1986). Unpublished Ph.D. dissertation, University of Montreal.

Meekers, D.
1992 The process of marriage in African societies. *Population and Development Review* 18(1):61-78.

Montalieu, T., and P. Plane
1993 *Chocs et Ajustement de la Balance des Paiements; un Modèle Balassa Révisé.* Working Paper. Clermont-Ferrand, France: Centre de Recherches pour le Développement International.

Moore, D.G., G.G. Tappan, S.M. Howard, R.W. Lietzow, C.A. Nadeau, W. Renison, J. Olsson, and R. Kite
1992 *Geographic Modeling of Human Carrying Capacity from Rainfed Agriculture: Senegal Case Study.* USAID PASA No. AFR-0510-P-IC-7022. Washington, D.C.: Office of Technical Resources, Bureau for Africa, U.S. Agency for International Development; Sioux Falls, South Dakota: EROS Data Center.

National Research Council
1982 *The Estimation of Recent Trends in Fertility and Mortality in Egypt.* Panel on Egypt, Committee on Population and Demography, Report No. 9. Washington, D.C.: National Academy Press.

Ndiaye, K.L.
1985 Polygamie et fécondité. Pp. 59-72 in Y. Charbit, L. Guèye, and S. Ndiaye, eds., *Nuptialité et Fécondité au Sénégal.* Paris: Institut National d'Etudes Démographiques, Presses Universitaires de France.

Ndiaye, S.
1992 Niveaux et Tendances de la Fécondité. Preliminary Report. Direction de la Statistique, Dakar. Restricted.

Ndiaye, S., I. Sarr, and M. Ayad
1988 *Enquête Démographique et de Santé au Sénégal, 1986.* Dakar: Ministère de l'Economie et des Finances, Direction de la Statistique, Division des Enquêtes et de la Démographie; Columbia, Md.: Institute for Resource Development/Westinghouse.

Ndiaye, S., P.D. Diouf, and M. Ayad
1994 *Enquête Démographique et de Santé au Sénégal (EDS-II), 1992/93.* Dakar: Divi-

sion des Statistiques Démographiques, Direction de la Prévision et de la Statistique; Calverton, Md.: Macro International, Inc.

OCCGE-Muraz
1990 *Evaluation du Programme Elargi de Vaccination (PEV) au Sénégal.* B. Floury, coordinator of study. Project of OCCGE-Muraz, Bobo Dioulasso, Burkina Faso.

Ogbu, O., and M. Gallagher
1992 Public expenditures and health care in Africa. *Social Science and Medicine* 34(6):615-624.

Osmanski, R., J. DuMoulin, N.P. Harris, C.C. Hart, P. Kelly, A. Lagace, S. Maher, and B. Pillsbury
1991 *Senegal Health and Population Sector Assessment.* Report No. 90-082-117. Washington, D.C.: U.S. Agency for International Development.

Pillsbury, B.
1990 Socio-cultural factors influencing the delivery and use of health and family planning services in Senegal (with special attention to women's health). Pp. 10-i-10-40 in R. Osmanski, J. DuMoulin, N.P. Harris, C.C. Hart, P. Kelly, A. Lagace, S. Maher, and B. Pillsbury, *Senegal Health and Population Sector Assessment.* Report No. 90-082-117. Washington, D.C.: U.S. Agency for International Development.

Pison, G.
1978 Etudes démographiques de la région du Sine Saloum (Sénégal): La reprise de l'enquête à passages répétés de Nayokhème en 1977. *Méthodes d'Enquêtes et Premiers Résultats.* Dakar: ORSTOM.
1986 La démographie de la polygamie. *Population* 41(1):93-122.
1989 La nuptialité en Afrique au sud du Sahara: Changements en cours et impact sur la fécondité. *Population* 44(4-5):949-959.

Pison, G., and A. Desgrées du Loû
1993 Bandafassi (Sénégal): Niveaux et tendances démographiques 1971-1991. *Dossier et Recherches* No. 40. Paris: Institut National d'Etudes Démographiques.
Forth-coming Bandafassi: A 22 year prospective community study in rural Senegal. In M. Das Gupta, P. Aaby, M. Garenne, G. Pison, eds., *Prospective Community Studies in Developing Countries.* Oxford: Clarendon Press.

Pison, G., J.F. Trape, M. Lefebvre, and C. Enel
1993 Rapid decline in child mortality in a rural area of Senegal. *International Journal of Epidemiology* 22(1):72-80.

Pison, G., A. Langaney, M. Lefebvre, and C. Enel
1991 The Bandafassi and Mlomp Studies in Sénégal. Paper prepared for the seminar on Socio-Cultural Determinants of Morbidity and Mortality in Developing Countries: The Role of Longitudinal Studies. The Anthropological Demography Committee of the International Union for Scientific Study of Population. Saly Portudal, Senegal, October 7-11.

Preston, S.H., and N.G. Bennett
1983 A census-based method for estimating adult mortality. *Population Studies* 37(1):91-104.

Projet Niakhar
1992 *Population et Santé à Niakhar: Niveaux et Tendances des Principaux Indicateurs Démographiques et Epidémiologiques de la Zone d'Etude 1984-1991.* Dakar: ORSTOM, 76 pp.

République du Sénégal
1964 *Résultats de L'Enquête Démographique 1960/1961, Données Régionales.* Dakar: Ministère du Plan et du Développement, Service de la Statistique.

1974 *Enquête Démographique National 1970-1971, Série A.* Dakar: Ministère des Finances et des Affaires Economiques, Direction de la Statistique.

1981 *Enquête Sénégalaise sur la Fécondité, 1978: Rapport National d'Analyse,* Volume 1, *Analyse des Résultats Définitifs,* and Volume 2, *Résultats Définitifs.* Dakar: Ministère de l'Economie et des Finances, Direction de la Statistique.

1982a *Recensement Général de la Population d'Avril 1976: Résultats Définitifs Région du Cap-Vert.* Ministère de l'Economie et des Finances, Direction de la Statistique, Bureau National du Recensement.

1982b *Recensement Général de la Population d'Avril 1976: Résultats Définitifs Région de Casamance.* Ministère de l'Economie et des Finances, Direction de la Statistique, Bureau National du Recensement.

1982c *Recensement Général de la Population d'Avril 1976: Résultats Définitifs Région de Diourbel.* Ministère de l'Economie et des Finances, Direction de la Statistique, Bureau National du Recensement.

1982d *Recensement Général de la Population d'Avril 1976: Résultats Définitifs Région du Fleuve.* Ministère de l'Economie et des Finances, Direction de la Statistique, Bureau National du Recensement.

1982e *Recensement Général de la Population d'Avril 1976: Résultats Définitifs Région de Louga.* Ministère de l'Economie et des Finances, Direction de la Statistique, Bureau National du Recensement.

1982f *Recensement Général de la Population d'Avril 1976: Résultats Définitifs Région de Sénégal Oriental.* Ministère de l'Economie et des Finances, Direction de la Statistique, Bureau National du Recensement.

1982g *Recensement Général de la Population d'Avril 1976: Résultats Définitifs Région du Sine Saloum.* Ministère de l'Economie et des Finances, Direction de la Statistique, Bureau National du Recensement.

1982h *Recensement Général de la Population d'Avril 1976: Résultats Définitifs Région de Thiès.* Ministère de l'Economie et des Finances, Direction de la Statistique, Bureau National du Recensement.

1988 *Situation Economique.* Dakar: Direction de la Prévision et de la Statistique.

1989 *Les Principaux Résultats Provisoires du Recensement de la Population de l'Habitat du Sénégal.* Présidence de la République, Sécrétariat Général, Délégation de la Prévision et de la Statistique. December.

1990 *Programme National de Planification Famililale.* Dakar: Ministère de l'Economie et des Finances et du plan, Direction de la Planification.

1991 *Déclaration de la Politique de Population.* Dakar: Ministère de l'Economie et des Finances et du Plan, Direction de la Planification.

1992a *Population du Sénégal: Structure par Sexe et par Age en 1988 et Projections de 1989 à 2015.* Dakar: Ministère de l'Economie, des Finances et du Plan, Direction de la Prévision et de la Statistique.

1992b *Recensement Général de la Population et de l'Habitat de 1988, Rapport Régional (Résultats Définitifs) Dakar.* Dakar: Ministère de l'Economie, des Finances et du Plan, Direction de la Prévision et de la Statistique.

1992c *Recensement Général de la Population et de l'Habitat de 1988, Rapport Régional (Résultats Définitifs) Diourbel.* Dakar: Ministère de l'Economie, des Finances et du Plan, Direction de la Prévision et de la Statistique.

1992d *Recensement Général de la Population et de l'Habitat de 1988, Rapport Régional (Résultats Définitifs) Fatick.* Dakar: Ministère de l'Economie, des Finances et du Plan, Direction de la Prévision et de la Statistique.

1992e *Recensement Général de la Population et de l'Habitat de 1988, Rapport Régional*

(Résultats Définitifs) Kaolack. Dakar: Ministère de l'Economie, des Finances et du Plan, Direction de la Prévision et de la Statistique.

1992f *Recensement Général de la Population et de l'Habitat de 1988, Rapport Régional (Résultats Définitifs) Kolda.* Dakar: Ministère de l'Economie, des Finances et du Plan, Direction de la Prévision et de la Statistique.

1992g *Recensement Général de la Population et de l'Habitat de 1988, Rapport Régional (Résultats Définitifs) Louga.* Dakar: Ministère de l'Economie, des Finances et du Plan, Direction de la Prévision et de la Statistique.

1992h *Recensement Général de la Population et de l'Habitat de 1988, Rapport Régional (Résultats Définitifs) Saint-Louis.* Dakar: Ministère de l'Economie, des Finances et du Plan, Direction de la Prévision et de la Statistique.

1992i *Recensement Général de la Population et de l'Habitat de 1988, Rapport Régional (Résultats Définitifs) Tambacounda.* Dakar: Ministère de l'Economie, des Finances et du Plan, Direction de la Prévision et de la Statistique.

1992j *Recensement Général de la Population et de l'Habitat de 1988, Rapport Régional (Résultats Définitifs) Thiès.* Dakar: Ministère de l'Economie, des Finances et du Plan, Direction de la Prévision et de la Statistique.

1992k *Recensement Général de la Population et de l'Habitat de 1988, Rapport Régional (Résultats Définitifs) Ziguinchor.* Dakar: Ministère de l'Economie, des Finances et du Plan, Direction de la Prévision et de la Statistique.

no date *Recensement Général de la Population d'Avril 1976: Analyse des Résultats Nationaux.* Ministère de l'Economie et des Finances, Direction de la Statistique, Bureau National du Recensement.

République Tunisienne

1982 *Enquête Tunisienne sur la Fécondité 1978, Vol. 1 & 2.* Office National du Planning Familial et de la Population. République Tunisienne: Enquête Mondiale sur la Fécondité.

Rodriguez, G., and J.N. Hobcraft

1980 Illustrative analysis: Life table analysis of birth intervals in Columbia. *World Fertility Survey Scientific Reports.* No. 16. London: International Statistical Institute.

Rosetta, L.

1989 Breast feeding and post-partum amenorrhea in Serere women in Senegal. *Annals of Human Biology* 16(4):311-320.

Rouis, M.

1994 Senegal: Stabilization, partial adjustment, and stagnation. Pp. 286-351 in I. Husain and R. Faruqee, eds., *Adjustment in Africa: Lessons from Country Case Studies.* Washington, D.C.: The World Bank

Russell, S.S.

1993 International migration. Pp. 297-349 in K.A. Foote, K.H. Hill, and L.G. Martin, eds., *Demographic Change in Sub-Saharan Africa.* Panel on the Population Dynamics of Sub-Saharan Africa, Committee on Population, National Research Council. Washington, D.C.: National Academy Press.

Rutstein, S.O.

1983 Infant and child mortality: Levels, trends and demographic differentials. *Comparative Studies No. 24, World Fertility Survey.* Voorburg, Netherlands: International Statistical Institute.

Sadio, A.

1985 Fécondité générale et fécondité légitime: Analyse différentielle. Pp. 15-36 in Y. Charbit, L. Guèye, and S. Ndiaye, *Nuptialité et Fécondité au Sénégal.* Paris: Presses Universitaires de France.

Schultz, T.P.
1981 *Economics of Population.* Reading, Mass.: Addison-Wesley Publishing Company.
1994 Human capital, family planning and their effects on population growth. *American Economic Review* 84(2):255-260.

Shryock, H.S., J.S. Siegel, and Associates
1976 *Studies in Population: The Methods and Materials of Demography.* Condensed Edition by E.G. Stockwell. San Diego, Calif.: Academic Press, Inc.

Smith, D.P., E. Carrasco, and P. McDonald
1984 *Marriage Dissolution and Remarriage.* World Fertility Survey Comparative Studies No. 34. London: World Fertility Survey.

Sow, B.
1994a Déterminants des intervalles intergénésiques. Pp. 197-209 in Y. Charbit and S. Ndiaye, eds., *La Population du Sénégal.* Paris: Centre d'Etudes et de Recherches sur les Populations Africaines et Asiatiques.
1994b Allaitement, abstinence, et aménorrhée post-partum. Pp. 211-230 in Y. Charbit and S. Ndiaye, eds., *La Population du Sénégal.* Paris: Centre d'Etudes et de Recherches sur les Populations Africaines et Asiatiques.

Sow, F.
1985 Nuptialité et fécondité des femmes rurales. Pp. 129-132 in Y. Charbit, L. Guèye, and S. Ndiaye, eds., *Nuptialité et Fécondité au Sénégal.* Paris: Institut National d'Etudes Démographiques.

Stoto, M.A.
1993 Models of the demographic effect of AIDS. Pp. 350-379 in K.A. Foote, K.H. Hill, and L.G. Martin, eds., *Demographic Change in Sub-Saharan Africa.* Panel on the Population Dynamics of Sub-Saharan Africa, Committee on Population, National Research Council. Washington, D.C.: National Academy Press.

Sy, M.
1991 Les raisons de migrer des Sénégalaises déterminées par l'appartenance ethnique et le statut social. *Pop Sahel* 16(April):29-35.

Timæus, I.M.
1991 New estimates of adult mortality from DHS data on the timing of orphanhood relative to marriage. Pp. 857-874 in *Proceedings of Demographic and Health Surveys World Conference, Washington, D.C., 1991*, Vol. 2. Columbia, Md.: Institute for Resource Development/Macro International, Inc.
1993 Adult mortality. Pp. 218-255 in K.A. Foote, K.H. Hill, and L.G. Martin, eds., *Demographic Change in Sub-Saharan Africa.* Panel on the Population Dynamics of Sub-Saharan Africa, Committee on Population, National Research Council. Washington, D.C: National Academy Press.

United Nations
1983a *Manual X: Indirect Techniques for Demographic Estimation.* Population Studies No. 81. New York: United Nations, Department of International Economic and Social Affairs.
1983b Marriage and fertility in Africa. *Nuptiality and Fertility (A comparative analysis of WFS data).* Africa Population Studies Series, No. 5. Addis Ababa, Ethiopia. New York: United Nations Economic Commission for Africa.
1991 *World Population Prospects 1990.* Population Studies No. 120. New York: Department of International Economic and Social Affairs, United Nations.

Valette, A.
1991 *Enjeux et Réalités d'une Politique Publique: La Nouvelle Politique Industrielle Sénégalaise.* Bordeaux: ORSTOM.

van de Walle, E.

1968 Marriage in African censuses and inquiries. Pp. 183-238 in W. Brass, A.J. Coale, P. Demeny, D.F. Heisel, F. Lorimar, A. Romaniuk, and E. van de Walle, eds., *The Demography of Tropical Africa.* Princeton, N.J.: Princeton University Press.

1993 Recent trends in marriage ages. Pp. 117-152 in K.A. Foote, K.H. Hill, and L.G. Martin, eds., *Demographic Change in Sub-Saharan Africa.* Panel on the Population Dynamics of Sub-Saharan Africa, Committee on Population, National Research Council. Washington, D.C: National Academy Press.

van de Walle, E., and A.D. Foster

1990 *Fertility Decline in Africa: Assessment and Prospects.* World Bank Technical Paper No. 125, Africa Technical Department Series. Washington, D.C.: The World Bank.

Vandemoortele, J.

1991 Labour market informalisation in sub-Saharan Africa. Pp. 81-113 in G. Standing and V. Tokman, eds., *Towards Social Adjustment.* Geneva: International Labour Office.

Verrière, L.

1965 La Population du Sénégal: Aspects Quantitatifs. Unpublished doctoral thesis. Faculté de Droit et des Sciences Economiques, Université de Dakar.

Waltisperger, D.

1974 *Le Fichier de Population de Ngayokhème: Analyse des Données 1963-1970.* Dakar: ORSTOM.

Waterlow, J.R., R. Buzina, W. Keller, J. Lane, M. Nichaman, and J. Tanner

1977 The presentation and use of height and weight data for comparing the nutritional status of groups of children under the age of five years. *Bulletin of the World Health Organization* 55:489.

Willis, R.J.

1973 Economic theory of fertility behavior. Pp. 25-75 in T.W. Schultz, ed., *Economics of the Family: Marriage, Children and Human Capital.* Chicago: University of Chicago Press for the National Bureau of Economic Research.

Working Group on Demographic Effects of Economic and Social Reversals

1993 *Demographic Effects of Economic Reversals in Sub-Saharan Africa.* Panel on the Population Dynamics of Sub-Saharan Africa, Committee on Population, National Research Council. Washington, D.C.: National Academy Press.

Working Group on Kenya

1993 *Population Dynamics of Kenya.* W. Brass and C.L. Jolly, eds. Panel on the Population Dynamics of Sub-Saharan Africa, Committee on Population, National Research Council. Washington, D.C.: National Academy Press.

Working Group on the Social Dynamics of Adolescent Fertility

1993 *Social Dynamics of Adolescent Fertility in Sub-Saharan Africa.* C.H. Bledsoe and B. Cohen, eds. Panel on the Population Dynamics of Sub-Saharan Africa, Committee on Population, National Research Council. Washington, D.C.: National Academy Press.

World Bank

1982 *World Development Report 1982.* New York: Oxford University Press.

1988 *Education in Sub-Saharan Africa: Policies for Adjustment, Revitalization, and Expansion.* Washington, D.C.: The World Bank.

1993a *Senegal: Macroceonomic Update Report.* Report no. 11041-SE. Washington, D.C.: The World Bank.

1993b *World Development Report 1993: Investing in Health.* Oxford: Oxford University Press.

Index

A

Abortion, 77, 102–105 (*see also* Index of induced abortion)
Abstinence, 96–99 (*see also* Index of postpartum infecundability)
Accidents
  and adult mortality, 175
Acquired immunodeficiency syndrome (AIDS), 178–180
Administrative divisions, 9–10, 11 *(see also* Departments; Regions; *and specific departments and regions)*
Adolescence
  and age at marriage, 85
Adoption effect (*see* Orphanhood method)
Africa *(see also specific countries)*
  age at marriage in, 198–199
  demand for children in, 199
  demographic transition in, 7, 45, 198–201
  family planning in, 197
  fertility decline in, 3, 7, 198–199
  illegitimacy in, 3, 107, 198–199
  mortality decline in, 7, 113
Africa, north (*see also* Tunisia)
  age at marriage in, 3, 199–200
  contraceptive use in, 3, 107, 200
  fertility decline in, 107, 199–200
  fertility in, 3, 107, 109
  ideal family size in, 3, 200
Africa, sub-Saharan
  contraceptive use in, 3
  fertility decline in, 7, 45, 56, 107
  marriage and fertility in, 3
  mortality trends in, 113
  population growth in, 45
Age
  and adult mortality, 161–180, 184
  of child, and child mortality, 130–135
  data quality for, 32, 115, 163
  and desired family size, 103
  exaggeration, 161, 163, 168, 223–224
  and fertility (*see* ASFRs)
  at first marriage (*see* Age at marriage)
  heaping in censuses, and mortality estimation, 159
  and internal migration, 37, 40
  and life expectancy, 5, 161–163, 165, 166–175, 175, 180, 184
  misreporting, 32, 159, 161, 163
  of mother, and child mortality, 152–154
  and polygyny, 91–95
  and proportions never married, 80–85, 86–87

sex ratios by, 33
and stunting, 137, 142–143
and wasting, 137, 140–141
Age at first birth *(see also specific areas)*
and age at marriage, 88–91
changes in, 68
in Dakar, 91
and education, 200
by ethnicity, 90–91
Age at marriage, 80–85 *(see also* Marriage; Proportions never married; *and specific areas and ethnic groups)*
and adolescence, 85
and age at first birth, 88–91
and ASFRs, 77
and birth interval, 111
and education, 2, 83, 85, 106
by ethnicity, 83, 90–91
and fertility, 80–85, 92, 95
and fertility decline, 2, 3, 77, 106–107, 197–201
by grand region, 83–84
and internal migration, 83
rise in, 3, 89, 91, 106
singulate mean age at marriage (SMAM), and socioeconomic indicators, 74
in small-scale studies, 63, 90, 91
by urban/rural residence, 83, 85
Age distribution
of Dakar, 34, 36
and intercensal growth rates, 161
stationary ($_5L_x$), 166–167
of total country, 31–32
Age-specific fertility rates (*see* ASFRs)
Age-specific mortality rates (ASMRs), 163–164, 166–167
AIDS (acquired immunodeficiency syndrome), 178–180
Amenorrhea (*see* Postpartum amenorrhea)
Anovulatory interval (*see* Index of postpartum infecundability)
Antimalarial campaign, 186–187
ASFRs (age-specific fertility rates) *(see also* Fertility; *and specific areas)*
and age at marriage, 77
from census and other sources, compared, 64, 66
changes in, 2, 58, 106
in Dakar, 68, 70, 210
by department, 59–61, 210–219
by education, 70–72, 73
by ethnicity, 70–71
by grand region, 57–59, 60
national, 209
by region, 210–219
in small-scale studies, 62–67
and TFR, 51–52, 55, 57, 72–75
by urban/rural residence, 69, 209–219
from various sources, compared, 51
ASMRs (age-specific mortality rates), 163–164, 166–167

B

B_{60} (censored parity progression ratios), 55–57, 108
Bakel (department)
child mortality in, 127–129, 128, 130, 149–150
Bambey (department)
child mortality in, 127–129
Bandafassi (study area)
adult mortality in, 168–170, 173, 175, 184
and age at marriage and age at first birth, 90–91
ASFRs in, 62–66
birth intervals in, 98–99
fertility in, 49, 62–63
life expectancy at ages 15 or 20 in, 169, 175, 184
life tables for, 173
sterility in, 106
survey of, 62, 204, 205
vaccination coverage in, 191–193
Bandafassi, child mortality in
by age, 131–135
causes of, 138–139, 144, 145
by ethnicity, 151
and infant mortality, 116, 117
in rural areas of, 123
by sex, 134, 136
Basse Casamance (region) (*see* Ziguinchor)
BCG vaccine (*see* Tuberculosis)
Bedik (ethnic group) (*see also* Ethnicity)
and age at marriage and age at first birth, 90–91
fertility of, 63
Beds, hospital
distribution and numbers of, 185, 187
Birth histories
data sources with, 204–206

and fertility estimation, 47, 50, 53–54
and mortality estimation, 115
as source of mortality data, 119–122
Birth intervals *(see also specific areas)*
and abstinence, amenorrhea, and breastfeeding, 95–99
and age at marriage, 111
and child survival, 97
and fertility, 2
and fertility decline, 2
by urban/rural residence, 98–99
Birth order
and child mortality, 152–154
Birth registers, 46
Botswana
family planning program in, 197
fertility decline in, 3, 45, 55, 107, 198–199
illegitimacy in, 3, 198–199
teenage marriage in, 3, 198–199
Brass Growth Balance Method for estimating coverage of adult deaths, 222–224
Brass orphanhood method (*see* Orphanhood method)
Brass P/F ratio fertility estimating technique, 47–50, 53, 54
Breastfeeding, 78 *(see also* Index of postpartum infecundability; *and specific areas)*
and abstinence, amenorrhea, and birth intervals, 95–99
and anovulatory intervals, 96
and contraception, 112
and education, 112
by urban/rural residence, 97–98
Burkino-Faso
emigration to, 41–42, 43
Burundi
fertility decline in, 45

C

C_a (*see* Index of induced abortion)
Cap-Vert (Dakar) Fertility Survey, 205
Casamance (region), 10 (*see also* Kolda; Ziguinchor)
age at marriage in, 106
C_c (*see* Index of contraception)
Censored parity progression ratios (*see* B_{60})
Census (*see* Population census)
Central region (*see* Grand regions)
Child mortality (*see* Mortality, child)
Child survival
and birth intervals, 97
preceding, and child mortality, 152, 154
Children, demand for (*see* Ideal family size)
Chloroquinization (antimalarial program), 187
Cholera
and adult mortality, 175
C_i (*see* Index of postpartum infecundability)
Circulatory system
diseases of, 175
C_m (*see* Index of marriage)
Coale-Demeny model life tables (*see* Model life tables)
Coitus, frequency of, 77
and polygyny, 91–92
Community health workers
in new health policy, 188
Composite facilities indicator (*see also* Electricity; Housing quality; Latrine facilities; Socioeconomic indicators; Water)
defined, 23, 75
by department, 24–25, 75–76
and fertility, 75
and nuptiality, 76
by region, 24–25, 28
Condoms (*see* Contraception)
Consensual unions, 111
Construction, good (*see also* Housing quality)
defined, 29
by region, 23–26
Contraception
effectiveness of methods of, 110
knowledge of modern methods of, 100, 101
Contraceptive use (*see also* Index of contraception)
and breastfeeding, 112
in Dakar, 3
and education, 100, 101, 112
effectiveness of, 110
factors affecting, 108
and fertility decline, 106–108, 197
levels of, 2–3, 100–101, 106, 200
and MCH, 3–4
in north Africa, 3, 107, 200
in other African countries, 3, 198–199, 200

by parity, 72
and urban/rural residence, 100, 101
Correlations between socioeconomic indicators
and adult mortality, 183
and child mortality, 155
and fertility and nuptiality, 74
Côte d'Ivoire
emigration to, 42, 43

D

Dagana (department), child mortality in, 127–129
by urban/rural residence, 128, 149
Dakar
adult mortality in, 176, 177, 181, 182
age at first birth in, 91
age at marriage in, 2, 3, 106
age distribution of, 34, 36
ASFRs in, 68, 70, 210
concentration of health infrastructure in, 187
contraceptive use in, 3
distance from, and child mortality, 125–126
distance from, and socioeconomic status, 28
dominant ethnic group in, 32
fertility and marriage in, 91
fertility decline in, 2, 3
fertility in, 2, 48–49, 60, 68, 109
fertility survey of, 205–206
health infrastructure in, 185
health personnel in, 185, 187
HIV prevalence in, 178–179
immigrants in, 41
and migration, temporary, 39, 40
migration to and from, 34, 36, 37, 38
population density of, 34
population size and growth of, 31, 32–33, 34
proportion of total population, 34
proportions never married in, 81, 85, 87, 91
sex ratio in, 32
socioeconomic indicators for, 23–29
urbanization in, 34
and urban/rural comparisons of child mortality, 146
vaccination coverage in, 191–193
vital registration system in, 12
Dakar, child mortality in, 4, 118–124, 156
by age, 130–131, 132
by migrant status, 120–121
Dakar-Pikine Survey, 207
Data quality
in 1988 census, 65–67, 115–117, 208–209
for adult mortality, 194
for age, 32, 159, 161, 168, 173, 223–224
for child mortality, 118, 133
and estimates of population growth, 32–33
for fertility, 50–54, 108
and period parity distribution, 52
and P/F ratio, 47
and reference period error, 108
Data sources, 7–8, 8, 46 (*see also* DHS; DS; NDS; Population census; Small-scale studies; WFS)
for abortion, 102–104
for adult mortality, 157, 159
for child mortality, 114–122
for fertility, 46–47
historical, 12
listed and described, 203–206
for migration, internal, 35–36
DDT
use in antimalarial campaign, 186–187
Death
age at, data quality for, 115, 163
causes of, among adults, 169–175
causes of, among children, 138–139, 144, 145
registration of, 12, 175
Deaths
in previous year, and mortality estimation, 163–164, 166, 178, 184
Demand for children, 109 (*see also* Desired family size)
in other African countries, 199
Demographic and Health Surveys (*see* DHS)
Demographic indicators
and child mortality, 139–151, 152, 153
correlations of, with socioeconomic indicators, 74
Demographic Survey (*see* DS)
Demographic transition in Africa, 7, 45, 198–201
Density, population, 9
by region, 34, 35

Departments, administrative, 9–10, 11 *(see also specific departments)*
adult mortality in, 177
ASFRs in, 59–61, 210–219
composite facilities indicator in, 24–25, 75–76
fertility in, 59–61, 72–75, 210–219
HIV prevalence in, 178–179
infant and child mortality in, 116, 117
nuptiality in, 75–76
socioeconomic indicators for, 24–25
Departments, administrative, child mortality in, 127–130, 149–150
and infant mortality, 116, 117
by urban/rural residence, 128, 149
Depo-Provera (*see* Contraception)
Desired family size (*see also* Ideal family size)
by age, 103
decline in, 107, 200–201
by education, 200–201
and fertility decline, 107, 196–197
level of, 101–102
by parity, 101–102
Development assistance
and economic reforms, 20
and family planning, 100
and GDP, 19
and mortality decline, 156
DHS (Demographic and Health Surveys)
and B_{60}, 55–57
child mortality estimates from, 116, 118–122, 127
child nutrition estimates from, 137
data on vaccinations from, 189, 193–194
described, 204, 205
fertility data from, 1, 48–54, 56–59
regions in, 6
as source for abortion data, 105
as source for fertility data, 46–47, 50
as source for nuptiality data, 85
as source for vaccination data, 193–194
as source of child mortality data, 115
Diahanor (study area)
birth intervals in, 98–99
survey of, 204, 206
Diarrhea
and adult mortality, 175
and child mortality, 138–139
Diffusion
of fertility trends, 76
Digestive system
diseases of, 175
Digit preference
and mortality estimation, 159, 161, 163
Diola (ethnic group), 32 (*see also* Ethnicity)
and age at marriage and migration, 83
fertility of, 49, 70–71
polygyny among, 95
temporary migration of, 41
Diourbel (region), 10 (*see also* Louga)
adult mortality in, 6, 176, 178
ASFRs in, 211
dominant ethnic group in, 32
and migration, temporary, 40
migration to and from, 37, 38
population density of, 34
population size and growth of, 32–33
proportions never married in, 81
socioeconomic indicators for, 23–27
vaccination coverage in, 191–192
Diphtheria, 188 (*see also* DPT)
Dispensaries
and child mortality, 130
distance from, and vaccination coverage, 193
distribution and number of, 185–187
under EPI, 188
Divorce (*see* Marital disruption; Marital stability)
Doctors
distribution of, 185, 187
DPT (diphtheria, pertussis, tetanus)
vaccination levels of, 189, 190
DS (Demographic Survey), 203
fertility data from, 47–48, 53, 55
as source of child mortality data, 114–115
as source of fertility data, 46

E

Economic indicators, 22 (*see also* Socioeconomic indicators)
Economic policy, 5, 14–15, 155–156
Economic setting, 13–29
Education, 13 (*see also* School enrollment)
and adult mortality, 180–183
and age at first birth, 200
and age at marriage, 2, 83, 85, 106
and ASFRs, 70–72, 73
and breastfeeding, 112

and child mortality, 5, 139, 146–150, 152–157
and contraceptive use, 100, 101, 112
and demographic indicators, 74
and desired family size, 200–201
and fertility, 2, 3, 50, 67, 70–74, 77, 107, 196–197
and fertility decline, 2, 3, 107–108, 197
and formal sector employment, 110
level of, 13, 17, 23–26
and marital stability, 88
and marriage, 74
and mortality decline, 198
and polygyny, 93, 95, 112
and population growth, 13
and proportions never married, 81–83, 85, 86
quality of, 13
by region, 24–27
and stunting, 137–138, 142
and wasting, 137–138, 140

Egypt
age at marriage in, 3
desired family size in, 3
fertility decline in, 3, 107, 199

Electricity (*see also* Composite facilities indicator; Socioeconomic indicators)
and adult mortality, 180, 183
and demographic indicators, 74
by region, 23–26

Emigration
data on, 42
destinations of, 41–42, 43

Employment
in formal sector and education, 110
and marital stability, 88
public-sector, 14, 20, 21

Enquête Sur les Priorités (structural adjustment survey), 205

Enrollment (*see* School enrollment)

EPI (Expanded Programme on Immunization), 187–194, 198
and decline in child mortality, 5
impacts of, 114
results of, 139, 155

Ethnic groups (*see also specific ethnic groups*)
composition of, 43
major, 32
wealth of, and child mortality, 130

Ethnicity
and age at first birth, 90–91
and age at marriage, 83, 90–91
and ASFRs, 70–71
and child mortality, 146, 150–151, 152–153
and fertility, 49, 63, 68–71, 93
and life expectancy at age 20, 169
and marital stability, 88
and marriage process, 110–111
and migration, 83
and migration, temporary, 41
and polygyny, 95
and proportions never married, 82

European contact, 10–12

e(x) (*see* Life expectancy)

Exchange rate, 22

Expanded Programme on Immunization (*see* EPI)

Expectation of life (*see* Life expectancy)

Exports, 14, 15, 19

F

Fakao (study area)
birth intervals in, 98–99
survey in, 204, 206

Family planning
clinics, number of, 185
demand for, 101–102
and fertility decline, 196–197
and foreign assistance, 100
growth in, 100
and ideal family size, 101–102, 104
in other African countries, 197

Family size (*see also* Desired family size; Ideal family size)
and measles, 131

Fatick (department), child mortality in, 127–129
and infant mortality, 116, 117

Fatick (region)
adult mortality in, 6, 176, 177
antimalarial campaign in, 186–187
ASFRs in, 212
demographic survey of, 206
dominant ethnic group in, 32
and migration, temporary, 39, 40–41
migration to and from, 37, 38
population size and growth in, 32–33, 34
proportions never married in, 81

socioeconomic indicators for, 24–28
urbanization in, 34
vaccination coverage in, 192
Fertility, 1–4, 45–112 *(see also* ASFRs; Proximate determinants; TFR; *and specific areas)*
and abortion, 105
African fertility transition, 198–199
and age at marriage, 80–85, 92, 95
and birth intervals, 2
control of (*see* Contraception)
in Dakar, 2, 48–49, 60, 68, 91, 109
data quality, 50–54, 108
data sources, 46–47
by department, 59–61, 72–75, 210–219
and education, 2, 3, 50, 67, 70–74, 77, 107, 196–197
estimates of, from censuses, 46, 51–53, 59–61, 64–67, 109, 208–219
estimating techniques, 47, 208–209
by ethnicity, 49, 68–70, 71
by grand region, 48, 57–60, 61, 77
and housing quality, 74
illegitimate (*see* Illegitimacy)
increase in, 53–55, 76, 106
and infertility, 55
levels of, 46–57, 106
and marital stability, 55, 88
and marriage, 3, 77–95
new home economics model of, 67, 109
policies, 3–4, 107–108
and polygyny, 91–95
and population growth, 196
premarital (*see* Illegitimacy)
and proportions never married, 92
by region, 48, 57–67, 77, 210–219
by socioeconomic characteristic, 67–76
teenage, 89–91, 90
transition in, 198–201
trends in, 46–57, 76, 106
and urbanization, 2. 3, 74, 197
by urban/rural residence, 49, 59, 60, 68, 69, 107, 197
Fertility decline *(see also specific areas)*
by age, 2, 106 (*see also* ASFRs)
and age at marriage, 2, 3, 77, 91, 106–107, 197–201
and birth intervals, 2
and child mortality, 196–197
conditions for, 196–197
and contraceptive use, 106–108, 197
contrasted with other African countries, 3, 7
in Dakar, 2, 3
and desired family size, 107, 196–197
detecting, 55–59
diffusion of, 76
and education, 2, 3, 107–108, 197
factors affecting, 2–4, 196–197
and family planning, 196–197
and ideal family size, 2–3, 106, 196
and illegitimacy, 107
and income, 67
and mortality, 196–197
in north Africa, 107
policies regarding, 3–4, 107–108
by region, 57–59
in rural areas, 197
in Senegal compared with Tunisia, 199–201
in sub-Saharan Africa, 7, 45, 56, 107
and urbanization, 2, 3, 197
by urban/rural residence, 107
First births (*see* Age at first birth)
Fissel (study area)
abstinence, amenorrhea, and breastfeeding in, 98–99
child mortality in, 123–125, 151
survey of, 204, 207
Formal sector
and education, 110
Foundiougne (department)
child mortality in, 127–129
France
migration to and from, 42
French
presence of, 10–12
Frequency of intercourse, 77
and polygyny, 91–92

G

Gambia, The
migration to and from, 42, 43
struggle over, 12
GDP (gross domestic product)
change in, 13–14
and development assistance, 19
growth in, 20, 21, 22
General Growth Balance Method for estimating coverage of adult deaths, 222–224

GNP (gross national product) (*see also* Per capita GNP)
and external debt, 19
Grand regions
and age at marriage, 83–84
ASFRs in, 57–59, 60
child mortality in, 4, 126, 149, 152–153
defined, 6, 57, 108, 194, 204
fertility in, 48, 57–60, 61, 77
proportions never married in, 81, 83, 84, 85
Gross domestic product (*see* GDP)
Gross national product (*see* GNP; Per capita GNP)
Growth (*see also* Population growth)
of children, and nutrition, 134–138, 140–143
Growth Balance Method for estimating coverage of adult deaths, 164, 222–223
Guinea
immigration from, 41, 42
Guinea-Bissau
migration to and from, 41, 42, 43

H

Hazard models (*see* Multivariate analysis)
Hazards of child mortality
in Poisson regression method of analysis, 220–221
Health centers
distribution and number of, 185, 187
MCH centers, operation of, 188
Health infrastructure, 185–186, 187
decentralization of, 126, 185, 188
and mortality decline, 155, 197–198
Health knowledge
and mortality decline, 197–198
Health personnel
distribution and number of, 185, 187
Health policy, 126, 155, 185
impacts of, 138, 198
reform of, in 1978, 114, 188
Health programs, 186–194 (*see also* EPI)
Health services (*see also* Primary health care)
availability of, and distance from Dakar, 125
and child mortality, 130, 132–133
decentralization of, 126, 185, 188
development of, 113–114
expenditures on, 15
Height of children (*see* Stunting; Wasting)
HIV (human immunodeficiency virus)
prevalence rates of, 178–180
Hospitals and hospital beds
distribution and number of, 185, 187
Household size
and child mortality, 151
Housing quality (*see also* Composite facilities indicator; Socioeconomic indicators)
and adult mortality, 180, 183
and child mortality, 151, 154
by demographic indicator, 74
by department, 24–25
and fertility, 74
good construction defined, 29
and marriage, 74, 75, 76
by region, 23–26
by urban/rural residence, 26

I

Ideal family size
and family planning, 101–102, 104
and fertility decline, 2–3, 106, 197
in north Africa, 3, 200
Illegitimacy
in Africa, 3, 107, 198–199
difficulty in defining, 111
and fertility decline, 107
levels of, 88–90
rise in, 111
Immigration, 41, 42
and population growth, 196
IMR (infant mortality rate), 16 (*see also* Mortality, child; ${}_1q_0$)
estimates from various sources, 116
underestimation of, 108
Income
distribution of, 14, 21–22
and fertility decline, 67
and mortality decline, 197–198
and urban/rural residence, 14
Index of contraception (C_c), 78, 79, 100–102, 110 (*see also* Contraceptive use)
Index of induced abortion (I_a), 78, 79, 105, 110 (*see also* Abortion)
methods of calculating, 112
Index of marriage (C_m), 78, 79–95, 110 (*see*

also Age at marriage; Marital stability; Marriage; Polygyny; Proportions never married)
Index of postpartum infecundability (C_i), 78, 79, 110
and breastfeeding, 96–97
methods of calculating, 112
Index of potential fertility (TF), 78
Index of sterility (I_p), 78, 79, 105–106, 110
Indicators (*see* Composite facilities indicator; Demographic indicators; Economic indicators; Socioeconomic indicators)
Infant mortality rate (*see* IMR)
Infectious and parasitic diseases (*see also specific diseases*)
and adult mortality, 175
and household size, 151
Infecundity (*see* Index of postpartum infecundability)
Infertility (*see also* Sterility)
and fertility trends, 55
levels of, 106
Informal sector, 19, 21
Intercensal survival methods of estimating adult mortality, 157–163, 184
Intercourse, frequency of, 77
and polygyny, 91–92
Intermediate variables (*see* Proximate determinants)
Intrauterine device (IUD) (*see* Contraception)
Investment, domestic, 22
I_p (*see* Index of sterility)
Islam, 10
and postpartum abstinence, 96
IUD (Intrauterine device) (*see* Contraception)

J

Le jebalé (traditional waiting period before marriage consummation), 110–111

K

Kaffrine (department)
child mortality in, 128, 149
Kaolack (city)
HIV prevalence in, 178–179
Kaolack (department)
child mortality in, 127–129, 130, 149
Kaolack (region), 10
adult mortality in, 6, 176, 177
ASFRs in, 213
demographic survey of, 206
dominant ethnic group in, 32
and migration, temporary, 39–41
migration to and from, 37, 38
population size and growth in, 32–33, 34
proportions never married in, 81
socioeconomic indicators for, 24–28
tetanus vaccination coverage in, 193
vaccination coverage in, 191–192
Kébémer (department)
child mortality in, 127–129
low mortality of, 194
Kédougou (department)
infant and child mortality in, 116, 117
Kenya
family planning program in, 197
fertility decline in, 3, 45, 55, 107, 198–199
illegitimacy in, 3, 198–199
reasons for choice as case study, 7
teenage marriage in, 3, 198–199
Khombole (rural area)
abstinence, amenorrhea, birth intervals, and breastfeeding in, 98–99
MCH center in, 123, 188
Kolda (department)
child mortality in, 128, 149
Kolda (region)
adult mortality in, 5, 176, 177
ASFRs in, 214
dominant ethnic group in, 32
immigrants in, 41
and migration, temporary, 40, 41
migration to and from, 37, 38
population size and growth in, 32–33, 34
proportions never married in, 81
socioeconomic indicators for, 24–28
vaccination coverage in, 191–192
La Korité (Muslim holiday)
and fertility estimation, 51, 108, 207
and mortality estimation, 115, 116, 163, 207

L

l(x) (proportion surviving from birth to age x)
  from census estimates, 166–167
$_5L_x$ (stationary age distribution), 166–167
Latrine facilities for households (*see also* Composite facilities indicator; Socioeconomic indicators)
  and child mortality, 154–155, 156
  and demographic indicators, 74
  by region, 23–26
Leprosy
  control efforts, 186
Life expectancy
  by age and sex, 161–175, 180, 184
Life tables
  functions of, estimated from census, 166–167
  for small-scale studies, 171–174
Linguère (department)
  child mortality in, 128, 149–150
Literacy (*see* Education)
Living conditions (*see* Housing quality)
Louga (department)
  child mortality in, 127–129, 149
Louga (region), 10
  adult mortality in, 6, 176, 177
  ASFRs in, 215
  dominant ethnic group in, 32
  immigrants in, 41
  and migration, temporary, 40
  migration to and from, 37, 38
  population size and growth of, 32–33
  proportions never married in, 81
  socioeconomic indicators for, 23–29
  vaccination coverage in, 191–192
Lung diseases
  and adult mortality, 175

M

$_4M_1$ (death rate for ages 1-4) (*see also* Mortality, child)
  compared with $_{45}q_{15}$, 178, 179
Major Endemic Diseases Department, 186
Malaria
  and adult mortality, 175
  campaign against, 186–187
  and child mortality, 127–128, 131–132, 138–139, 145, 157
  factors affecting, 131–132
Malawi
  fertility decline in, 45
Mali
  migration to and from, 42, 43
Malinké (ethnic group), 43 (*see also* Ethnicity)
  and age at marriage and age at first birth, 90
  child mortality of, 151
  life expectancy at age 20 in, 169
Malnutrition
  of children, 134–138, 139
  and postpartum amenorrhea, 97
Mandingo (ethnic group), 43 (*see also* Ethnicity)
  child mortality of, 146, 150, 151, 152–153
  fertility of, 49, 70, 71
  polygyny among, 95
Marital disruption, 85
  and fertility, 55
Marital stability, 85–88
  compared with other countries, 85–87
  and fertility, 88
  by socioeconomic characteristics, 87–88
Marriage (*see also* Age at marriage; Index of marriage; Polygyny; Proportions never married)
  consensual unions, 111
  in Dakar, 91
  definitions of, 111
  by department, 75–76
  and education, 74
  and fertility, 3, 77–95
  forms of, 111
  and housing quality, 74, 75, 76
  as process, 110–111
  and socioeconomic indicators, 72, 74
  teenage, 89, 90
  and urbanization, 74
Matam (department)
  child mortality in, 127–129, 149–150
Maternal and child health (*see* MCH)
Maternal mortality
  in small-scale studies, 175
Maternity clinics
  after health policy reform, 188
  number of, 185, 186

Mauritania
  migration to and from, 42, 43
Mbacké (department)
  child mortality in, 127–129
Mbour (department)
  child mortality in, 127–129
MCH (maternal and child health) centers, 123, 188
MCH services
  and contraceptive use, 3–4
  history of, 186
Measles
  and child mortality, 131–132, 134, 138, 145
  factors affecting, 131–132
  and family size, 131
  vaccinations for, 130, 187–192
Medical technology
  and mortality decline, 197–198
Meningitis
  vaccinations for, 187
Midwives
  distribution of, 185, 187
Migration, internal, 34–43 *(see also specific areas)*
  by age and sex, 37, 40
  and age at marriage, 83
  and child mortality, 120–122
  to Dakar, 34, 36–40
  data sources for, 35–36
  defined, 35
  and development, 43
  effects of, 35, 41
  lifetime, 36–37
  net, 37–39
  north to south, 34
  and orphanhood data, 176
  recent, 36–38
  by region, 38
  rural-urban, 34, 37–39
  seasonal, 39–41
  by sex, 37, 40
  temporary, 36–37, 39–41
  by urban/rural residence, 37
Migration, international, 41–42
Minimum wage (SMIG), 21–23, 29
Mlomp (study area)
  adult mortality in, 168–169, 174, 175, 176
  age at marriage in, 63, 90
  ASFRs in, 65–66
  birth intervals and abstinence in, 98–99
  fertility in, 49, 63–65
  life expectancy at age 15 in, 175
  life tables for, 174
  and migration, temporary, 63
  mortality decline in, 198
  survey of, 62, 204, 206
Mlomp, child mortality in, 4–5
  by age, 131–135
  causes of, 130, 138–139, 144, 145
  decline in, 4–5
  and infant mortality, 116–117
  rural areas of, 125, 130
  by sex, 136
Mobile health teams, 186–189, 193
Model life tables, 166–167
  and adult mortality estimates, 158–163, 164–178
  and applicability to Senegal data, 194
  child mortality in, 134
  and estimates of ${}_{45}q_{15}$, 176–178
  in intercensal survival methods, 157–163
  in orphanhood method, 164–165
  survivorship ratios from, 160
Mortality, 4–6, 113–198
Mortality, adult, 5–6, 157–184 *(see also* Life expectancy; ${}_{45}q_{15}$; *and specific areas)*
  by age, 161–180, 184
  by cause, 169–175
  in Dakar, 176, 177
  data quality, 159, 161, 163, 194
  data sources, 157, 159
  by department, 177
  estimates of, from censuses, 157–169, 176–180, 184
  estimates of, from small-scale studies, 165–176
  methods for calculating, 157–163
  by region, 5–6, 176–184
  by sex, 161–184, 194
  and socioeconomic factors, 6, 180–183
Mortality, child, 118–157, 198 *(see also* IMR; ${}_{1}q_{0}$; ${}_{4}q_{1}$; *and specific areas)*
  and age of child, 130–135
  and age of mother, 152–154
  analysis methodology, 220–221
  and birth order, 152–154
  causes of, 138–139, 144, 145
  in Dakar, 4, 118–124, 130–131, 132, 156
  data quality for, 118, 133
  data sources for, 114–122

and demographic indicators, 139–151, 152, 153
by department, 127–130, 149–150
and distance from Dakar, 125–126
and education of mother, 5, 139, 146–150, 152–157
and EPI program, 5
estimates of, from 1988 census, 127–130, 149–150, 154–155
estimation methods, 117–118
by ethnicity, 146, 150–151, 152–153
and fertility decline, 196–197
by grand region, 4, 126, 149, 152–153
and health policy, 5, 155
and health services, 130, 132–133
and household size, 151
and housing quality, 151, 154
and income growth, 198
levels and trends of, 113, 117–126, 155–156
and malaria, 127–128, 131–132, 138–139, 145, 157
and measles, 131–132, 134, 138, 145
measures of, 114
by migrant status, 120–122
multivariate analysis of, 146–149, 151–155, 220–221
and NGOs, 156
north-south gradient in, 127, 149
and nutrition, 138–139, 151
and population growth, 196
and rainfall, 127
by region, 4, 126, 149–150, 152–153
in rural areas, 122–133, 135, 139
by sex, 133–134, 136, 194
and socioeconomic factors, 139–155
and structural adjustment policies, 5, 155–156
and urbanization, 5
by urban/rural residence, 4, 122, 124, 127–130, 139, 146–150, 152–157
and vaccinations, 134

Mortality, neonatal (*see also* Mortality, child)
causes of, 138, 144

Mortality, postneonatal (*see also* Mortality, child)
causes of, 138–139, 145

Mortality decline, 4–6, 12 *(see also specific areas)*
in Africa, 7, 113
factors affecting, 113, 197–198
and fertility, 196–197
and foreign assistance, 156
and health care, 155, 197–198
and income, 197–198
and medical technology, 197–198
and population growth, 196

Mortality rates, age-specific (ASMRs), 163–164, 166–167

Multivariate analysis of child mortality, 146–149, 151–155
methodology of, 220–221

N

Namibia
fertility decline in, 45

National Vaccination Coverage Surveys, 205

Natural increase, rate of, 196

Ndemene (study area)
child mortality in, 151
survey of, 204, 206

NDS (National Demographic Survey), 203
and child mortality data, 115
and fertility, 46, 54
as source of fertility data, 47

Neonatal mortality, 138, 144 (*see also* Mortality, child)

Neonatal tetanus (*see* Tetanus)

New home economics model of fertility, 67, 109

Ngayokhème (*see* Niakhar/Ngayokhème)

NGOs (nongovernmental organizations)
and child mortality, 156

Niakhar/Ngayokhème (study area)
adult mortality in, 168–175
age at marriage in, 91
age exaggeration in, 168
ASFRs in, 63–67
birth intervals and breastfeeding in, 98–99
changing boundaries of, 194
fertility in, 48, 54, 62
infant and child mortality in, 117
life expectancy at age 15 in, 169, 175, 184
life tables for, 171, 172
maternal mortality in, 175
polygyny and fertility in, 93
survey of, 62, 204, 206

Niakhar/Ngayokhème, child mortality in
by age, 130–132, 135
causes of, 138–139, 144, 155
and infant mortality, 116, 117
rural areas of, 123, 124
by sex, 133–134, 136
Nigeria
fertility decline in, 45
Nioro du Rip (department)
child mortality in, 128, 149–150
Nongovernmental organizations (NGOs)
and child mortality, 156
Norplant (*see* Contraception)
Northeastern region (*see* Grand regions)
Nuptiality (*see* Marriage)
Nurses
distribution of, 185, 187
Nutrition and Health Protection Program, 186
Nutritional status of children
and growth, 134–138, 140–143
and mortality, 138–139, 151

O

Odds ratios (*see* Multivariate analysis)
Orphanhood method of estimating adult mortality, 158, 164–165, 168–169, 177
adoption effect in, 165
effect of migration on, 176
Oussouye (department)
child mortality in, 127–129, 130, 149–150
infant and child mortality in, 116, 117

P

Paos Koto/Ndemene
birth intervals and breastfeeding in, 98–99
fertility in, 49
survey of, 204, 206
Parental survivorship
estimating adult mortality from, 164–165, 168–169, 176–178, 184
Parity
and desired family size, 101–102
and fertility control, 72, 96
Parity progression ratios (*see* B_{60})
Per capita GNP, 14, 15, 16, 21
Period parity distribution
and data quality, 52
Person-years lived in life table (${}_5L_x$)
estimated from census data, 166
Pertussis (*see also* DPT)
and child mortality, 139, 145
vaccinations for, 188
Peul (ethnic group), 43 (*see also* Ethnicity)
and age at marriage and age at first birth, 90
child mortality of, 151
fertility of, 63
P/F ratio technique for estimating fertility, 47–50, 53, 54
Pharmacists
distribution of, 185, 187
Pikine (*see also* Dakar)
abortion in, 105
child mortality in, 120–122, 124, 148–149
survey of, 204, 207
Pill, contraceptive (*see* Contraception)
Place of residence (*see* Urban/rural residence)
Pneumonia
and child mortality, 138, 145
Podor (department)
low mortality of, 194
Poisson regression (*see* Multivariate analysis)
Polio
vaccinations for, 188–190
Political divisions, 9–10, 11
Polygyny, 91–95, 111
and coital frequency, 91–92
and education, 93, 95, 112
and fertility, 91–93, 95
and socioeconomic characteristics, 93, 95
Population census, 12
Population census (1976), 207
adult mortality estimates from, 157–163, 184
coverage rates of, 163, 18463
as source of fertility data, 46
Population census (1988), 207
adult mortality estimates from, 157–165, 166–169, 176–178, 184
ASMR estimates from, 163–164
child mortality estimates from, 127–130, 149–150, 154–155

correcting fertility estimates from, 208–219
coverage rates of, 163, 184
data quality of, 51–53, 65–67, 115–117, 208–209
death reporting in, completeness of, 115–117, 164, 222–224
fertility estimates from, 51–53, 59–61, 64–67, 109
life-table estimates from, 178, 180
as source of fertility data, 46
as source of mortality data, 115–118
Population density, 9, 34, 35
Population distribution (*see also* Migration, internal)
changes in, 10, 34
Population growth
causes of, 1
in Dakar, 31, 34
and data quality, 32–33
and decline in child mortality, 196
and education, 13
and fertility, 196
and immigration, 196
rates of, 14, 30–31, 196
by region, 32–33, 34
in sub-Saharan Africa, 45
Population policies, 3–4, 107–108
Population projections, 1
Population pyramid (*see* Age distribution)
Population size
and health infrastructure, 186
by region, 32–33
Postneonatal mortality, 138–139, 145 (*see also* Mortality, child)
Postpartum abstinence, 96, 97, 98–99 (*see also* Index of postpartum infecundability)
Postpartum amenorrhea, 96–99 (*see also* Index of postpartum infecundability)
Postpartum infecundity (*see* Index of postpartum infecundability)
Potential fertility (TF), 78
Poular (ethnic group), 32 (*see also* Ethnicity)
age at marriage of, 83
child mortality of, 146, 151, 152–153
fertility of, 49, 70, 71
marital stability of, 88
marriage process of, 110–111
polygyny among, 95
PPR (Parity Progression Ratio) (*see* B_{60})
Pregnancies, unwanted, 105 (*see also* Abortion)
Prematurity
and neonatal mortality, 138, 144
Preston-Bennett method of estimating adult mortality, 158, 159–163
Primary health care, 113–114
and decline in child mortality, 155
history of, 185–186
policy and mortality decline, 198
and policy reform of 1978, 188
Proportions married, 77, 88
correlations of, with socioeconomic indicators, 72, 74
Proportions never married, 80–85, 88 (*see also* Age at marriage)
by age, 80–85, 86–87
in Dakar, 81, 83, 87, 91
by education, 81–83, 85, 86
by ethnicity, 82
and fertility, 92
by grand region, 81, 83, 84, 85
by region, 81, 84
by sex, 80–83
for small-scale studies, 81–82
by urban/rural residence, 82, 85, 87, 92
Proximate determinants of fertility, 77–106 (*see also* Index of contraception; Index of induced abortion; Index of marriage; Index of postpartum infecundability; Index of sterility; Potential fertility)
levels of, 79
model of, 78, 110
Public health (*see* Health)

Q

${}_5q_0$ (probability of dying before fifth birthday), 114 (*see also* Mortality, child)
${}_1q_0$ (probability of dying before first birthday) (*see also* IMR; Mortality, child)
comparisons from various sources, 116–118
relationship of, to ${}_4q_1$, 130–133, 134, 135, 194
${}_4q_1$ (probability of dying between 1st and 5th birthdays) (*see also* Mortality, child)
comparisons from various sources, 116–118
by department, 127–130

factors affecting, 131
and malaria, 131–132
and measles, 131–132
relationship of, to $_1q_0$, 130–133, 134, 135, 194
$_{45}q_{15}$ (probability of dying between 15th and 60th birthdays), 165, 175 (*see also* Mortality, adult)
compared with $_4M_1$, 178, 179
by region, 5–6, 176–178, 179, 180, 181
by sex, 175, 176–178, 179, 180, 181, 184

R

Ramadan (*see* Korité)
Reference point error
in 1988 census, 115
in birth histories, 47
Regions, administrative, 9–10, 11 *(see also* Grand regions; *and specific regions)*
abstinence, amenorrhea, birth intervals, and breastfeeding in, 96–99
adult and child mortality in, 178, 182
adult mortality in, 5–6, 165–184
age at marriage in, 106
antimalarial campaign in, 186–187
ASFRs in, 210–219
child mortality in, 4, 126, 131, 132, 149–150, 152, 153
composite facilities indicators for, 24–25, 28
dominant ethnic group in, 32
education in, 23–28
fertility decline in, 57–59
fertility in, 48, 57–67, 77, 210–219
good construction in, 23–26
health care system in, 28
immigrants in, 41
migration, temporary, in, 41
migration to and from, 37–38
nuptiality and economic status in, 7
population density of, 34, 35
population size and growth of, 32–33, 34
proportions never married in, 81, 84
quality of data on, 108
socioeconomic indicators for, 6, 23–29
surveys of, 205–207
urbanization in, 24–25, 34
vaccination coverage in, 191–193
Regression analysis (*see* Multivariate analysis)
Religion (*see* Islam)
Remarriage, 85, 88 (*see also* Marital stability)
and polygyny, 92
Remittances
and balance of payments, 19
and health investment, 130
Residence (*see* Rural residence; Urban/rural residence)
Respiratory infections
and child mortality, 138–139, 145
Ross-Mauldin Index of family planning program effort, 197, 201
Rural residence (*see also* Urban/rural residence)
and child mortality, 122–133, 135, 139
and fertility decline, 197
and HIV prevalence, 180

S

Saint-Louis (city)
causes of death in, 175
child mortality in, 122–124
HIV prevalence in, 178–179
registration of deaths in, 175
vital registration in, 12, 116–117, 122
Saint-Louis (region)
adult mortality in, 6, 176, 177
ASFRs in, 216
child mortality in, 131, 132
and migration, temporary, 40
migration to and from, 37, 38
population size and growth in, 32–33, 34
proportions never married in, 81
socioeconomic indicators for, 24–28
vaccination coverage in, 191–192
Sanitation (*see* Latrine facilities)
School enrollment (*see also* Education)
and fertility, 3
levels and trends of, 3, 17, 29
by region, 23–25
Seasonal migration, 36–37, 39–41
Sédhiou (department)
child mortality in, 127–129
Serer (ethnic group), 32 (*see also* Ethnicity)
and age at marriage and migration, 83
child mortality of, 146, 151, 152–153
fertility of, 70, 71, 93
identification by, with Wolof, 109

and migration, temporary, 41
polygyny among, 95
Sex
and adult mortality, 161–184, 194
and child mortality, 133–134, 136, 194
and life expectancy, 161–167
and migration, 37, 40
and proportions never married, 80–83
and socioeconomic characteristics and adult mortality, 180
Sex ratios, 32, 33
Sexually transmitted diseases, 105–106 (*see also* AIDS)
Sine-Saloum (region), 10 (*see also* Fatick; Kaolack)
abstinence, amenorrhea, breastfeeding, and birth intervals in, 96–99
quality of data on, 108
survey of, 206
Singulate mean age at marriage (SMAM) (*see also* Age at marriage)
correlations with socioeconomic indicators, 74
Smallpox, 186, 187
Small-scale studies (*see also* Bandafassi; Mlomp; Niakhar/Ngayokhème)
abstinence, amenorrhea, birth intervals, and breastfeeding in, 98–99
adult mortality in, 165–176, 184
age at first birth in, 90–91
age at marriage in, 63, 90–91
age exaggeration in, 168
ASFRs in, 62–67
boundaries of, 194
causes of death in, 169–175
fertility in, 48–49, 54, 62–67
infant and child mortality in, 116, 117
life expectancy at ages 15 or 20 in, 169, 175, 184
life-tables for, 171–174
location of sites, 204
maternal mortality in, 175
proportions never married in, 81–82
${}_{45}q_{15}$ in, 175
sterility in, 106
surveys of, 62, 204–207
vaccination coverage in, 191–193
Small-scale studies, child mortality in, 4–5
by age, 130–135
causes of, 130, 138–139, 144, 145, 155
decline in, 4–5
by ethnicity, 151
and infant mortality, 116, 117
in rural areas of, 123, 124, 125, 130
by sex, 133–134, 136
SMAM (singulate mean age at marriage) (*see also* Age at marriage)
correlations with socioeconomic indicators, 74
Socioeconomic factors
and adult mortality, 6, 180–183
and child mortality, 139–155
and marital stability, 87–88
and polygyny, 93, 95
and stunting, 137, 142–143
Socioeconomic indicators, 23–29 (*see also* Composite facilities indicator)
correlations of, with adult mortality, 183
correlations of, with child mortality, 155
correlations of, with fertility and nuptiality indicators, 74
by department, 24–25
and distance from Dakar, 28
by region, 6, 23–29
Soninke (ethnic group) (*see also* Ethnicity)
wealth of, and child mortality, 130
South Africa
fertility decline in, 45
Southern region (*see* Grand regions)
STDs (sexually transmitted diseases), 105–106 (*see also* AIDS)
Sterility, 78, 105–106 (*see also* Index of sterility)
Sterilization (*see* Contraception)
Structural adjustment
and child mortality, 5, 155–156
policies, 5, 14, 155–156
survey of, 205
Stunting (low height for age), 134–138, 142–143
Sub-Saharan Africa (*see* Africa, sub-Saharan)
Surveillance systems (*see* Small-scale studies)
Survey on Child Mortality in the Sahel (EMIS), 124, 207
Surveys (*see* Data sources)
Survival, child
and birth intervals, 97
preceding, and child mortality, 152, 154

Survivorship
- estimating adult mortality with, 157–163, 164–168, 169, 176–178, 184

T

Tambacounda (region)
- adult mortality in, 5, 176, 177
- ASFRs in, 217
- dominant ethnic group in, 32
- and migration, temporary, 40
- migration to and from, 37, 38
- population density of, 34
- population size and growth of, 32–33, 34
- proportions never married in, 81
- socioeconomic indicators for, 24–28
- vaccination coverage in, 191–193

Tanzania
- fertility decline in, 45

Technology, medical
- and mortality decline, 197–198

Temporary migration, 36–37, 39–41

Tetanus (*see also* DPT)
- and neonatal mortality, 138, 144
- vaccinations for, 188, 193

TF (potential fertility), 78

TFR (total fertility rate) (*see also* ASFRs; Fertility)
- defined, 108
- levels and trends of, 1–2, 16, 47–50, 196, 199, 200

Thiénaba (study area)
- abstinence, amenorrhea, birth intervals, and breastfeeding in, 98–99
- child mortality in, 123–125, 151
- survey in, 204, 207

Thiès (department)
- child mortality in, 127–129, 149

Thiès (region)
- adult mortality in, 6, 176, 177
- antimalarial campaign in, 186–187
- ASFRs in, 218
- child mortality in, 149
- dominant ethnic group in, 32
- and migration, temporary, 40
- migration to, 37
- population density of, 34
- population size and growth of, 32–33
- proportions never married in, 81
- socioeconomic indicators for, 24–28
- vaccination coverage in, 192

Tivaouane (department)
- child mortality in, 127–129, 149

TMFR (total marital fertility rate), 79

Toilet facilities for households (*see also* Composite facilities indicator; Socioeconomic indicators)
- and child mortality, 154–155, 156
- and demographic indicators, 74
- by region, 23–26

Total fertility rate (*see* TFR)

Tuberculosis
- vaccinations for, 188–190

Tunisia
- demographic transition in, 199–201
- fertility decline in, 3, 107, 199–201

U

Unwanted pregnancies, 105 (*see also* Abortion)

Urbanization
- and child mortality, 5
- definitional problems, 43–44
- and demographic indicators, 74
- by department, 24–25
- and fertility, 74
- and fertility decline, 2, 3, 197
- level of, 16
- by region, 24–25, 34

Urban/rural residence (*see also* Rural residence)
- and abortion, 104
- and access to clean water and electricity, 26
- and age at first birth, 68, 200
- and age at marriage, 83, 85
- and ASFRs, 69, 209–219
- and birth intervals, 98–99
- and breastfeeding, 98–99
- and child mortality, 4, 122, 124, 127–130, 139, 146–150, 152–157
- and contraceptive use, 100, 101
- and fertility, 49, 60, 68, 69, 107, 197
- and housing quality, 26
- and income, 14
- and marital stability, 88
- and migration, 37
- and polygyny, 93, 95
- and postpartum amenorrhea, 97, 98
- and proportions never married, 82, 85, 87, 92

and stunting, 137, 142
and vaccination coverage, 114, 191–192
and wasting, 140

V

Vaccination coverage
differentials in, 5
and distance from dispensaries, 193
before EPI, 187–188
under EPI, 5, 114, 189–194
methods of estimating, 190–191
by region, 191–193
in small-scale studies, 191–193
surveys of, 205
uneven, 189
by urban/rural residence, 114, 191–192
Vaccinations *(see also specific diseases)*
and child mortality, 134
complete, defined, 195
programs of, before 1978, 187–188
Verbal autopsies
and causes of death, 169
Vital registration systems, 12, 175

W

Wages, 21–23, 29
Wasting (low weight for height), 134–138, 140–141
Water supply for households (*see also* Composite facilities indicator; Socioeconomic indicators)
and adult mortality, 180, 183
and child mortality, 148–149, 151, 154
by region, 23–26
Weaning
and stunting, 137
Weight of children (*see* Wasting)
Western region (*see* Grand regions)
WFS (World Fertility Survey of 1978), 2, 204
ASFRs from, 57, 58
child mortality estimates in Dakar from, 119–122
data quality of, 108
fertility estimates from, 46–50, 51, 57, 58
regions in, 6
as source of abortion data, 104
as source of child mortality data, 115
as source of nuptiality data, 85
Wolof (ethnic group), 12, 32, 43 (*see also* Ethnicity)
child mortality of, 146, 151, 152–153
fertility of, 49, 70, 71
polygyny among, 95
Serer identifying as, 109
World Fertility Survey (*see* WFS)

Y

Yellow fever
vaccinations for, 187, 190

Z

Zambia
fertility decline in, 45
Ziguinchor (city)
HIV prevalence in, 178–179
Ziguinchor (department)
nuptiality and socioeconomic status in, 75
Ziguinchor (region), 10
adult mortality in, 6, 176, 177
ASFRs in, 219
dominant ethnic group in, 32
educational indicators in, 28
health care system in, 28
level of urbanization in, 34
and migration, temporary, 39, 40–41
migration to and from, 37, 38
nuptiality and socioeconomic status in, 76
population size and growth in, 32–33, 34
proportions never married in, 81
socioeconomic indicators for, 23–27
vaccination coverage in, 191–192
Zimbabwe
family planning program in, 197
fertility decline in, 3, 45, 55, 107, 198–199
illegitimacy in, 3, 198–199
teenage marriage in, 3, 198–199